TSRA Review of Cardiothoracic Surgery

Edited by:

Carlos M. Mery, MD, MPH
Cardiothoracic surgery fellow
University of Virginia
Charlottesville, VA
President TSRA 2010 – 2011

Joseph W. Turek, MD, PhD
Congenital cardiac surgery fellow
Children's Hospital of Philadelphia
Philadelphia, PA
President TSRA 2009 – 2010

Thoracic Surgery Residents Association
www.tsranet.org

TSRA Review of Cardiothoracic Surgery

TSRA / TSDA
633 N. Saint Clair Street
Suite 2320
Chicago, IL 60611
www.tsranet.org

ISBN-13: 9781530804160
ISBN-10: 1530804167
Library of Congress Control Number (LCCN): 2011903676

Cover artwork by: Carmina Mery, Ramón Mery, and Mari Pili Guzmán (age 3)

To all cardiothoracic surgery residents, present and future.

Foreword

The Thoracic Surgery Directors Association (TSDA) is dedicated to the education of all cardiothoracic surgery residents and has spent considerable time and resources to create a comprehensive curriculum to help residents develop their surgical knowledge bases. Cardiothoracic surgery residents represent the future of our specialty and this unique book, developed by residents for residents, is a shining example of why we are so proud to be cardiothoracic surgeons. The 83-chapter compendium, developed and written by members of the Thoracic Surgery Residents Association (TRSA), provides superb individual summaries of important cardiothoracic surgery topics and should be an invaluable asset to cardiothoracic surgeons in every stage of training.

The review book's contributors, including editors Carlos Mery, MD and Joseph Turek, MD, should be congratulated for their vision, contribution to educational resources for residents, and combined resolve to improve resident education. As President of the TSDA, I thank each of them for this considerable effort and I challenge every cardiothoracic resident to incorporate this body of knowledge into their daily activities for the benefit of our patients.

George L. Hicks, Jr., MD
President
Thoracic Surgery Directors Association

March 2011

Preface

As the field of cardiothoracic surgery continues to evolve, the amount of knowledge that a cardiothoracic surgeon must acquire continues to increase. There are several excellent and established textbooks in cardiothoracic surgery. However, there is a clear scarcity of review books that can serve as a concise analysis of the field.

The goal of this book, edited by the Thoracic Surgery Residents Association (TSRA) and authored by more than 50 cardiothoracic surgery residents from different programs around the country, is to synthesize the breadth of information that a cardiothoracic surgeon has to be familiar with into a few hundred pages. This brief review book is not intended to be exhaustive, but rather to relay essential information in cardiothoracic surgery to residents and established surgeons alike.

The material is organized into four different sections: General Thoracic Surgery, Adult Cardiac Surgery, Congenital Cardiac Surgery, and Cardiothoracic Trauma and Critical Care. The material included in each of the chapters is well known to anyone familiar with the topic and can be found in most cardiothoracic surgery textbooks. The books and journal articles that served as source material are listed at the end of the book.

We would like to thank the Thoracic Surgery Directors Association (TSDA) for their support with this project and all other initiatives. We would particularly like to thank the TSRA committee members and the multiple contributors that made possible the creation of this book.

Carlos M. Mery

Joseph W. Turek

March, 2011

Contributors

Ibrahim Abdullah, MD
Children's Hospital Boston
Palliative operations, Total anomalous pulmonary venous return, Truncus arteriosus and aortopulmonary window

Carlos J. Anciano, MD
University of Pittsburgh
Esophageal cancer

Nicholas D. Andersen, MD
Duke University Medical Center
Cardiac tumors, Hypoplastic left heart syndrome

Ashok Babu, MD
University of Colorado
Cardiac anatomy, Cardiopulmonary bypass, Postoperative care and perioperative neurological complications

Keki R. Balsara, MD
Duke University Medical Center
Double outlet right ventricle

Bryan M. Burt, MD
Brigham and Women's Hospital
Pulmonary metastatic disease, Malignant pleural effusions and malignant pleural mesothelioma, Aortic valve disease, Cardiac trauma, Ventricular septal defects

Shamus R. Carr, MD
University of Pittsburgh
Paraesophageal hernias

George M. Comas, MD
Columbia University Medical Center
Cardiac transplantation

Mani A. Daneshmand, MD
Duke University Medical Center
Thoracoabdominal aortic aneurysms

Elizabeth A. David, MD
The University of Texas M.D. Anderson Cancer Center
Surgery for emphysema

Daniel J. DiBardino, MD
University of Michigan
Cardiac embryology and segmental approach, Pediatric cardiac intensive care

Lucas M. Duvall, MD
University of Texas Health Sciences Center - San Antonio
Tricuspid valve repair and replacement, Thoracic trauma

Leo M. Gazoni, MD
University of Virginia
Mechanical complications of coronary artery disease, Left ventricular aneurysms

Ravi K. Ghanta, MD
Brigham and Women's Hospital
Pulmonary metastatic disease, Malignant pleural effusions and malignant pleural mesothelioma, Aortic valve disease, Cardiac trauma, Ventricular septal defects

Shawn S. Groth, MD, MS
University of Minnesota
Early stage non-small cell lung cancer, Tracheal tumors

Kendra J. Grubb, MD, MHA
University of Virginia
Mediastinal masses, Coronary artery disease

John C. Haney, MD, MPH
Duke University Medical Center
Thoracic and pulmonary anatomy

Matthew G. Hartwig, MD
Duke University Medical Center
Locally advanced lung cancer, Thoracic infections and hemoptysis

James M. Isbell, MD, MSCI
University of Virginia
Lung transplantation, Anatomy and surgical approaches to the mediastinum

J. Chad Johnson, MD, MS
Duke University Medical Center
Aortic dissection

Zain Khalpey, MD, PhD, MRCS
Brigham and Women's Hospital
Endocarditis, Low cardiac output

Ahmet Kilic, MD
University of Virginia
Combined valve / coronary artery bypass grafting, Tricuspid atresia

T. K. Susheel Kumar, MD
University of Michigan
Cardiac embryology and segmental approach

John C. Lin, MD
Cedars-Sinai Medical Center
Congenital cardiac evaluation and physiology, Interrupted aortic arch and aortic coarctation, Transposition of the great arteries

Gabriel Loor, MD
Cleveland Clinic Foundation
Diseases of the pericardium

Robroy H. MacIver, MD, MPH
University of Washington
Paraneoplastic syndromes, Benign pleural disease, Patent ductus arteriosus

Ryan A. Macke, MD
University of Pittsburgh
Anatomy and physiology of the esophagus

Jenifer Marks, MD
The University of Texas M.D. Anderson Cancer Center
Pulmonary physiology and pulmonary function tests, Pulmonary carcinoid tumors and other primary lung tumors

Jeremiah T. Martin, MD
University of Kentucky
Chest wall deformities, Congenital diseases of the esophagus, Esophageal diverticula

Stephen H. McKellar, MD, MSc
Mayo Clinic
Combined carotid and coronary artery surgery, Ascending aortic aneurysms, End-stage heart failure

Robert A. Meguid, MD, MPH
University of Washington
Chest wall tumors

Serguei I. Melnitchouk, MD, MPH
Columbia University Medical Center
Acute and chronic pulmonary embolism

Carlos M. Mery, MD, MPH
University of Virginia
Other esophageal tumors, Atrial septal defects, Tetralogy of Fallot, Ebstein's anomaly

Bret A. Mettler, MD
Children's Hospital Boston
Palliative operations, Total anomalous pulmonary venous return, Truncus arteriosus and aortopulmonary window

Stephanie Mick, MD
Brigham and Women's Hospital
Benign tumors of the lung, Atrioventricular septal defects, Vascular rings, pulmonary artery sling, and associated tracheal anomalies

Daniela Molena, MD
Memorial Sloan-Kettering Cancer Center
Lung cancer overview and preoperative evaluation, Diseases of the diaphragm, Esophageal motility disorders

Jennifer S. Nelson, MD
University of Michigan
Aortic stenosis and left ventricular outflow tract obstruction

Tom C. Nguyen, MD
Columbia University Medical Center
Mitral regurgitation, Mitral stenosis

Aundrea L. Oliver, MD
Brigham and Women's Hospital
Esophageal reflux disease

Theolyn Price, MD
Mayo Clinic
Post-pneumonectomy complications, Congenital lung diseases, Interstitial lung disease

Siva Raja, MD, PhD
Cleveland Clinic Foundation
Esophageal reflux disease

Keshava Rajagopal, MD, PhD
Duke University Medical Center
Pacemakers and defibrillators

Ramesh Singh, MBBCh, MRCS
University of Colorado
Cardiac anatomy, Cardiopulmonary bypass, Postoperative care and perioperative complications

Chad N. Stasik, MD
University of Texas Health Sciences Center - San Antonio
Arrhythmia surgery

Matthew D. Taylor, MD
University of Virginia
Thoracic outlet syndrome

Joseph W. Turek, MD, PhD
The Children's Hospital of Philadelphia
Cardiac tumors, Hypoplastic left heart syndrome, Coronary artery anomalies

Immanuel I. Turner, MD
Duke University Medical Center
Coronary artery anomalies

Benjamin Wei, MD
Duke University Medical Center
Locally advanced lung cancer, Thoracic infections and hemoptysis

Bryan A. Whitson, MD, PhD
University of Minnesota
Early stage non-small cell lung cancer, Tracheal tumors, Thoracic sympathectomy

Daniel C. Wiener, MD
Brigham and Women's Hospital
Esophageal injury

Jason A. Williams, MD
Duke University Medical Center
Thoracic and pulmonary anatomy, Aortic dissection, Thoracoabdominal aortic aneurysms

Samuel J. Youssef, MD
Yale University
Chylothorax, Tracheal stenosis and postintubation injury, Pulmonary failure

Abbreviations

ABG: Arterial blood gas
ACC: American College of Cardiology
ACE: Angiotensin-converting enzyme
ACS: American College of Surgeons
ACT: Activated clotting time
AFP: Alpha fetoprotein
AHA: American Heart Association
AI: Aortic insufficiency
ARB: Angiotensin-receptor blocker
ARDS: Acute respiratory distress syndrome
ASD: Atrial septal defect
ATLS: Advanced Trauma Life Support
ATP: Adenosine triphosphate
β-HCG: Beta human chorionic gonadotropin
bpm: Beats per minute
BMI: Body mass index
BSA: Body surface area
CABG: Coronary artery bypass graft surgery
CAD: Coronary artery disease
CHF: Congestive heart failure
CMV: Cytomegalovirus
CNS: Central nervous system
COPD: Chronic obstructive pulmonary disease
CPB: Cardiopulmonary bypass
CSF: Cerebrospinal fluid
CT: Computed tomography
CTA: Computed tomographic angiography
CVP: Central venous pressure
CXR: Chest X-ray
DLCO: Diffusing capacity of the lung for carbon monoxide
DM: Diabetes mellitus
EBUS: Endobronchial ultrasound
EBV: Ebstein-Barr virus
ECMO: Extracorporeal membrane oxygenation
EF: Ejection fraction
EGD: Esophagogastroduodenoscopy
EKG: Electrocardiogram
EUS: Endoscopic ultrasound
FAST: Focused assessment with sonography in trauma
FDG-PET: 2-Fluoro-2-deoxy-D-glucose positron emission tomography
FEV_1: Forced expiratory volume in the first second

FiO_2: Inspired fraction of oxygen
FNA: Fine needle aspiration
FVC: Forced vital capacity
GI: Gastrointestinal
GM-CSF: Granulocyte and monocyte colony stimulating factor
H&P: History & physical exam
HBV: Hepatitis B virus
HIV: Human immunodeficiency virus
HLA: Human leukocyte antigen
IABP: Intra-aortic balloon pump
ICU: Intensive care unit
IFN: Interferon
IL: Interleukin
IV: Intravenous
IVC: Inferior vena cava
IVF: Intravenous fluids
IVIG: Intravenous immunoglobulin
LA: Left atrium
LAD: Left anterior descending artery
LDH: Lactate dehydrogenase
LES: Lower esophageal sphincter
LLL: Left lower lobe
LUL: Left upper lobe
LV: Left ventricle
LVOT: Left ventricular outflow tract
MAP: Mean arterial pressure
MI: Myocardial infarction
MR: Mitral regurgitation
MRA: Magnetic resonance angiography
MRI: Magnetic resonance imaging
NGT: Nasogastric tube
NPO: *Nil per os* (nothing by mouth)
NSCLC: Non-small cell lung cancer
NYHA: New York Heart Association (classification of heart failure)
PA: Pulmonary artery
$PaCO_2$: Partial pressure of carbon dioxide in arterial blood
PaO_2: Partial pressure of oxygen in arterial blood
PAP: Pulmonary artery pressure
PCI: Percutaneous coronary intervention
PDA: Patent ductus arteriosus
PE: Pulmonary embolus
PECLA: Pumpless extracorporeal lung assistance
PEEP: Positive end-expiratory pressure

PET: Positron emission tomography
PFO: Patent foramen ovale
PFT: Pulmonary function test
PGE_1: Prostaglandin E_1
PGE_2: Prostaglandin E_2
PTFE: Polytetrafluoroethylene
PVD: Peripheral vascular disease
PVR: Pulmonary vascular resistance
Qp:Qs: Ratio of pulmonary blood flow to systemic blood flow
RA: Right atrium
RANTES: Regulated upon Activation, Normal T-cell Expressed, and
    Secreted chemokine
RCA: Right coronary artery
RLL: Right lower lobe
RML: Right middle lobe
RUL: Right upper lobe
RV: Right ventricle
RVOT: Right ventricular outflow tract
RT: Radiation therapy
SaO_2: Oxygen saturation of the blood
SCLC: Small cell lung cancer
SLE: Systemic lupus erythematosus
SUV: Standardized uptake value
SVC: Superior vena cava
SVR: Systemic vascular resistance
TB: Tuberculosis
TBNA: Transbronchial needle aspiration
TEE: Transesophageal echocardiography
TGF: Transforming growth factor
TPN: Total parenteral nutrition
TNF: Tumor necrosis factor
UNOS: United Network for Organ Sharing
US: Ultrasound
V/Q: Ventilation/perfusion
VAD: Ventricular assist device
VATS: Video-assisted thoracic surgery
VSD: Ventricular septal defect
WBC: White blood cell
WHO: World Health Organization

Table of Contents

I. General Thoracic Surgery

1. Thoracic and pulmonary anatomy

John C. Haney, Jason A. Williams

Thorax

The bony thorax serves to protect the organs of the chest and facilitate respiration by changing volume. The thorax is comprised of 12 paired ribs connecting the thoracic vertebral bodies with the sternum. Each rib has a head that articulates with the same-numbered vertebral body, a tubercle, which articulates with the vertebral transverse process, and a neck that terminates in an anterior articulation. The upper seven (true) ribs articulate directly with the sternum; ribs 8-10 (false) articulate with the costal cartilage, and ribs 11-12 have no anterior articulations (floating). Along the inferior aspect of each rib is a costal groove containing the neurovascular bundle.

The sternum is divided into the manubrium (which contains the articulation of the clavicle and first rib), the body, and the xyphoid process. The second rib articulates at the junction of the manubrium and sternal body, a junction that can be palpated on the chest wall as the sternal angle or angle of Louis. The insertion of the posterior scalene muscle and the origin of the pectoralis major muscle also indicate the site of the second rib. This roughly corresponds with the level of the carina.

The diaphragm muscle is the primary muscle of inspiration, contracting downward to increase intrathoracic volume. It includes crural fibers that arch around the diaphragmatic hiatus, costal fibers that connect to the ribs, and a central tendon. In the setting of extreme effort or disease, secondary muscles of inspiration include the scalenes and external and parasternal intercostals, which serve to elevate the thorax. Expiration is primarily a passive process depending on the innate elasticity of the lung. In pathophysiologic states, the transversus abdominus may help compress the thorax and assist expiration.

There are three larger apertures in the diaphragm and several smaller ones. From posterior to anterior, the diaphragmatic apertures and the structures that traverse them are:

- *Aortic hiatus (T12):* aorta, azygos vein, and thoracic duct

- *Esophageal hiatus (T10):* esophagus and anterior (left) and posterior (right) vagal trunks

- *Caval hiatus (T8):* IVC and branches of the right phrenic nerve

A mnemonic to remember hiatal levels is "I ate 10 eggs at 12" (I8, 10E, A12). Several smaller openings carry branches of the splanchnic nerves and the hemiazygos vein (left). Posterior to the diaphragm runs the sympathetic trunk along the lateral aspect of the vertebral column. Immediately behind the sternum, the superior epigastric artery branches from the internal mammary and runs through the foramen of Morgagni.

At the thoracic inlet, the relationships of the vessels and nerves to the scalene muscles are of importance. The brachial plexus can be found between the anterior and middle scalene muscles and over the first rib, and it is in this space that hypertrophy or connective tissue may impinge on the nerve bundles. The subclavian vein runs over the first rib and beneath the clavicle, anterior to the scalene muscle. The phrenic nerve descends over the anterior scalene within its fascial sheath. The subclavian artery overlies the first rib but runs behind the anterior scalene.

The chest wall is also the source of several muscles utilized as tissue coverage either for reconstruction of chest wall defects or for intrathoracic tissue buttressing. The pectoralis major, supplied by the pectoralis branch of the thoracoacromial artery, may be rotated to cover superior chest wall defects. The latissimus dorsi, with blood supply based off of the thoracodorsal bundle, can be rotated to cover a variety of chest wall defects. The serratus anterior may be harvested in similar fashion, its pedicled blood supply also based off the thoracodorsal artery, and used as a tissue buttress for airway or esophageal defects within the chest. Pedicled intercostal muscle flaps may also be used for intrathoracic coverage or airway defects. From the abdomen, rectus abdominus may be harvested as a transverse rectus abdominus myocutaneous (TRAM) flap and rotated cephalad to cover lower anterior chest wall defects. Its blood supply is based off of the superior epigastric artery, thus it is not an appropriate choice if the ipsilateral internal mammary artery has been harvested for CABG.

Tracheobronchial tree

The tracheobronchial tree contains 23 generations of branches, the first 6 of which are purely conductive. The trachea averages 10-11 cm in length, 5 cm of which are above the suprasternal notch starting at the inferior border of the larynx. The trachea has 17-21 incomplete anterior cartilaginous rings that give the trachea an elliptical shape; the posterior or membranous trachea lies in contact with the esophagus. The proximal airway is lined with ciliated columnar mucosa with intermittent mucus-secreting goblet cells. These are responsible for the mucociliary elevator. The trachea bifurcates into right and left mainstem bronchi at the carina at approximately the level of the sternal angle. The blood supply to the trachea consists primarily of supply from the inferior thyroid artery with an anastomotic arcade on the posterolateral aspect of the trachea. Inferiorly, bronchial arterial branches feed the carina.

Regional lymph nodes

Tracheobronchial lymph nodes are the key to staging lung cancer. Since 1997, the mediastinal lymph node classification system of Mountain and Dresler has been most widely utilized. Lymph node stations are classified from 1-14.

Single-digit levels (1-9) are classified as *mediastinal* nodes contained within the mediastinal pleura and signify at least N2 disease. Level 1 nodes are supraclavicular, located between cricoid and clavicles. Superior mediastinal nodes are defined as levels 2-4. Levels 2 (upper paratracheal nodes above the aortic arch) and 4 (lower paratracheal, below the aorta) are accessible with cervical mediastinoscopy. Level 3 nodes are not immediately adjacent to the trachea but are prevascular or prevertebral. Levels 5 and 6 are aortic nodes, level 5 aortic window nodes are located between the aortic arch and PA, and level 6 nodes sit anterior to the aortic arch. These are accessible by anterior or extended mediastinoscopy only. Inferior mediastinal nodes are defined as levels 7-9. Level 7 subcarinal nodes are accessible via cervical mediastinoscopy. Level 8 nodes are paraesophageal and level 9 nodes lie along the pulmonary ligament.

Pulmonary nodes (levels 10-14) are all classified (ipsilaterally) as N1 disease. These nodal stations (hilar, interlobar, lobar, segmental and subsegmental, respectively) are all located within the reflection of the visceral pleura.

Sampling regional lymph node stations is critical for appropriate staging. Cervical mediastinoscopy provides reliable access and good tissue sampling of stations 2, 4 and 7 (defining N2 or N3 disease). Anterior mediastinoscopy (Chamberlain procedure) provides additional access to level 5 and 6 nodes. More recently, EBUS has allowed for FNA of nodes through the tracheobronchial tree. EBUS allows access to nodal stations 1, 2, 3, 4, 7, 10, and 11. Most significantly are the addition of stations 10 and 11, which can define N1 disease. Level 8 nodes may also be accessed with EUS via the esophagus.

Pulmonary anatomy

The lungs are divided into bronchopulmonary segments – the smallest anatomic segment with preserved airway, vascular and lymphatic supply. Within the right lung, 10 segments are defined:

- *RUL:* apical, anterior, and posterior segments

- *RML:* medial and lateral segments

- *RLL:* superior, anterior basal, posterior basal, medial basal, and lateral basal segments

The left lung is similar with three major exceptions: the lingula takes the place of the middle lobe but is part of the upper lobe, the upper lobe apical and posterior segments are usually combined, and the anterior and medial basal segments of the lower lobe are usually combined. This leaves the left lung with 8 segments:

- *LUL:* apicoposterior, anterior, superior lingular, and inferior lingular segments

- *LLL:* superior, anteromedial basal, posterior basal, and lateral basal segments.

In reality, some variability persists from patient to patient. The most consistent landmark for pulmonary resection remains the intersegmental pulmonary vein.

Pulmonary vasculature

The PA conveys deoxygenated blood from the right ventricle to the lungs. On the right, the right pulmonary artery courses behind the ascending aorta and SVC and in front of the right bronchus. At the hilum, the right PA gives off the truncus anterior branch to the RUL. This divides into two branches to the anterior and posterior segments. The posterior segmental artery branches again to form the apical and posterior arteries. In most individuals, an additional artery supplies the RUL, the posterior ascending artery arising from the interlobar portion of the ongoing PA and crossing over the bronchus intermedius. This posterior ascending branch runs behind the RUL pulmonary vein and may be damaged inadvertently while encircling the vein during a right upper lobectomy and can be a problematic source of bleeding during dissection. The middle lobe artery then branches from the ongoing right PA at the level of the fissures, bifurcating after its takeoff. The blood supply to the RLL then consists of a superior segmental artery, arising posteriorly often at the level of the middle lobe artery, a medial basal segmental artery and an ongoing common basal trunk.

The left PA runs in front of the descending aorta and left bronchus. Superiorly, it is attached to the aortic arch by the ligamentum arteriosum, on the left of which is the left recurrent laryngeal nerve. Typically, four branches arise to supply the LUL, but may range from 2-7. These usually include an anterior and an apical artery as well as several posterior arteries. In the interlobar segment, the lingular artery arises anteriorly, providing the total supply to the lingular segment in 80% of individuals. Posteriorly, within this interlobar segment, a superior segmental artery supplies the lower lobe. The common basal trunk then commonly divides into two branches to supply the rest of the lower lobe.

The pulmonary veins carry oxygenated blood from the lungs back to the LA and lie anterior and inferior to the PAs and bronchi. On the right, the superior pulmonary vein crosses anterior to the bronchus intermedius, giving off three branches to the RUL (apical, anterior, posterior) and a single branch to the RML. The right inferior pulmonary vein gives off a superior segmental branch that runs posterior to the RLL bronchus as well as a common basal vein running anteriorly. On the left, the superior pulmonary vein gives off three branches – apical, anterior, and lingular. The inferior vein gives off a superior segmental vein that runs posterior to the bronchus (as on the right) and a common basal vein anteriorly.

2. Pulmonary physiology and pulmonary function tests

Jenifer Marks

Pulmonary physiology

Gas exchange of oxygen and carbon dioxide is the primary function of the lungs. Large volumes of air are brought into the chest via the chest wall muscles and conducting airways. The alveolar surface then provides a large area for diffusion of oxygen into the blood and for the elimination of carbon dioxide. Ventilation (air volumes) and perfusion (blood volumes) are matched in the healthy lung. Four major factors determine the alveolar gas composition: inspired gas composition, mixed venous gas composition, alveolar ventilation, and alveolar perfusion. In the normal lung, alveolar and blood pO_2 and pCO_2 equilibrate within the first third of the capillary. Any number of disease processes can affect this exchange such that diffusion will not be complete when the blood is leaving the capillary.

Lung inflation and deflation occur due to changes in the dimensions of the chest wall. These changes are due to the elastic properties of the bony and soft tissue structure of the thorax and by the muscles of the respiratory system. The lung itself is a volume container that tends to deflate itself. The deflation force exerted by the lung is the elastic recoil pressure. Lung recoil pressure is positive, expiratory, and equals the pressure difference between the alveolar lumen and the pleural space. The chest wall also exerts a passive recoil pressure in the opposite direction, proportional to its volume of expansion. The lungs and chest wall are mechanically coupled by the pleural fluid such that at the end of expiration, the inspiratory chest wall recoil balances the expiratory recoil of the lung. The compliance of the chest wall is normally high enough that respiratory motion is not restricted. In a healthy system, the lungs and chest wall contribute equally to the total compliance over a normal tidal volume range. The FVC is the most frequently used objective clinical tool to assess the mechanical characteristics of the lungs.

Lung volume measurements

- *Vital capacity (VC):* maximum volume expired after a maximum inhalation

- *Total lung capacity (TLC):* Volume in lungs after maximal inhalation

- *Residual volume (RV):* Volume remaining in lungs after maximal exhalation

- *Functional residual capacity (FRC):* volume in lungs at end of normal exhalation

- *Tidal volume (TV):* volume of spontaneous breath

- Inspiratory capacity: maximum volume inspired from resting end expiratory position to total lung capacity

- *Expiratory reserve volume:* volume expired from spontaneous end expiratory position

- *Inspiratory reserve volume:* Volume that can still be inspired from a spontaneous end inspiratory position

Pulmonary function testing

The most commonly performed test uses the forced expiratory vital capacity maneuver: maximal inhalation followed by rapid and complete exhalation. For any given individual during expiration there is a unique limit to the maximal flow that can be reached at any lung volume. This flow is very sensitive to the most common diseases affecting the lung (i.e., COPD, chronic bronchitis, asthma, and pulmonary fibrosis). A decrease in FVC may be due to the lung itself, pleural cavity disease, chest wall restriction, or abnormal function of the respiratory muscles.

FEV_1 is also a very useful measurement. FEV_1 decreases in direct proportion to the disease process causing the airway obstruction or restriction. The FEV_1/FVC ratio ranges from 75-85% for normal adults and decreases with age. Children have higher flows for their size and thus ratios up to 90%. A low FEV_1 with a normal ratio usually indicates a restrictive process. A low FEV_1 and decreased ratio indicate an obstructive process.

Maximal voluntary ventilation (MVV) is a test done where the patient is instructed to breathe as hard and fast as possible for 10 to 15 seconds and the result is then extrapolated to 60 seconds and reported in liters/minute. Low MVV can occur in both obstructive and restrictive processes and is very non-specific but can be useful in estimating the patients' ability to undergo a major pulmonary resection.

DLCO is another commonly obtained value that estimates the transfer of carbon monoxide (CO) across the alveolar capillary membrane. The area of the alveolar capillary membrane, the thickness of the membrane, and the driving pressure for each gas all affect the amount of gas transferred.

Bronchodilators are often administered during pulmonary function testing. A positive response is defined as one in which the FEV_1 or FVC increases by both 12% and 200ml.

Pulmonary preoperative evaluation

PFTs are useful because they provide objective data on lung function and help to initially screen the high-risk patient. They should be done prior to any pulmonary resection. A room air ABG also provides useful information. Preoperative resting hypoxemia (pO_2 < 60 mmHg) is not an absolute contraindication to resection because the lung to be resected may be a contributing factor. Resting hypercapnea (pCO_2 > 50mm Hg) indicates advanced lung disease and correlates with increased perioperative morbidity.

Predicted postoperative PFTs can be calculated based on the amount of lung volume to be resected and provide a good measurement of risk. The calculation is performed by multiplying the preoperative value of the test by the fraction of functional segments remaining postoperatively. Obstructed segments are eliminated from the equation. A V/Q scan can be used to assess the contribution of the different areas of the lung in case of heterogeneous disease. A calculated predicted postoperative FEV_1 ($ppoFEV_1$) < 40% is indicative of high risk with values < 20% being prohibitive. Similarly, a calculated postoperative DLCO (ppoDLCO) < 40% indicates high risk and < 20% is prohibitive for resection.

The best method to determine the risk for complications after major lung resection is the measurement of maximum oxygen consumption (VO_{2max}) during exercise. Patients with values < 10 mL/kg/min are at prohibitive risk for resection while those patients with values 10-15 mL/kg/min are considered high risk.

The following values are considered high risk or prohibitive for pulmonary resection: $ppoFEV_1$ < 0.8L or < 40% predicted, FVC < 1.5L or < 30% predicted, FEV_1/FVC ratio < 50%, resting pO_2 < 45 mmHg, resting pCO_2 > 50, ppoDLCO < 40% predicted, VO_{2max} < 10 mL/kg/min. Patients that are unable to climb 1 flight of stairs, have a resting oxygen saturation of < 90%, or desaturate > 4% during exercise oximetry are generally not operative candidates.

3. Lung cancer overview and preoperative evaluation

Daniela Molena

Lung cancer is the leading cause of cancer death among both men and women. The American Cancer Society estimated 222,520 new cases and 157,300 deaths from lung cancer in 2010. When compared to all types of cancer, lung cancer will account for 15% of new cancer cases and 28% of all cancer deaths in 2010. The overall chance of developing lung cancer in a lifetime is about 8% for a man and 6% for a woman. Despite improvement in diagnosis and treatment, the incidence has decreased only about 1.8% per year over the last 20 years among men and increased about 0.5% per year among women. The prevalence is significantly higher for African-American males and for lower socioeconomic classes.

Risk factors

Cigarette smoking is the most important risk factor and it is estimated to directly cause about 85% of lung cancers. The risk is directly correlated to the quantity of cigarettes and the duration of smoking and inversely correlated to the starting age. An active smoker has a 16-fold higher risk of developing lung cancer and the risk is doubled in those who started smoking before age 16. Cigar, pipe smoking and secondhand smoke have been independently associated with increased risk. The damage of smoking to the lungs is partially reversible and a 30-50% reduction in cancer mortality risk has been reported after 10 years of smoking cessation. Several other environmental carcinogens have been identified (i.e. asbestos, radon, tar, soot, arsenic, chromium and nickel), but they only account for approximately 10% of lung cancers altogether. Moreover, cigarette smoking interacts synergistically with these substances to increase the risk. Air pollution, alcohol and low fiber diet have been associated with increased cancer risk as well. Recent studies about genetic mapping suggest that certain families are at higher risk to develop lung cancer and higher mortality rates have been reported in relatives of lung cancer patients. Strong evidence exists that inherited cancer susceptibility may be linked to a genetic marker on chromosome 6.

In addition to the aforementioned risk factors, a number of genetic markers have been identified to correlate with various lung cancers. Probably one of the best-studied oncogenes is k-*ras*. Mutations of k-*ras* are associated with earlier distant metastasis and worse prognosis in NSCLC. Mutations in the epidermal growth factor receptor (EGFR) have been observed in lung adenocarcinomas in smokers and non-smokers that respond more favorably to tyrosine kinase inhibitors. Finally, c-*myc* mutations have been linked to SCLC.

Screening

Due to the unfavorable natural history of the disease, the high costs associated with management of affected patients and the poor outcome despite aggressive multimodality treatment, screening tools for lung cancer have been investigated for decades. Several controlled clinical trials have evaluated the role of CXR and sputum cytology as screening tools in the general population and in the population at risk due to heavy smoking or professional exposure to carcinogens. Although lung cancer was typically detected at an earlier stage in the screened population, no significant benefit in terms of decreased mortality was shown in these studies. More recently, CT, which has a higher sensitivity than CXR in detecting lung nodules, has been considered as a screening test for lung cancer. Several observational trials and a randomized controlled trial sponsored by the National Cancer Institute are ongoing. Very recent preliminary data from the National Lung Screening Trial showed 20.3% fewer lung cancer deaths among high-risk subjects screened with low-dose helical CT compared to conventional chest radiograph. The trial Data and Safety Monitoring Board recommended ending the study and final results should be available shortly.

Pathology

Lung cancer is a very heterogeneous malignancy with many histologic types often present in the same tumor. The World Health Organization in cooperation with the International Association for the Study of Lung Cancer has proposed a very extensive classification of lung and pleural tumors. Briefly, lung cancer can be divided into three main categories: NSCLC, SCLC and rare mixed epithelial types. The most frequent histologic type is NSCLC, accounting for 85% of all cases. NSCLC can be further divided into adenocarcinoma, squamous cell carcinoma, and large cell carcinoma. Adenocarcinoma is now the predominant subtype among NSCLC, is the most frequent histologic type in non-smokers, is peripherally distributed in the lung parenchyma, and is positive for cytokeratin 7 and thyroid transcription factor-1 (TTF-1). Bronchioalveolar carcinoma is an indolent, non-invasive, clinicopathologically discrete variant of adenocarcinoma. Squamous cell carcinoma usually arises in the major bronchi, has a distinct dose-response relationship to smoking, is associated with necrosis and cavitary lesions and is characterized by the presence of keratin pearls on histology. Large cell carcinoma accounts for 10-15% of lung cancers and usually presents as a large peripheral mass on chest radiograph. SCLC accounts for 15-20% of all lung cancers, is usually metastatic at diagnosis and carries a poor prognosis. SCLC can be considered one extreme of the spectrum of neuroendocrine tumors of the lung, with typical carcinoid tumors being at the opposite extreme.

Clinical presentation

The majority of all lung cancers patients are symptomatic. Symptoms may be related to the primary tumor or metastatic disease and are often associated with generalized complaints like weight loss and fatigue. The most common pulmonary symptoms are cough, dyspnea, and hemoptysis. Post-obstructive pneumonia and lung abscess are often seen with proximal tumors obstructing the main bronchi. Adjacent structures like chest wall, diaphragm, and mediastinum can be invaded or compressed by the tumor mass causing chest pain, dyspnea, nerve dysfunction, venous obstruction, fistulas, and effusions. Paraneoplastic syndromes are rare and more common with SCLC and squamous cell carcinoma. SVC syndrome can be caused by bulky upper lobe tumors (most commonly in SCLC). Neurologic symptoms and bone pain are the most common metastatic symptoms.

Diagnosis and staging

The history, physical exam, and CXR represent the mainstay of the diagnostic process. Reviewing prior CXR is very useful to assess the risk for malignancy in an incidentally found lung nodule. CT is the next step to further characterize a suspicious lung mass, evaluate the location within the parenchyma and the relationship with the surrounding structures. Histologic confirmation is mandatory since benign conditions and metastasis from other primary sites can mimic lung cancer. Tissue samples can be obtained with sputum cytology, bronchoscopy with biopsy, FNA, or cytology, CT-guided biopsy or FNA, and finally with surgery. The choice of technique depends on tumor factors (size, type and location), patient's variables (operative risk, respiratory function, lung parenchyma) and operator's skills.

Once the diagnosis is made, it is important to evaluate the stage of the disease in order to plan the appropriate treatment and predict patient prognosis. Lung cancer is staged according to the size of the tumor, spread to lymph nodes and distant metastasis (TNM classification, Table 3-1).

Assessment for mediastinal involvement and distant metastasis are essential steps for clinical staging. Mediastinoscopy has been considered the "gold standard" for mediastinal staging but this paradigm is being challenged by the development of new technologies such as PET, combined PET-CT and endobronchial/esophageal US-guided biopsy. For clinical suspicion of metastatic disease or for advanced stages under consideration of aggressive treatment, bone scan and brain imaging should be performed to rule out distant metastasis, as the most common site of distant metastasis in NSCLC is the brain. Adrenal metastasis should also be assessed and can be done with high sensitivity (86%) utilizing CT. Pathologic staging is determined after surgical resection.

Preoperative risk assessment

Preoperative risk assessment includes perioperative morbidity and mortality as well as long-term pulmonary disability risks. Patients overall functional status, presence of comorbidities and baseline pulmonary function should be assessed. Cardiovascular risk should be evaluated since cigarette smoking predispose to atherosclerosis. Spirometry is the initial test to evaluate pulmonary function and suitability for surgery. Older studies have shown a mortality rate of less than 5% when the FEV_1 was > 1.5 L before lobectomy or > 2 L before pneumonectomy. Subsequently, preoperative DLCO was shown to have a higher correlation with postoperative deaths than FEV_1. In patients with compromised lung function preoperatively (FEV_1 or DLCO <80% predicted), postoperative pulmonary function should be estimated either by anatomic calculation of functioning lung parenchyma removed, or by mean of quantitative CT scan, ventilation and/or perfusion scan. Patients with postoperative FEV_1 and/or DLCO <40% predicted are at increased risk of perioperative death and cardiopulmonary complications and should undergo preoperative cardiopulmonary exercise testing (CPET). The most specific predictor of postoperative pulmonary complications related to lung resection is the measurement of maximal oxygen consumption (VO_2 max). Patients with VO_2 max greater than 15 mL/kg/min can undergo surgical resection with an acceptably low mortality rate. Patients with postoperative FEV_1 and DLCO less than 40% predicted and VO_2 max less than 15 mL/kg/min have a very high risk of postoperative complications and/or death. Alternative non-operative treatment should be considered for these patients. When CPET is not available, the shuttle-walk test, the stair-climb test or the 6-min walk test can be used.

Table 3-1. International staging of lung cancer *(Adapted with permission from Sobin L, Gospodarowicz M, Wittekind C. TNM Classification of Malignant Tumours. 7th edition. Oxford: Wiley-Blackwell; 2009).*

TNM Descriptors	
T – Primary Tumor	
Tx	Primary tumor cannot be assessed or tumor proven by malignant cells in sputum or bronchial washings but not visualized by imaging or bronchoscopy
T0	No evidence of primary tumor
Tis	Carcinoma *in situ*
T1	Tumor ≤ 3 cm surrounded by lung or visceral pleura, not invading more proximal than lobar bronchus
T1a	Tumor ≤ 2 cm
T1b	Tumor > 2 cm but ≤ 3 cm
T2	Tumor > 3 cm but ≤ 7 cm, or tumor with any of the following features: - Involvement of main bronchus, 2 cm or more distal the carina - Invasion of visceral pleura - Atelectasis or obstructive pneumonitis not involving the entire lung
T2a	Tumor > 3 cm but ≤ 5 cm
T2b	Tumor > 5 cm but ≤ 7 cm
T3	Tumor > 7 cm or tumor with any of the following features: - Invasion of chest wall, diaphragm, phrenic nerve, mediastinal pleura, parietal pericardium - Involvement of main bronchus < 2 cm from the carina (no involvement of the carina) - Atelectasis or obstructive pneumonitis of the entire lung - Separate tumor nodules in the same lobe
T4	Tumor that invades mediastinum, heart, great vessels, trachea, recurrent laryngeal nerve, esophagus, vertebral body, carina, or separate tumor nodules in a different ipsilateral lobe
N – Regional Lymph Nodes	
NX	Regional lymph nodes cannot be assessed
N0	No regional lymph node metastasis
N1	Metastasis in ipsilateral peribronchial and/or hilar nodes and intrapulmonary nodes
N2	Metastasis in ipsilateral mediastinal and/or subcarinal nodes
N3	Metastasis in contralateral mediastinal or hilar nodes, ipsilateral or contralateral scalene or supraclavicular nodes
M – Distant Metastasis	
M0	No distant metastasis
M1	Distant metastasis
M1a	Separate tumor nodules in a contralateral lobe, tumor with pleural nodules, or malignant pleural or pericardial effusion
M1b	Distant metastasis

Stage	T	N	M
Occult carcinoma	TX	0	0
0	Tis	0	0
IA	1a, 1b	0	0
IB	2a	0	0
IIA	2b	0	0
	1a, 1b	1	0
	2a	1	0
IIB	2b	1	0
	3	0	0
IIIA	1a, 1b, 2a, 2b	2	0
	3	1, 2	0
	4a	0, 1	0
IIIB	4	2	0
	Any	3	0
IV	Any	Any	1

4. Early stage non-small cell lung cancer

Shawn S. Groth, Bryan A. Whitson

Epidemiology

Of the estimated 222,250 patients in the United States who will be diagnosed with lung cancer in 2010, about 13% will have early stage (stage I [T1N0M0] or stage II [T2N0M0]) NSCLC. Smoking is the leading risk factor for developing NSCLC, followed by exposure to radon gas and asbestos.

Early detection

Most NSCLC patients present with locally advanced or metastatic disease. In an attempt to increase detection at an earlier stage, a number of studies over the last 40 years have evaluated the role of screening (with CXR, chest CT, and/or sputum cytology) patients at high risk (i.e., from heavy tobacco abuse) for developing lung cancer. None of these studies demonstrated a mortality benefit for screening. Preliminary results from the National Lung Screening Trial (NLST) suggest a 20% improvement in cancer specific mortality and a 7% decrease in all-cause mortality with low-dose helical CT as compared with CXR. The final results have yet to be published.

Pretreatment Staging

Based on current National Comprehensive Cancer Network (NCCN) guidelines, a CT scan of the chest and abdomen (through the adrenals) and PET/CT should be obtained for patients with biopsy-proven (or suspected) early stage NSCLC. Mediastinal lymph nodes (MLNs) that are greater than 1 cm in long-axis diameter or are hypermetabolic on PET (max SUV $\geq$ 2.5) are considered abnormal. Though the adrenals are a common site of metastasis, all adrenal masses detected on CT should be assessed to ascertain whether they are a functional primary adrenal tumor. Nonfunctional adrenal masses should be biopsied. Patients with clinical stage Ib or greater should also undergo a brain MRI.[1]

All primary tumor biopsy specimens should undergo pathologic review to ascertain the histological subtype and to assess for molecular abnormalities that may dictate adjuvant treatment (i.e., EGFR, KRAS, ELM4/ALK, and ERCC1).

All patients should undergo bronchoscopy. Because current imaging modalities lack sufficient sensitivity and diagnostic accuracy, all radiographic MLN findings should be confirmed histologically. Potential options include mediastinoscopy (which allows access to MLN stations 1, 2, 3, 4, and 7), EBUS-TBNA (which allows access to stations 2, 3, 4, 7, 10, and 11), and EUS-FNA (which allows to stations 2R, 2L, 4L, 7, 8, and 9). EUS-FNA can also be used to biopsy left adrenal masses. Though a direct head-to-head comparison has not been performed, mediastinoscopy and EBUS-TBNA likely have comparable sensitivity, specificity, and diagnostic accuracy in experienced hands.

Treatment

Surgery

A number of observational studies have compared lobar and sublobar resection for early stage NSCLC. Most studies demonstrate that patients who undergo lobectomy have a more favorable 5-year overall and cancer-specific survival rate as compared with patients who undergo sublobar resection. For patients who undergo sublobar resection, segmentectomy is associated with tmore favorable local recurrence and 5-year survival rates as compared with wedge resection (Table 4-1).

Table 4-1. Long-term results after resection for NSCLC.

	Wedge resection	Segmentectomy	Lobectomy
Local recurrence	16-31%	2.2-23%	1.3-11.5%
5-Year survival	26-69%	43-93%	67-90%

The only prospective, multi-institutional, randomized trial comparing lobectomy and sublobar resection for stage I NSCLC was published by the Lung Cancer Study Group in 1995.[2] There was no difference in morbidity or long-term preservation of pulmonary function between the two groups. As compared with lobectomy, a 3-fold increase in local recurrence rates after wedge resection and a 2.4-fold increase in local recurrence rates after segmentectomy were noted. Tumor size (even if less than 1 cm) did not affect local recurrence rates; sublobar resection was associated with higher local recurrence rates. Until the results of other randomized trials provide evidence to the contrary, lobectomy should be considered the standard of care for early stage NSCLC.

A sublobar resection (preferably a segmentectomy) with margins equal to the size of the primary tumor may be a reasonable alternative for patients who are not lobectomy candidates due to poor cardiopulmonary fitness or other major medical co-morbidities.

Proximal tumors may be difficult to resect with a lobectomy. In these cases, a sleeve resection is preferred over a pneumonectomy, if possible.

The key for an optimal sleeve anastomosis is a well-approximated tension-free repair. The anastomosis should be wrapped with additional tissue such as intercostal muscle, omentum, or pericardium to improve healing and decrease the risk of fistulization between the PA and the bronchus.

The treatment of bronchioalveolar carcinoma (BAC), an indolent type of adenocarcinoma that originates from type II pneumocytes (Clara cells), depends on presentation but relies on complete surgical resection, if possible. BAC can present as a solitary peripheral nodule, as a pulmonary infiltrate, or as multifocal disease. Lobar resection is used if the patient has adequate pulmonary reserve and the lesion is localized. Multifocal BAC may be treated with several wedge resections as long as the burden of disease is not significant. If there are too many lesions, chemotherapy may be used (EGFR inhibitors are used for the 25% of patients with EGFR mutations).

Complete MLN evaluation is a critical adjunct to lobectomy. All abnormal appearing MLNs should be removed. For right-sided tumors, all lymphatic tissue from stations 2R, 4R, 7, 8, 9, and 10R to 14R should be sampled or removed. For left sided tumors, all lymphatic tissue from stations 2L, 4L, 5, 6, 7, 8, 9, and 10L to 14L should be sampled or removed.

In addition to the extent of resection, the approach may also be important. Based on recent meta-analyses, a VATS lobectomy is associated with lower morbidity, improved quality of life, and improved survival as compared with an open lobectomy.

Postoperative complications occur in 30% of patients undergoing pulmonary resections. Complications include arrhythmias, prolonged postoperative air leaks, pneumonia, respiratory failure, wound infections, and alterations in mental status. A unique complication that can present after right upper lobectomy is torsion of the RML due to lack of tethering of the middle lobe once the minor fissure is divided and the upper lobe removed. In order to prevent this complication, the middle lobe is attached to the lower lobe with stitches or staples. If this complication is suspected based on postoperative CXR, the diagnosis should be expeditiously made with bronchoscopy. If the diagnosis is in doubt, CT can be helpful. Reoperation is mandatory.

Adjuvant therapy

Based on current NCCN guidelines, patients with stage Ia disease who undergo R0 resection do not require adjuvant therapy. Patients with stage I or II NSCLC who undergo an R1 resection should undergo re-resection (preferred) or adjuvant RT. Chemotherapy is indicated for patients with high-risk stage Ib tumors and patients with stage II tumors. First-line chemotherapy is cisplatin-based. For patients who are unable to tolerate cisplatin and patients with comorbidities, carboplatin combined with paclitaxel is a reasonable alternative.[1]

Patients who are not surgical candidates

Patients who are medically inoperable are treated with definitive chemo-radiation therapy. Radiofrequency ablation (RFA) is a potential alternative to patients with early stage NSCLC who lack sufficient cardiopulmonary reserve to tolerate pulmonary resection.

Post-treatment surveillance

Based on current guidelines, patients should be followed by a routine history and physical exam and non-contrast chest CT every 4 to 6 months for the first 2 years and annually thereafter. PET is not indicated for routine follow-up. NSCLC survivors should continue to undergo routine health maintenance.

Prognosis

Untreated, patients with early stage NSCLC have a median survival of 17 months (0% survival at 5 years). For patients who undergo lobectomy, 5-year survival rates of 55% to 90% have been reported.

5. Locally advanced lung cancer

Benjamin Wei, Matthew Hartwig

Diagnosis and staging

Locally-advanced lung cancer can be defined as NSCLC that has invaded adjacent structures, and represents about 5-10% of newly diagnosed lung cancers in the US. Patients with locally advanced lung cancer may present with chest pain related to chest wall invasion or obstructive symptoms related to compression of the airways or great vessels within the chest, but up to 25% of them are asymptomatic.

Diagnosis is facilitated by cross-sectional imaging. CT is effective for evaluating invasion of the ribs and intercostal muscles, while MRI is the preferred modality for assessing involvement of the spinal cord and vascular structures. Neither CT nor MRI, however, is sensitive enough for detecting pleural invasion, which can often only be discovered at the time of surgery or at pathological examination of the specimen.

Locally advanced lung cancer can be considered T3 or T4 tumors according to the TNM system (Table 3-1), depending on which organs they invade. Tumors that invade chest wall, diaphragm, phrenic nerve, parietal pleura, pericardium, or main stem bronchus < 2 cm from the carina but without involvement of the carina are T3 lesions. Tumors that invade the contents of the mediastinum (i.e., heart, great vessels, trachea/carina, recurrent largyngeal nerve, esophagus) or vertebral body are T4 lesions. It is important to note that the T3 and T4 classification also contains cancers that would not traditionally be considered "locally invasive." T3 tumors include tumors 7 cm or larger, tumors that result in obstructive atelectasis or pneumonitis of the entire lung, and 2 or more tumors within the same lobe. T4 tumors include 2 or more tumors in different ipsilateral lobes.

The spectrum of locally advanced cancer is broad; patients with locally advanced lung cancer may be anywhere between Stage IIB and IV under the current staging guidelines. Patients with T3N0 disease are considered stage IIB. Patients with T4N2 disease or T3 or T4 and N3 disease are considered stage IIIB. All other patients with T3 or T4 disease (T3N1, T3N2, T4N0, T4N1) are considered stage IIIA. Prior to contemplating surgery for the patient with locally advanced lung cancer, it is important to rule out the presence of metastatic disease. This should include surgical staging of the mediastinum, PET and CT imaging of the chest and abdomen through the level of the adrenals, as well as neurological evaluation with a head CT or MRI.

Treatment

Prior to consideration of surgery for a patient with locally advanced lung cancer, it is essential to consider tumor resectability, patient fitness, nodal status, and the specific surgical considerations relevant to the tumor.

Resectability

The goal of surgery is to achieve an R0 resection, or resection with grossly and microscopically negative margins. T4 lesions, with the exception of invasion of the carina or vertebral bodies have classically been considered unresectable and the dominant therapeutic option for these patients is palliative chemoradiation. Highly selected patients with invasion of the SVC, PA, and aorta have been treated surgically in the context of multimodality therapy.

Patient fitness

The patient with locally advanced cancer should undergo a thorough preoperative evaluation including pulmonary function, cardiac evaluation, and a nutritional assessment. The addition of a chest wall or diaphragmatic resection is likely to compromise the patient's respiratory physiology beyond what is entailed by the pulmonary resection alone. Although it is difficult to quantify the effect, this should be taken into account when deciding what extent of pulmonary resection to perform.

Nodal status

The treatment strategy for locally advanced lung cancer depends on the extent of lymph node involvement. Non-invasive modalities such as CT, MRI, or PET scans are often first used to assess nodal status; however, surgical staging with mediastinoscopy remains the gold standard. EBUS is a newer method for staging mediastinal lymph nodes. If these studies do not suggest mediastinal lymph node involvement, and the above criteria of fitness and resectability are met, the surgeon can proceed to the operating room for resection. Special caution is advised in evaluating the nodal status for LUL tumors, as these lesions notoriously have the most inconsistent lymph node positivity.

The mediastinoscopy and subsequent resection can occur in the same setting if the mediastinal nodes are negative for malignancy on frozen section. Positive ipsilateral bronchial or perihilar nodes (N1 disease) are often hard to reach by mediastinoscopy, but may be more readily accessible by EBUS. In either case, N1 patients with locally advanced cancer (i.e., T3N1) should generally be offered surgery. For the most part, N2 patients are offered induction platinum-based chemotherapy. The possibility of surgical resection exists if their disease responds favorably on repeat cross-sectional imaging. In this regard, patients with a single N2 node demonstrate a superior prognosis to those with multinodal involvement. Patients with contralateral mediastinal node disease (N3) are generally candidates for palliative chemoradiation only, and should not be offered surgery.

Chest wall invasion

The approach for most patients with chest wall invasion is through a posterolateral thoracotomy. The interspace for entry should be at least one rib and one intercostal space above or below the margin of the tumor. Ideally, tumors involving the chest wall should be resected *en bloc* with the overlying structures into which the cancer is invading. Usually the skin is spared, unless the lesion has eroded into or through the skin. Removal of tissue to include one uninvolved rib above and one below the tumor is general practice. A margin of 2 cm is considered adequate. Reconstruction of the chest wall is often done if the defect is larger than 5 cm, though it may be omitted if it is protected by the scapula. The defect can be reconstructed with tissue flaps (latissimus dorsi, serratus anterior, and rectus abdominus flaps) or synthetic material (PTFE, polypropylene with methylmethacrylate, and Vicryl). The presence of an infected or contaminated space favors the use of autogenous tissue.

Spinal invasion

Tumors with invasion of the vertebra require a partial or complete vertebrectomy with spinal reconstruction, at times spanning multiple levels. Tumors extending into the intervertebral foramen may require laminectomy and/or rib disarticulation to access the nerve roots. Induction chemoradiotherapy should be considered in these patients. Surgery involving the spine may result in a CSF leak, which can cause meningitis and subarachnoid or ventricular air leak and necessitate reoperation.

Superior sulcus tumors

Superior sulcus tumors are located at the uppermost aspect of the costovertebral gutter in the chest cavity. In addition to invading the chest wall and spine, these tumors can invade any of the structures of the thoracic inlet, which is divided into anterior, middle, and posterior compartments. The compartments contain the following structures:

- *Anterior:* platysma, sternocleidomastoid muscle, subclavian vein

- *Middle:* phrenic nerve, anterior scalene muscle, subclavian artery, brachial plexus, middle and posterior scalene muscles

- *Posterior:* sympathetic ganglia, long thoracic nerve, external branch of spinal accessory nerve, subscapular artery.

Pancoast syndrome refers to the triad of shoulder pain, atrophy of the intrinsic hand muscles, and Horner's syndrome (ptosis, myosis (pupillary constriction), anhydrosis), usually caused by tumors invading the posterior compartment.

The treatment for malignant superior sulcus tumors is induction chemoradiation followed by resection. Traditional contraindications to resection include N2 or greater disease, involvement of brachial plexus beyond C8-T1, and invasion of the spinal cord. Resection can be performed via the anterior or posterior approaches. The tumor is resected as an upper lobectomy *en bloc* with the involved structures. Removal of the T1 nerve root alone is well-tolerated, but removal of C8 causes atrophic paralysis of the muscles of the hand and forearm (Klumpke paralysis), and may not be acceptable to a prospective surgical candidate. The phrenic nerve should be preserved if possible. The subclavian vein should be resected and the ends ligated if part of it is involved by tumor. The subclavian artery may be partially resected, with primary anastomosis or grafting with PTFE if necessary.

Bronchoplastic procedures

The bronchi may be resected and reconstructed in the process of performing a sleeve lobectomy or bilobectomy; the carina may be resected as part of a sleeve or carinal pneumonectomy. Compared to pneumonectomy, sleeve lobectomy has been shown to have a decreased risk of operative morbidity and mortality, comparable local recurrence rates, and similar if not better long-term survival rates. Sleeve pneumonectomy is used when lung cancer has invaded the carina. Important concepts when performing these sleeve resections include confirmation of negative proximal and distal bronchial margins, ensuring a tension-free anastomosis, and wrapping the anastomosis with a pericardial, pleural, or intercostal muscle flap.

Anastomotic dehiscence can occur, and in the case of a sleeve lobectomy it usually requires completion pneumonectomy if the dehiscence is large, total, or associated with empyema. A small dehiscence with no bronchopleural fistula may be treated non-operatively. Late anastomotic stricture is related to ischemia or partial dehiscence.

Lung cancers involving the carina can be resected with acceptable mortality at specialized centers. The approach to a right carinal pneumonectomy is via a right posterolateral thoracotomy. The approach to a left carinal pneumonectomy is via a median sternotomy, left thoracotomy, or bilateral thoracotomies/clamshell incision. It is difficult to visualize the carina from the left chest due to the aortic arch, however the left lung cannot be removed via a right thoracotomy alone, which accounts for the variety of approaches taken. To get to the carina via a median sternotomy, the posterior pericardium between the SVC and the ascending aorta needs to be opened. For carinal pneumonectomies, tension on the anastomosis can be reduced by 1) immediate preoperative mediastinoscopy, which loosens the tissue, 2) maintaining the neck in a flexed position, and 3) intrapericardial release.

Ipsilateral metastases

As mentioned earlier, patients with multiple cancers located in the same lobe are deemed T3, while patients with cancers in different lobes of the ipsilateral lung are deemed T4. These patients have been shown to have a 40-50% five-year survival rate after pulmonary resection, which compares favorably to patients with metastases to the contralateral lung, who are deemed to have M1 disease. After assessment of nodal status to confirm the absence of N2 disease, these patients may be offered surgery with reasonable outcomes.

6. Paraneoplastic syndromes
Robroy H. MacIver

Approximately 2% of lung cancer patients develop paraneoplastic syndromes. Size of the cancer does not appear to correlate with the potential for developing a paraneoplastic process. In some cases, the paraneoplastic symptoms will preclude identification of a primary tumor. Common paraneoplastic syndromes include:

- *Hypercalcemia.* Results from either metastatic bone destruction or resorption from ectopic and excessive PTH secretion. 10% of lung cancer patients will have hypercalcemia. It is more common in squamous cell cancer. Symptoms are those of hypercalcemia such as constipation, anorexia, polydipsia and irritability.

- *Syndrome of inappropriate secretion of antidiuretic hormone (SIADH).* Patients present with hyponatremia that can result in symptoms of nausea, seizures and altered mental status. SIADH is more common in SCLC and in women. A diagnosis is made in the setting of hyponatremia with a high urinary sodium. Initial treatment is fluid restriction. Medical treatment includes demeclocycline, which blocks the receptor for antidiuretic hormone in the kidney.

- *Cushing's syndrome.* Most commonly in SCLC. Unlike classical Cushing's syndrome, the classic symptoms do not develop as the ACTH levels rise too rapidly. The symptoms are usually edema and muscle weakness. A key finding in the diagnosis is that the ACTH is produced autonomously, so ACTH levels are not suppressed by dexamethasone.

- *Bone changes.* Clubbing can be found with NSCLC, mostly squamous cell. Patients can also present with hypertrophic pulmonary osteoarthropathy, a process that frequently affects the radius, ulna, tibia, and fibula. The new bone formation and inflammation at the end of these bones can cause significant pain. This process can precede the diagnosis of cancer. Treatment, outside of cancer therapy, is with non-steroidal anti-inflammatory agents.

- *Neuropathy.* Common in lung cancer patients. Although multifactorial, it is often secondary to brain or neurologic metastases. Circulating antibodies have also been implicated in paraneoplastic neuropathies. The neuropathies frequently precede the diagnosis of cancer.

- *Myopathy.* Frequently causes proximal muscle weakness. Two theories exist regarding the etiology. One is that the weakness is a manifestation of a myositis with general degeneration of the muscle fibers. The other is that there is a defect in the neuromuscular transmission. Lambert-Eaton syndrome is more commonly associated with SCLC. In this syndrome antibodies are formed against voltage-gated calcium channels. In turn, this inhibits presynaptic release of acetylcholine at the motor endplate.

- *Anemia.* Common in lung cancer patients. The cause is multifactorial and includes decreased life span of red cells, decreased iron stores, and decreased iron binding capacity.

- *Hypercoagulability.* Like solid organ cancer, lung cancer is associated with hypercoagulability and vascular thrombosis. Thrombosis can be resistant to anticoagulation. Treatment of the tumor may reverse the hypercoagulable state.

- *Dermatologic changes.* Manifestations include dermatomyositis, erythema gyratum and lanuginoa acquisita. Skin manifestations can develop very quickly. Cutaneous manifestations are most commonly associated with adenocarcinoma.

7. Post-pneumonectomy complications
Theolyn Price

Mortality for pneumonectomy can vary from as low as 3% to as high as 30%, but with a standard pneumonectomy for lung cancer the range is 3-12%. There is significantly higher mortality with right-sided pneumonectomies due primarily to a higher incidence of bronchopleural fistula (BPF), empyema, and pulmonary edema. Other factors that are thought to increase the risk of pneumonectomy are older age, induction therapy, completion pneumonectomy, resection for infectious or inflammatory disease, extended procedures such as carinal pneumonectomy and extrapleural pneumonectomy. The morbidity of pneumonectomy ranges from 15-75%. Some of the most frequently seen complications are respiratory failure, pneumonia, BPF, empyema, arrhythmias, MI, and PE. Some more lethal complications that are less frequently seen are cardiac herniation, and post-pneumonectomy pulmonary edema.

Post-pneumonectomy syndrome

More commonly seen in children, but occasionally seen in adults, this is progressive post-pneumonectomy mediastinal shift, which can result in stretching or compression of the trachea or remaining bronchus by the PA, aorta, or vertebral column. Theories for this extensive shift include hyperinflation of the remaining lung, hyperplasia, size of the pneumonectomy space, elasticity of the mediastinal tissues, chest wall and diaphragmatic changes. This is primarily seen after right pneumonectomy (counterclockwise rotation), but can also be seen after left pneumonectomy (clockwise rotation) and can result in severe respiratory compromise, tracheobronchial malacia, recurrent infections, bronchiectasis, and parenchymal destruction. Children tend to present early, but adults usually develop late symptoms, including dyspnea, stridor, recurrent infections, and orthopnea. Some will not develop symptoms for years, at which time tracheomalacia has developed. Bronchoscopy and CT are diagnostic. Treatment involves thoracotomy and placement of prosthetic devices within the ipsilateral hemithorax, most commonly saline breast implants, which will restore anatomic position and relieve airway obstruction. Occasionally, expandable airway stents are also required.

Cardiac herniation

This is a rare complication seen equally after right and left sided pneumonectomies and occasionally after extended lobectomy. However, it remains the most significant complication after an intrapericardial pneumonectomy. Herniation can be avoided on the left side by opening the pericardium to the diaphragm, but this is ineffective on the right side. The mechanism of hemodynamic collapse is unique for each side. On the left, the LV herniates through the defect then strangulates, causing impairment of diastole, systole, and coronary perfusion. On the right, there is torsion of the LV anteriorly and to the right through the defect, occluding inflow from the SVC and IVC. Both result in catastrophic circulatory failure with an approximate 50% mortality rate. It usually occurs within the first 72 hours after surgery and can be triggered by a change in patient position. Patients may develop cyanosis, elevated CVP, hypotension, tachycardia, a displaced cardiac impulse, and rapid deterioration. CXR and EKG may be helpful but a high index of suspicion may be life saving. If prior right pneumonectomy was performed, the patient should be positioned left side down and returned immediately to the OR for reduction via a redo-thoracotomy, and patch repair of the defect.

Post-pneumonectomy pulmonary edema

This is a complex complication that occurs in 2-5% of cases and is nearly impossible to predict, prevent, or treat successfully. If unrecognized, this complication is lethal, but even with early detection the mortality rate is 60-90%. It is more frequently seen after right-sided pneumonectomy and those with extensive resection such as a carinal pneumonectomy. Clinically and histologically it is very similar to ARDS with endothelial injury, an increased gradient across the pulmonary microcirculation, and hyperpermeability that result in diffuse alveolar damage. The causal mechanisms thought to contribute are excess fluid administration, interruption of major lymphatics to the remaining lung, immunologic reaction to blood products (e.g., fresh frozen plasma), increase in extent and duration of operation, use of an underwater seal drainage system vs. a balanced system, and mechanical factors (e.g., hyperinflation, air-blocking). A typical presentation would be rapidly progressive dyspnea, hypoxemia, and radiographic signs of pulmonary edema in a patient with normal PFTs, and an unremarkable 12-24 hour post-operative course after right pneumonectomy. As this is a diagnosis of exclusion, it is imperative to rule out other causes of deterioration, such as cardiogenic shock, PE, sepsis, BPF, aspiration or infectious pneumonitis, and treat empirically until reliably eliminated. The patients should have invasive right heart monitoring, CT, pan-cultures, and bronchoscopy. It is often refractory to standard therapies, but when treated early, mortality is reduced. The treatment algorithm should include IVF restriction, early use of diuretics, pain control, use of pressors for hypotension once fluid resuscitation is adequate, and avoiding barotrauma by limiting high pressure ventilation. Inhaled nitric oxide has also been shown to improve oxygenation and decrease mortality. Steroids are thought to be beneficial, but their role is still controversial.

Bronchopleural fistula (BPF)

Incidence varies from 1-10%, is more common after pneumonectomy than lesser resections, and is more common after a right-sided pneumonectomy. Mortality ranges from 30-50% (as low as 16%, to as high as 72%), with most deaths secondary to sepsis, respiratory failure, malnutrition, and rarely, from bronchovascular fistula. With this in mind, prevention is key. Risk factors include right pneumonectomy, completion pneumonectomy, resection for infection/inflammation (especially TB with positive sputum), previous mediastinal/hilar RT, prolonged mechanical ventilation, DM, post-pneumonectomy empyema or infected post-resection space, residual tumor at the stump, and technical factors (devascularization, incomplete closure, long bronchial stump). Other factors that are also thought to contribute are old age, steroid use, malnutrition, preoperative chemotherapy, and partial-dose RT.

If the BPF develops early (usually 1-2 days, but can be within 2 weeks) after surgery, it is likely due to technical factors, may manifest as a massive air leak, progressive subcutaneous air, or respiratory insufficiency, and requires reoperation. If the BPF develops later in the post-operative course, it is likely due to inadequate healing or rupture of an empyema through the bronchial stump. These patients may present febrile, with a productive cough (purulent sputum, blood, or frothy serosanguineous fluid), and are in danger of flooding the remaining lung. With any deterioration, the patient should be place with the operative side down, head elevated, and immediate drainage of the pleural space should be performed with tube thoracostomy or re-opening of the thoracotomy.

An occult BPF occasionally occurs, is usually asymptomatic to minimally symptomatic, and is suspected due to a fall in the pleural space fluid level (swallowed or absorbed through parietal pleura). Confirmation is most commonly via bronchoscopy, but may also require further investigation with injection of methylene blue into the pneumonectomy space, or use of inhaled radionucleotide. Management may be close observation as long as the patient remains asymptomatic with no clinical signs of infection. Antibiotics are not necessary. Should any signs or symptoms of infection develop, prompt drainage of the pleural space should ensue.

Treatment of a clinically evident BPF depends on the underlying cause, and the timing of presentation. For early presentation (within 2 weeks), patients require antibiotics, reoperation, repair and coverage of the bronchial stump (omentum, pericardial fat pad, muscle). In those associated with severe empyema, an open flap may be a better alternative for drainage than chest tubes. For late presentation a more aggressive approach is required to close the fistula and manage the associated empyema. Recommendations are for antibiotics, chest tube or open drainage (Eloesser flap, Eloesser modification, or re-opening of the original thoracotomy), cleansing of the pleural space, re-closure of the bronchial stump along with vascularized flap coverage (omentum or muscle), and sterilization of the pleural space with the Clagett procedure, a modification thereof, or open thoracic window. If this fails, pleural space obliteration with muscle flaps may be required. If the distal stump cannot be removed it is imperative to transpose a muscle flap between the divided ends to avoid re-fistulization.

Empyema

The incidence of post-pneumonectomy empyema ranges from 2-16%, but is 5-7% in most series. A BPF is frequently associated, with the risks factors being concordant. A patient can present anywhere along the spectrum of systemic toxicity, with an elevated WBC count, anorexia, and failure to thrive. A diagnosis should be secured with sampling of the pleural fluid, and when confirmed, initiation of the appropriate antibiotics and drainage. The remaining treatment algorithms for empyema depend on whether there is an associated BPF, the chronicity of infection, adequacy of drainage, size of any remaining space, and the prognosis unrelated to the infection. Early empyemas with no associated BPF are uncommon, and are best managed by VATS drainage, tube irrigation, and systemic antibiotics. Once sterilized (negative cultures), the space is filled with antibiotic solution and the chest tubes are removed. Most large infected spaces and essentially all postpneumonectomy empyemas will require open drainage, a Clagett procedure (or modification), space obliteration with flaps (muscle, omentum), thoracoplasty, or a combination of procedures. An individualized treatment approach is ideal. Maintaining adequate nutrition is crucial during the recovery phase of all these patients.

8. Pulmonary carcinoid tumors and other primary lung tumors

Jenifer Marks

Primary pulmonary carcinoid tumors comprise 0.4 to 3% of resected lung cancers and the lungs are the second most common site of origin for primary carcinoid tumors. The WHO classifies carcinoid tumors as typical (<2 mitotic figures/10 high-power fields, no necrosis) or atypical (2-10 mitotic figures/10 high-power fields, tissue necrosis or architectural disruption). Both typical and atypical tumors have the ability to metastasize and invade local structures and therefore are both considered malignant lesions. In most series of resected tumors, 15-20% are classified as atypical carcinoid tumors with the remainder being typical carcinoids. According to the WHO, carcinoid tumors are considered part of the histologic spectrum of neuroendocrine tumors: typical carcinoid tumor (low grade), atypical carcinoid tumor (intermediate grade), large-cell neuroendocrine tumor (high grade), and SCLC (high grade).

Clinical presentation

The median age at presentation is 48 years, with bimodal peaks at 35 and 55 years of age. Patients older than 50 years of age have a higher incidence of atypical lesions than those younger than 30 years of age (25% vs. 10%). The gender distribution is approximately even. One third of patients are asymptomatic. Among those with symptoms, recurrent pneumonia, cough, and hemoptysis are the most common presenting symptoms. Carcinoids may release ectopic hormones such as ACTH, vasopressin, insulin, and 5-hydroxytryptophan. Carcinoid syndrome is uncommon in the setting of localized disease; however approximately 5% of patients will develop Cushing's syndrome with localized disease.

Diagnosis and staging

CXR findings are non-specific and related to the location of the tumors. Fifty percent of atypical and 71% of typical carcinoid tumors are central in location, with 75% of these being found in a lobar or segmental bronchus. CT findings of carcinoid tumors are characteristic, with peripheral carcinoids having a smooth, rounded, homogenous appearance and central lesions with an obvious airway component and post-obstructive atelectasis or pneumonitis. Both PET and octreotide scans are often obtained in these patients, however the data are conflicting and neither can be recommended as routine studies in the diagnosis or staging of these patients.

Bronchoscopy and biopsy for tissue diagnosis is important for patients with central lesions, while needle-guided biopsy should be used for peripheral lesions. It is well established that these lesions can be biopsied safely. Despite adequate tissue, a diagnosis of carcinoid is only be made 70 to 80% of the time preoperatively; even less accurate is the distinction between typical versus an atypical lesion. Clinical factors, such as patient age, tumor location, and radiographic findings (including nodal status) often support the clinical diagnosis and histologic subtype of carcinoid even in the absence of a tissue diagnosis. Most peripheral and central carcinoid tumors without evidence of nodal disease will be typical carcinoid tumors and require no further evaluation prior to resection. In contrast, 50% of central carcinoids and 50-72% of peripheral carcinoid tumors with cN1 or cN2 disease will be of atypical histology and these patients should have a thorough staging workup for metastatic disease including mediastinoscopy prior to resection.

Treatment

Surgical resection is the main treatment for carcinoid tumors. A limited resection is acceptable for typical carcinoids as long as R0 status (no residual tumor) is achieved. Formal mediastinal lymph node dissection should be performed for any clinical nodal disease and atypical lesions. Even those with N2 disease have good survival with complete resection. Adjuvant chemotherapy, either preoperatively if N2 disease is detected during staging, or postoperatively for pathologic N2 disease, is given in some centers with response rates similar to that seen with NSCLC. The data supporting this approach is limited. Endo-bronchial resection of carcinoid tumors has been attempted for those patients unable to tolerate a parenchymal resection, however every effort should be made to attain a negative margin, as these patients will recur locally.

Tumorlets, typical carcinoid tumors < 5 mm in diameter, can be seen in up to 10% of patients with a primary carcinoid lesion or other types of NSCLC. They are more common in women and older patients. It is unclear whether these patients have a worse survival but the tumorlets should not be staged as metastatic disease and treatment should be based on the primary lesion.

Metastatic and unresectable carcinoid is often treated with chemotherapy, while the value of RT is less clear and not often reported on. Chemotherapy response rates vary from 20 to 38%, while as many as 30% will progress on therapy. Small-cell regimens seem to provide most of the responses. It is recommended that carcinoid patients be followed for twenty years due to the indolent nature of the disease.

Other primary malignant lung tumors

Adenoid cystic carcinoma is a tumor of the trachea and mainstem bronchi that is usually detected only with the onset of symptoms, often with a significant obstructive component. Submucosal extension beyond gross intraluminal tumor is the rule with these lesions and intra-operative frozen section of the bronchial margin to ensure complete resection is essential when resecting adenoid cystic carcinomas.

Other salivary gland-type tumors include mucoepidermoid and acinic cell carcinoma. These are all malignant lesions with a usually indolent course. However, local invasion and nodal metastasis are possible. These lesions account for 1% of all primary lung neoplasms and the mainstay of treatment is resection with negative margins.

Soft tissue sarcomas, pleomorphic, spindle-cell, and giant-cell carcinomas, pulmonary blastomas, and pulmonary lymphomas are other rare malignant tumors of the lung.

Benign lung tumors

The most common benign tumors of the lung include pulmonary hamartoma, inflammatory pseudotumor, sclerosing hemangioma, bronchogenic cyst, leiomyoma, and adenomas. Papillomas, soft tissue tumors including lipomas, inflammatory fibrous polyps, lymphatic lesions, clear cell tumor, teratoma, and thymoma are much less common but reported. Diagnosis may only be at the time of resection or with the treatment of any associated symptoms, although uncommon.

9. Pulmonary metastatic disease

Bryan M. Burt, Ravi K. Ghanta

Autopsy series have demonstrated that pulmonary metastases are present in 20-54% of all patients who die of cancer. Most patients who develop pulmonary metastases are not curable, owing to the presence of extrathoracic metastases and ineffective systemic chemotherapy. Pulmonary metastasectomy (PM) is the only curative option for most patients with pulmonary metastases and can improve survival in select patient groups. PM should be considered in patients with resectable intrathoracic disease, no extrathoracic disease and adequate cardiopulmonary reserve. There has never been a randomized trial to determine the survival advantage of PM, however a large volume of retrospective data substantiates a survival benefit of PM for many histologic subtypes of metastases.

Diagnosis

The majority of pulmonary metastases are diagnosed by surveillance imaging. The radiographic appearance of pulmonary metastases is nonspecific and there is no pathognomonic radiographic feature that distinguishes metastatic disease from primary lung cancer. Pulmonary metastases are predominantly subpleural and located in the outer third of the lung fields. When multiple nodules are present, the probability of metastatic disease rather than primary lung cancer increases significantly. Chest CT is the standard imaging technique for identifying and following lesions. PET-CT is critical in the work-up of metastatic disease and can identify unsuspected extrathoracic disease, and thereby improves patient selection for PM.

Principles of surgical resection

Two main principles direct the surgical approach for resection of pulmonary metastases: complete resection of malignancy and maximal sparing of normal lung tissue. Because of their largely peripheral location, most lesions are amenable to wedge resection. It appears that wedge resection, if feasible, is as effective as anatomic resection for the treatment of pulmonary metastases. For lesions that are more central, segmentectomy or lobectomy may be required.

Of the 5206 cases of PM in the International Registry of Pulmonary Metastases, 67% of patients underwent wedge resection, 21% lobectomy, 9% segmentectomy, and 3% pneumonectomy. The VATS approach to PM has the advantages of less postoperative pain, shorter length of stay, fewer adhesions at reoperation, and better compliance with adjuvant therapies. The argument against the use of the VATS approach to PM, centers on the belief that manual palpation of the deflated lung is essential to identifying all metastatic disease. There is, however, no evidence to suggest that the timing of resection of nodules that would be missed at VATS resection, which are usually < 5 mm, is critical to the final outcome. Moreover, many recent studies in several different cell types suggest that VATS resection of pulmonary metastases yields comparable survival to thoracotomy.

Although the standard accepted resection for primary lung cancer includes either complete lymphadenectomy or lymph node sampling, this is not true for the surgical treatment of pulmonary metastases. Hilar or mediastinal lymph node involvement is present in 5 to 30% of cases of resected pulmonary metastases and is more common with carcinoma rather than sarcomatous metastases. Hilar or mediastinal nodal involvement negatively impacts survival in the setting of various metastatic tumors, and although it remains questionable as to whether lymphadenectomy affords a survival benefit, it is championed by some groups owing to its prognostic and staging benefits. Data on the outcomes of adjuvant or neoadjuvant chemotherapy and RT for pulmonary metastases are limited.

Mortality rates of PM do not differ from those of resection for lung cancer and vary between 0.6% and 2%. Many retrospective series on PM report overall 5-year survival rates of 30% to 40%. Data from the International Registry of Lung Metastases demonstrate global overall survival of 36% at 5 years and 26% at 10 years following complete resection of pulmonary metastases. These data represent the gamut of epithelial, sarcoma, melanoma, and germ cell histologies, for which the benefit of resection was shown to vary depending upon specific pathology. Patients with germ cell tumors had by far the best survival (68% at 5 years) and melanoma the worst (21% at 5 years). The survival of patients with epithelial tumors (37% at 5 years) and those with sarcomas (31% at 5 years) were similar.

The most common primary histology for patients evaluated for PM is colorectal carcinoma, and 35% to 45% five-year survival can be attained with resection. Sarcoma is the second most frequent source of metastases to the lungs, and in up to 50% of patients, the lungs are the only site of metastatic disease. Five-year survival rates of 25% to 35% are seen for PM for sarcomatous metastases. Encouraging results are also seen in renal cell cancer (20% to 50% five-year survival), gynecologic cancers (33% to 76% five-year survival), and head and neck cancers (34% to 84% five-year survival). PM for metastatic breast cancer is controversial because of the availability of other effective systemic treatments such as chemotherapy, hormone therapy, and targeted molecular therapy.

Besides histology, factors associated with improved survival in patients undergoing PM include a prolonged disease-free interval from the time of resection of primary tumor to the appearance of pulmonary metastases and a lower number of pulmonary metastases. In almost all series the strongest predictor of survival is complete resection. Finally, repeat PM may be required when there are isolated recurrences in the lungs. Forty to eighty percent of patients undergoing PM will suffer a pulmonary recurrence. Repeat PM has been shown in the International Registry and several subsequent databases to afford a long-term survival advantage in patients that qualify for repeated procedures.

10. Congenital lung diseases
Theolyn Price

Embryology

There are 4 phases of intrauterine pulmonary development:

- *Embryonic phase (weeks 1-5).* This phase begins with foregut development from the embryonic endoderm on day 9. On day 22, the median pharyngeal groove develops. By week 4 the lung buds have formed and there is separation of the trachea from the esophagus. The lung buds form the trachea and bronchial buds, which then form the mainstem bronchi by week 5. Then over the next few weeks, the 5 lobes become evident.

- *Pseudoglandular phase (weeks 5-16).* This phase involves the development of the bronchial tree and pulmonary vasculature, with complete development of the bronchial tree and pulmonary arteries by week 16.

- *Cannicular phase (week 16-26).* This phase involves the development of the respiratory bronchioles and alveolar ducts. The pulmonary venous system develops by week 26.

- *Terminal sac phase (week 26-40).* The primitive alveoli proliferate while they become intimately involved with the surrounding capillaries. Surfactant is produced by type II pneumocytes in preparation for delivery.

Lung development continues postnatally with the continuation of acinar production until the age of 8. Rather than increasing in number, after age 10, the alveoli enlarge. Airway diameter continues to increase until age 5, and the pulmonary vasculature length and diameter continue to rapidly grow until 18 months.

Tracheobronchial esophageal fistula (TEF)

TEF is the most common anomaly of the trachea. The most commonly used classification (by Gross) is:

- *Type A (8%):* esophageal atresia without TEF

- *Type B (1%):* esophageal atresia with proximal TEF

- *Type C (87%):* esophageal atresia with distal TEF

- *Type D (1%):* esophageal atresia with proximal and distal TEF

- *Type E (4%):* TEF without esophageal atresia

Patients present with feeding difficulty, excessive salivation, cyanosis, or recurrent infections. Suspicion should be aroused with excessive air within the esophagus, stomach, and intestinal tract, and the inability to pass a NGT, with CXR confirmation. Surgical correction is performed via a right extrapleural thoracotomy, a right cervical incision, or a combination of both. The fistula is divided and the defect is repaired. An interposition muscle flap should be considered to reduce the chance of recurrence.

Sequestration

This is an abnormal segment of lung tissue that has no communication with the tracheobronchial tree. The arterial supply is from a systemic vessel, most frequently the thoracic aorta, but it can also come from the abdominal aorta, an intercostal artery, or from multiple sources. The arterial blood supply usually enters the sequestration away from the hilum, most often at the base of the lung. The venous return is most commonly into the pulmonary veins but can also be through the systemic venous system. There is a male predominance of 3:1. Since they arise from foregut tissue, there may be an associated esophageal fistula.

Twenty-five percent of sequestrations are *extralobar (ELS)*, which are distinct from the remaining lung, with their own visceral pleura. They are round soft tissue masses that typically lie just above the dome of the diaphragm, with 90% found at the base of the left lung. The venous return is more often systemic (azygos, hemiazygos) with only 20% draining into the pulmonary veins. ELS are associated with other anomalies (congenital diaphragmatic hernia (CDH), congenital cystic adenomatoid malformation (CCAM), pericardial cysts, cardiac defects, esophageal achalasia), may be found in various locations (pericardium, diaphragm, below the diaphragm retroperitoneally), and have been known to contain malignancies.

Intralobar sequestrations (ILS) comprise 75% of pulmonary sequestrations and are primarily found in the right and left lower lobes, with the most frequent location being the posterior segment of the LLL. They are cystic abnormalities located within the visceral pleural of the lung that communicate with the normal lung tissue through the pores of Kohn. Ninety-six percent of ILS will have venous drainage to the pulmonary veins. It is rarely associated with other anomalies, but may present antenatally as polyhydramnios.

The typical presentation is recurrent pulmonary infections and hemopty-sis. Work up includes CT, MRI (occasionally), upper GI studies (if con-cern for enteric communication), and rarely angiography (generally the feeding vessels can be identified on other imaging studies). Sometimes the segment alone may be removed, but in most cases a lobectomy is re-quired. Early identification and control of the arterial supply is impera-tive to avoid bleeding complications. As the venous return can also be aberrant, care should be taken to identify the venous return of the normal lung. Any communications with the GI tract should be identified and divided.

Bronchogenic cysts

Bronchogenic cysts are the result of abnormal budding of the trachea. They are the most common mediastinal cysts (60%) and are typically located along the right paratracheal area. They may be attached to the carina or lobar bronchus, but occasionally they may be intraparenchymal, below the diaphragm, in the pericardium, peristernal subcutaneous tis-sues, or skin. Bronchial communication is rare (more likely with intra-parenchymal cysts), and they have an inner lining of ciliated pseudostrati-fied respiratory epithelium with goblet cells. They are typically uniloc-ular (2-10cm) and may contain normal bronchial elements such as smooth muscle and cartilage (which differentiates them from enteric cysts). They can be filled with blood, mucus, milky material, or pus (if infected). There is a male predominance.

Most bronchogenic cysts are asymptomatic and found incidentally on CXR as an air-filled cyst, but some may cause symptoms secondary to compression of the PA or atrial fibrillation. The intraparenchymal cysts are more likely to present with infection (90%) as compared to the medi-astinal cysts (36%). The differential diagnosis includes sequestration, teratoma, lymphadenopathy, hemangioma, lipoma, hamartoma, neurogen-ic tumors, and foregut and pericardial cysts. Workup includes CT, MRI (occasionally), and EUS. Mediastinal cysts can be subcarinal and be con-fused with subcarinal lymph nodes on CT.

The cyst should be excised completely for diagnosis and to avoid compli-cations such as bleeding, rupture, infection, enlargement with compres-sion of the airway, and retained malignancy. Generally, the mediastinal cysts can be enucleated and the stalk ligated, but the intraparenchymal cysts may require a segmentectomy or lobectomy. The bronchial defect and any other associated communications should be repaired.

Congenital lobar emphysema

This defect makes up 50% of all congenital pulmonary anomalies. It is the obstruction of a lobar bronchus that results in expansion of the distal air spaces without alveolar destruction. There is upper airway predominance (LUL > RUL > RML > lower lobes), with normal pulmonary vasculature to the affected lobe. The remaining normal lung is often compressed and there is mediastinal shift away from the affected lung.

Intrinsic causes include a cartilaginous defect (25%), mucous plugging, and granulation tissue obstructing the airway. Extrinsic causes include tetralogy of Fallot, pulmonary stenosis, anomalies of the pulmonary veins, adenopathy, mediastinal tumors, and bronchogenic or duplication cysts. In greater than 50% of cases there is no apparent cause.

Most defects will be asymptomatic at birth but within days patients may develop cough, dyspnea, and wheezing. There is a male predominance of 3:1, it is occasionally bilateral (LUL and RML), and 80% of those affected will show symptoms by the age of 6 months. Associated anomalies include cardiac (14%), and rib or chest abnormalities. If treatment is not administered promptly when symptoms begin, 50% of patients will die within 1 week, and another 30-40% will die within 1 month. The acuity of the patient will determine the diagnostic work-up chosen but this may include CXR, CT, bronchoscopy, echocardiography, MRA, and V/Q scan.

Asymptomatic to mildly symptomatic patients may be observed, with half normalizing during infancy. For all symptomatic patients, the diseased tissue should be removed in its entirety, which often necessitates a lobectomy. The procedural mortality rate is 7%, with the greatest risk at the time of induction. Selective intubation will minimize overinflation of the emphysematous tissue and the surgeon should be prepared for immediate thoracotomy after induction.

Acquired lobar emphysema is an entirely different process resulting from complications of respiratory distress syndrome or prolonged intubation. It most frequently affects the RUL and will manifest with low flow to the affected tissue on perfusion scan. It is also treated with resection but post-operatively those patients will continue to have progressive respiratory problems. Balloon dilation of airway stenosis is an alternative possibility for treatment.

Congenital cystic adenomatoid malformation (CCAM)

CCAM is a hyper-proliferation of bronchi (cartilage, smooth muscle, bronchial glands, columnar and cuboidal epithelial cells) in the setting of normal pulmonary vasculature, and abnormal alveolar development. The diseased tissue does communicate with the tracheobronchial tree. It comprises 25% of all congenital pulmonary anomalies. Typically the lesions are single and localized to one lobe.

Polyhydramnios may be seen prenatally but a third of those diagnosed *in utero* will resolve prior to birth. CCAM presents as neonatal acute respiratory distress with multiple air fluid levels on CXR. CT may solidify the diagnosis. Associated anomalies are pectus excavatum (most common), cardiac and pulmonary vessel malformations.

CCAM can be classified (by Stocker) as follows:

- *Type I* (macrocystic, 60-70%). Large, widely spaced, irregular cysts that are > 2 cm. This type is rarely associated with polyhydramnios or other anomalies. Most patients will reach term but some are stillborn. Mediastinal shifting can be seen in 75% of patients with some associated cyanosis and grunting. Half will develop pneumonia during infancy or early childhood, but the overall prognosis is good.

- *Type II* (mixed, 20-40%). The cysts are smaller than 2 cm, have the appearance of more bronchioles with increased proliferation and less mediastinal shift. Patients tend to be premature or stillborn.

- *Type III* (microcystic, 10%). The cysts are very small, <0.5 cm, and the mass is firmer, appearing to encase the entire affected lobe (most commonly LLL). Prognosis is very poor with life expectancy of hours after birth.

Patients with asymptomatic CCAMs can be observed for the first 4-6 months with repeat imaging at the age of 6 months to assess for enlargement or malignant degeneration, followed by resection. This delayed intervention allows further growth of the child, reducing operative morbidity. All symptomatic lesions after birth should be resected without delay. Most of the time a lobectomy is required. After successful resection, long term outcomes are excellent.

Congenital tracheal stenosis

Congenital tracheal stenosis is classified in three types (by Cantrell and Guild):

- *Type 1:* involves the entire trachea

- *Type 2:* funnel shaped stenosis of the upper, lower, or the entire trachea

- *Type 3:* segmental stenosis of the lower trachea

The stenotic areas have circumferential cartilaginous rings that can range in number from 2-18 rings. Fifty percent of cases are associated with a pulmonary vascular sling or a vascular ring, and all types may be associated with pulmonary agenesis.

Patients present with exertional wheezing or stridor after birth. Workup includes CT, bronchoscopy, and echocardiography. These patients must be treated aggressively as there is a high risk of sudden death. Surgery is required with partial tracheal resection being the most common procedure performed. There are various options for reconstruction including primary anastomosis, pericardium, aortic homograft, costochondral graft, slide tracheostomy, and tracheal autograft. For complete repair of the stenosis and any associated vascular rings /slings, CPB and / or circulatory arrest may be required.

The neonatal trachea does not tolerate tension as the adult trachea does. Up to 50% of an infant trachea can be removed and still be closed primarily. When 8 or fewer rings are resected then primary repair is ideal. If resection requires more than 8 rings then an autograft should be considered for reconstruction. ECMO may be necessary to get the patient through the postoperative period, but long-term outcomes are good, with normal growth and development of these patients. For non-surgical candidates, various options for palliation include balloon dilation and split posterior tracheoplasty, stenting, local steroid injection, electroresection, and cryotherapy.

Bronchial atresia

This is the 2nd most common airway abnormality after TEF. A lobar or segmental bronchus ends blindly, but lung parenchyma distally will expand and become emphysematous due to air communication via the pores of Kohn. Two theories exist for the development: 1) the distal bronchial bud separated but continued to develop, or 2) there was a vascular insult to the atretic segments. Despite the bronchial abnormalities, the distal airway and lung tissues continue to develop normally.

The patients may present with respiratory distress within days to weeks of birth or they may present with wheezing, stridor, or repeated pulmonary infections. The frequency of lobes affected in descending order are LUL,

LLL, RUL, with a segmental bronchus more frequently atretic than a lobar bronchus. CT is used for further workup.

Indications for resection include enlargement and repeated pulmonary infections, although, some resect in the presence of abnormal tissue to prevent infection and complications. Usually a lobectomy is required.

Other pulmonary congenital anomalies

Congenital pulmonary lymphangiectasia is a very rare disease characterized by dilated lymphatics (with resultant pulmonary hypoplasia) due to intrauterine lymphatic obstruction. CXR shows a "soap bubble" appearance with diffusely granular parenchyma, hyperinflation, and a prominent interstitium. Treatment is supportive with drainage of effusions and a low-fat, high-protein diet with medium-chain fatty acids. However, prognosis is dismal.

Pulmonary hemangiomatosis is a rare benign vascular tumor characterized by proliferation of capillaries in the interstitium. Patients present with respiratory distress, pulmonary hypertension, and consumptive coagulopathy (Kasabach-Merritt syndrome). Treatment is supportive. Prognosis is grim but IFN and lung transplantation may be useful.

Pulmonary arteriovenous fistulas are also extremely rare malformations, sometimes associated with Osler-Weber-Rendu syndrome. Presentation varies depending on the number of vessels involved. Patients may be asymptomatic or may present with variable degree of respiratory distress, cyanosis, and cardiac failure. Pulmonary hemorrhages may occur. Complications include hemoptysis, cerebral thrombosis, brain abscesses, and pneumothorax. Diagnosis is made with ABGs (right-to-left shunt), CT (confluence of vessels), V/Q scan, echocardiography (bubble study confirming the intrapulmonary shunt), and pulmonary angiography (gold standard). Treatment is by embolization of focal lesions and wedge resection of larger lesions or those that have failed embolization.

11. Surgery for emphysema

Elizabeth A. David

Clinical presentation

Emphysematous changes of the lung are characterized by permanent enlargement of the distal airspaces and destruction of their walls without fibrosis, resulting in breathlessness, decreased exercise tolerance, oxygen dependence in some cases, respiratory failure, and eventually death. The degradation of the elastin-collagen matrix in the airway is believed to be responsible for the destruction of lung tissue due to a lack of elastic recoil, which limits airflow and respiratory mechanics. As these changes in the parenchyma are permanent and irreversible, surgical goals for these patients are only for palliation of symptoms and to improve survival.

Diagnosis

Clinically, patients with end-stage emphysema who demonstrate decreased FEV_1:FVC ratio, absolute decrease in FEV_1, hyperinflation of the lungs, flattening of the diaphragm, or increased work of breathing should be evaluated for lung volume reduction surgery (LVRS). Hypoxia is uncommon in these patients. Preoperative evaluation should include cardiopulmonary clearance for surgery as well as a rigorous pulmonary rehab program that includes weaning of steroids, optimizing bronchodilators, nicotine abstinence, and physical reconditioning. CT scanning can be helpful in characterizing the distribution of the disease.

Indications for surgery

Patient selection is critical and based on the appropriate balance of indications and lack of contraindications for each patient. Indications for surgery include patients with decreased FEV_1 ($\geq$ 15% or $\leq$ 40% of predicted), increased total lung capacity ($\geq$ 100% of predicted), significantly increased residual volume ($\geq$ 150% of predicted), and no hypoxia or hypercarbia. Patients should have acceptable cardiac risk, ability to comply with rigorous pulmonary rehabilitation both preoperative and postoperatively, and abstain from nicotine use for over 6 months prior to planned LVRS.

Contraindications to surgery

As LVRS is truly an elective operation for benign disease, it is crucial to ensure that contraindications to proceeding do not exist. Significant contraindications include bronchiectasis, hypercarbia (paCO2) $\geq$ 60 mmHg on room air, PA hypertension, prior lobectomy on ipsilateral side, interstitial lung disease, and ventilator dependence. Relative contraindications include chronic bronchitis or asthma, use of $\geq$ 20 mg prednisone daily, oxygen dependence, active smoking, and morbid obesity.

Treatment

Surgical therapy of emphysema has evolved from early techniques designed to enlarge the thoracic cavity including costochondrectomy, transverse sternotomies, and paravertebral thoracoplasties. Other historical techniques for palliation included diaphragmatic plication, pleurectomy to increase collateral circulation to the lung parenchyma from the chest wall, bullectomy, and lung transplantation. In the mid 1990s, Joel Cooper revolutionized LVRS by suggesting simultaneous removal of parenchyma from both lungs via median sternotomy would be appropriate. His ideas have shaped LVRS into what it is currently, involving non-anatomic resection of poorly perfused lung tissue by median sternotomy, thoracotomy, or VATS.

The principles of surgical therapy involve:

1. Inspect/palpate the entire lung

2. Observe and preserve areas of fastest desaturation and determine tissue for resection

3. Mobilize the entire lung – divide inferior pulmonary ligament

    a. Resect target areas with reinforced stapler

    b. Use Gore-Tex® or bovine pericardium to reinforce stapler

4. Avoid over-resection to minimize space problems and air leaks

5. Use synthetic glues/sealants, pleural tents, or pleurodesis to control air leaks

6. Place chest tubes to water seal immediately, early extubation, and aggressive pulmonary toilet with reestablishment of preoperative medical optimization with physical therapy and inhaled bronchodilator therapy. Avoid steroids. Use an aggressive bronchoscopy strategy for pulmonary hygiene.

Results of surgery

Multiple studies have shown that LVRS results in improved FEV_1, respiratory muscle function, exercise capacity, and dyspnea. Common postoperative complications include: prolonged air leaks, respiratory failure,

MI, pneumonia, and stroke. Perioperative mortality rates are usually quoted at 5-15%. No differences in functional outcomes have been demonstrated between median sternotomy and VATS for LVRS; however VATS patients are able to return to independent living sooner and have lower hospital costs than median sternotomy.

Most data on LVRS come from single-center studies, but a large, multi-center randomized study comparing LVRS with best medical therapy was published in 2003 by the National Emphysema Treatment Trial Research Group (NETT). Seventeen centers participated and collected data over 7 years on 1218 patients with a mean follow-up of 2 years. Patients with upper lobe predominant disease were found to have decreased symptoms and improved exercise tolerance with surgery when compared to medical therapy. Patients with homogenous distribution of disease were found to have decreased survival after LVRS.

Surgical alternatives

One-way endobronchial valves and the use of drug eluting stents as means of airway bypass are still investigational and there have been no studies to directly compare these bronchoscopic-based technologies directly with surgery. The recently released VENT trial of endobronchial valves does suggest that there are improvements in lung function, exercise tolerance, and symptoms but at the cost of more frequent COPD exacerbations, pneumonia and hemoptysis after implantation.

12. Benign tumors of the lung
Stephanie Mick

Benign tumors (defined as masses that neither metastasize nor invade surrounding tissue planes) of the lung are uncommon, making up <1% of all resected lung neoplasms and 2-5% of all primary lung tumors. There is no accepted classification scheme for this large, varied group of lesions, but they are generally discussed in terms of their location (endobronchial or parenchymal) and/or cell of origin. It is important to recognize that some benign tumors listed in textbooks alongside the more common tumors have been reported in only handfuls of patients; only the most common will be discussed here.

Radiologic considerations in the evaluation of solitary pulmonary nodules

A "solitary pulmonary nodule" (SPN) is a rounded lesion with well-demarcated margins ranging from a few millimeters to a few centimeters in size. In evaluating an SPN radiologically, it is useful to consider doubling time and calcification pattern. An SPN with a doubling time of <10 days or >450 days is most likely benign. In general, central, diffuse, speckled, laminar or "popcorn" calcifications suggest benign lesions and eccentric calcifications suggest malignancy.

CT scanning with 1mm cuts is ~91% sensitive in determining malignancy. CT characteristics of malignancy include ill-defined borders, spiculation and involvement of bronchi. CT guided core biopsy can provide a definitive diagnosis in ~82% of cases (compared to ~17% using FNA). FDG-PET scanning can distinguish benign from malignant lesions with >90% sensitivity when the nodule is ≥10mm in size, but this decreases for smaller lesions. Keeping these limitations in mind, a glucose-avid nodule with a SUV of ≥2.5 has a >90% chance of being malignant. Nodules >10mm with malignant characteristics or indeterminate by other means must be defined by surgical excision.

Hamartomas

Hamartomas, mixed lesions arising from epithelial and mesodermal cells, are the most common benign lesion of the lung; they comprise 75% of all benign lung tumors and 8% of all radiologic "coin lesions." Hamartomas are slow growing (~3-5mm/year) collections of mixed mature tissue normally found in the lung such as cartilage and adipose tissue. They occur more often in men and although they arise much earlier, are not usually found until the 6th or 7th decade. They are generally in peripheral paren-chymal locations but do also occur centrally or endobronchially.

They appear as 1-3cm smooth, lobulated, well-circumscribed, smoothly marginated peripheral lesions with mixed fat and soft tissue attenuation on CT (the presence of fatty tissue within such a lesion is highly sugges-tive of hamartoma, but this is present only about half the time.) On CXR, popcorn-like calcifications can be seen in 10-30% of cases. If they are stable (not growing), they can be observed. However, if they are not re-sected, they **must** be followed; there is a rare but real rate of malignant transformation.

Tumors of epithelial origin

Tumors of epithelial origin can be found endobronchially (e.g., papillo-mas, mucus gland adenomas) or intraparenchymally (e.g., mucinous cystadenoma, alveolar adenoma, pleomorphic adenoma).

Papillomas are relatively common. In adults, they are often solitary, pre-senting more often in men in their 50's and 60's with a smoking history. In children, they are often multiple and associated with vocal cord or tra-cheal involvement. Clara cells may be present on histology. Treatment is usually laser ablation or endoscopic removal as these lesions carry a risk of malignant degeneration. *Mucus gland adenomas* arise from submuco-sal mucus glands in lobar or segmental bronchi. They appear as coin-like lesions in these locations on CT.

Tumors with mesodermal origin

Endobronchial tumors of mesenchymal origin include such entities as benign endobronchial histiocytoma. Parenchymal lesions in this category include intrapulmonary fibrous tumor, hemangiomas (e.g., cavernous hemangiomas, sclerosing hemangioma, or pulmonary capillary hemangi-omatosis), chondromas, etc. Leiomyomas can occur in either location.

Intrapulmonary fibrous tumor (also called localized pleural mesothelio-ma, pleural fibroma, solitary fibrous tumor of the pleura) is a benign tu-mor arising from the visceral pleura usually presenting as a large, asymp-tomatic mass. On imaging, these lesions make an obtuse angle with the chest wall, revealing they arise from the pleura and not the lung. There are about 800 cases in the literature. These are not associated with asbes-tos exposure and are not related to mesothelioma. Three to four percent of patients suffer symptomatic hyperglycemia from insulin-like active substances elaborated from tumor. Other paraneoplastic syndromes can also occur.

The presence of *pulmonary cavernous hemangiomas* should raise the suspicion of hereditary hemorrhagic telangiectasia (Osler-Weber-Rendu syndrome). The presence of *pulmonary chondroma* should raise the suspicion of Carney's Triad, which is pulmonary chondroma, gastric GI stromal tumor (GIST), and extraadrenal paraganglioma, occurring more often in females.

Leiomyomas can occur endobronchially or intraparenchymally (about 50/50) and comprise 2% of all benign lung lesions. They are more common in females and young adults. Note that when pulmonary leiomyomas are observed in conjunction with uterine leiomyomas, they are considered "metastasizing" and can be fatal. Treatment requires surgical removal, chemotherapy and hormonal manipulation.

Tumors of miscellaneous origin

Endobronchial lesions in this category include granular cell tumors (presenting as sessile polyps within the trachea or central bronchi) that appear as coin lesions in these locations. Parenchymal tumors in this category include nodular amyloid and primary pulmonary thymoma.

Nodular amyloid (~3cm in size on average) is more commonly found in the lower lobes with both sexes equally affected. Histologically, they appear as eosinophilic deposits with "apple-green birefringence." When found, the suspicion of multiple myeloma should be raised as these conditions can be associated. Long-term follow-up is also necessary because of the association of nodular amyloid and macroglobulinemia and lymphoma. *Primary pulmonary thymoma* is the presence of thymic tissue in intrapulmonary locations. It is very rare and likely results from embryologic descent of thymic tissue to a position more inferior than normal.

Tumors of inflammatory origin

Parenchymal tumors of this type include inflammatory pseudotumor (inflammatory myofibroblastic tumor) and hyalinizing granuloma. Such lesions are neoplastic collections of inflammatory cells that develop as a response to infection or inflammation and are treated by excision.

13. Interstitial lung disease
Theolyn Price

Idiopathic interstitial pneumonia

This is a spectrum of pulmonary disorders with characteristic alveolitic change secondary to infiltration of immune cells into the pulmonary interstitium. Although there are multiple terms and classifications used to define the various forms, many would argue that this is arbitrary, because these disease categories are merely different stages or manifestations of the same disease. Excluding lung transplant and treatment of complications (effusion, pneumothorax), the role of the thoracic surgeon is primarily diagnostic. They have an alveolitic pattern of interstitial lung disease that is characterized by activated macrophages, T cells, and inflammatory cytokines that activate B cells to secrete more antibodies. The antibody/antigen complex is deposited in the lung parenchyma, activating the complement system, which causes an inflammatory reaction with injury to the local tissues. Unchecked, there is further destruction by neutrophils, macrophages (TNF, IL-1), prostaglandins, and cytokines, which can ultimately lead to increasing degrees of fibrosis, that can become irreversible.

The specifics of each entity will be discussed below, but the patients generally present with dyspnea and nonproductive cough that progress over months to years. Some are associated with constitutional symptoms. The overall patient evaluation includes a detailed H&P, ABG, PFTs, labs, bronchoscopy, high resolution CT, and usually surgical biopsy. With diffuse lung disease, a confident pathologic diagnosis can only be made in 25% of cases with transbronchial biopsy. A definitive diagnosis is established by obtaining a large enough tissue sampling (preferably from at least 2 lobes) via an open or VATS procedure. Confirmation of diagnosis prior to therapy is important to rule out other pathology, to obtain prognostic information, and to justify withholding treatment for end-stage disease, but there are some that would accept a diagnosis based on solid clinical grounds.

The treatment plan includes oxygen supplementation as needed, removal of any causative agents, and early intervention to prevent disease progression to fibrosis. Steroids are the cornerstone of therapy. A slow wean over months may be attempted if symptoms improve. Only 20% of those with idiopathic pulmonary fibrosis (IPF) will respond to steroids, so other agents that could be considered include cyclophosphamide, azathioprine, methotrexate, penicillamine, colchicine, cyclosporine, and IFN-γ. There are no known treatments that reverse pulmonary fibrosis once it has occurred. After failure of medical therapy the only option is lung transplantation. Single lung transplant is usually the procedure of choice, with the basic criteria in this setting as follows:

- Progressive dyspnea/hypoxia despite maximal medical therapy

- Vital capacity ≤60-70% predicted and/or a DLCO ≤50-60% predicted

- Age ≤ 60 for double lung transplant or ≤65 for single lung transplant

The 5-year survival after transplant is about 50-60%, which is significantly better than the 28 month median survival seen for IPF treated medically.

Usual interstitial pneumonia (UIP) / Idiopathic pulmonary fibrosis (IPF)

UIP / IPF consists of parenchymal changes defined by thickened fibrotic alveolar interstitium with lymphocytic and plasmacytic infiltration. It is characterized by patchy distribution, non-uniform histology (normal, inflammation, fibrosis), and chronicity. The pathologic diagnosis of UIP and the clinical diagnosis of IPF are often interchangeable. Encountered most frequently, the incidence is 5-20 per 100,000, with a male predominance. The etiology is unknown, but possible mediators include infectious (hepatitis C, Epstein-Barr virus), environmental (heavy metal dusts, solvents, cigarette smoking), genetic (HLA- B15, B8, B12), or immunologic (associated with rheumatoid arthritis, SLE, progressive systemic sclerosis). Patients are typically older than 50, up to 50% present with constitutional symptoms, with digital clubbing seen in more advanced disease. CT demonstrates mediastinal lymphadenopathy, lower lobe / subpleural predominance in a reticular or reticulonodular pattern with honeycombing cysts, and ground glass opacities. Surgical biopsy is required for definitive diagnosis. The treatment is high-dose steroid therapy, although most do not respond and the overall prognosis is poor. Favorable prognostic factors include young age, disease <1 year, active inflammation, lymphocytosis on bronchioalveolar lavage, and the presence of immune complexes. The 5-year survival is 43% in the responders and 20% in the non-responders.

Desquamative interstitital pneumonia (DIP)

DIP consists of parenchymal changes defined by mildly thickened interstitium, sparse infiltration of inflammatory cells, and mild fibrosis. It is characterized by diffuse distribution and uniform histology. Filling of alveoli by macrophages is a defining feature. Smokers between the ages of 40-50 years are most affected. Imaging studies reveal bilateral ground opacities in a linear pattern. The pathologic changes in DIP may also be seen focally in IPF, making it difficult to differentiate these entities. Some have even suggested that DIP may be the early phase and UIP the later phase of the same disease process, although DIP is more amenable to therapy than UIP. Steroids are the mainstay of treatment, but DIP is often progressive, and may require lung transplantation in its final stages.

Non-specific interstitial pneumonia (NIP)

NIP consists of parenchymal changes defined by mildly thickened interstitium, infiltration of inflammatory cells, and mild fibrosis. The distribution is patchy, and the histology is uniform. NIP is rare, and without gender predominance. When compared to UIP/IPF, NIP has an improved response rate with steroid therapy and a better overall survival.

Bronchiolitis obliterans organizing pneumonia (BOOP) / Cryptogenic organizing pneumonia (COP)

BOOP/COP is a rare disease process characterized by chronic inflammation of the alveoli, granulation tissue in the bronchioles/alveoli, and accumulation of macrophages within the alveoli. The distribution is patchy, and the histology is uniform (organizing pneumonia involving the alveoli/alveolar ducts, occasionally bronchiolar intraluminal polyps). Men and women present equally between the ages of 40-60. Imaging reveals an airspace disease with bilateral, diffuse ground glass opacities. Surgical lung biopsy is required for definitive diagnosis. Rapid resolution of the disease process is typical with steroid therapy. Although relapses do occur, they also respond favorably to steroids. The mortality rate is approximately 12%.

Lymphocytic interstitial pneumonia (LIP)

LIP is a lymphoproliferative disorder characterized by infiltration of lymphocytes and plasma cells into the lung parenchyma without alveolar damage. It is often associated with immune disorders like Sjögren's syndrome, SLE, myasthenia, and chronic active hepatitis. LIP is rare disorder that is most commonly seen in children (seen in 50% of HIV+ children with pulmonary disease), immunocompromised patients, and women between the ages of 40-80. Presentation may be similar to other interstitial pneumonias or may be due to symptoms of the underlying autoimmune disorder. Imaging will show a reticular / reticulonodular pattern and air space consolidation, with lymphadenopathy being unusual. Surgical biopsy is necessary to make a definitive diagnosis. The outcomes are variable, from spontaneous regression, to progression with fibrosis, or even the development of lymphoma. Some will have a great response to steroid therapy, others will progress despite treatment. One third to half with LIP will die within 5 years of diagnosis, and 5% will progress to lymphoma.

Sarcoidosis

This is a chronic systemic disorder of unknown etiology that is characterized by non-caseating granulomas within multiple organ systems. The incidence is 10-20 per 100,000, with higher prevalence and severity in females and those of African ancestry. It is rare in the Asian population and most commonly presents between the ages of 20-40. Causal theories include environmental (workplace clusters, pathologically identical to some inhalation injuries), infectious (lymphadenopathy, some suspect *Mycobacterium tuberculosis*), hereditary (familial clusters, HLA A1 and B8 involvement), and immunological (altered T-cell ratios, impaired systemic immunity, hyperactive B-cell lines, altered macrophage production of inflammatory cytokines IFN-γ and RANTES).

The lungs (cough, dyspnea, wheezing) are involved in 94% of cases, with the most common symptomatic extrapleural sites being the eyes (uveitis, conjunctivitis, retinitis) and skin (nodules, plaques). Occasionally, the liver (hepatomegaly), spleen (splenomegaly), synovial joints (arthralgias), CNS, larynx, salivary glands, and heart are also affected. It is sometimes seen in association with rheumatoid arthritis, SLE, progressive systemic sclerosis, or Lofgren's Syndrome. Thirty to fifty percent of patients are asymptomatic at presentation, but will have radiographic abnormalities (lymphadenopathy, upper lobe predominance, variable interstitial/acinar lesions, occasional nodules). Presentation can include elevated ACE levels in serum and bronchioalveolar fluid, restrictive lung function (occasionally obstructive), hypercalcemia, peripheral lymphopenia (lymphocyte accumulation in the lungs), hilar or mediastinal adenopathy (80%), or constitutional symptoms (fever, chills, malaise, weight loss).

Staging is determined radiographically:

- *Stage 0* (8%): Normal

- *Stage 1* (50%): Lymphadenopathy

- *Stage 2* (30%): Lymphadenopathy and parenchymal infiltrates

- *Stage 3* (12%): Parenchymal infiltrates only

- *Stage 4* (rare): End-stage honeycomb lung

Workup includes PFTs, diagnostic bronchoscopy (bronchioalveolar lavage, transbronchial biopsy), and high resolution CT. Diagnosis is confirmed by tissue and sometimes requires mediastinoscopy or VATS procedure to obtain adequate sampling. The histology will show non-caseating granulomas with elevated tissue ACE levels and a mononuclear cell infiltration.

Many patients will improve or remain stable without treatment, but 20% will suffer progressive pulmonary deterioration. The standard treatment is steroids, but other agents that have been used are methotrexate, cyclosporine, chlorambucil, and antimalarial drugs. Due to high remission rates, those who are asymptomatic with stage 1 or 2 disease and normal PFTs are managed expectantly. Treatment is begun with any deterioration, and for those with stage 3 sarcoidosis, those that are symptomatic with stage 2 sarcoidosis, and for those with significant extrapulmonary manifestations. The 5-year mortality is 4% with most deaths attributable to pulmonary involvement.

14. Lung transplantation
James M. Isbell

Candidate selection

Suitable candidates will have advanced to end-stage pulmonary disease with significant functional limitation resulting in a predicted life expectancy of less than 2 years (NYHA class III or IV). Recipients must have failed maximal medical therapy and have sufficient nutritional status and cardiac function. Patients who are generally considered ineligible for transplantation include those who:

- are over 65 years of age

- continue to smoke (within the last 6 months)

- have organ failure in addition to their pulmonary dysfunction

- have a history of malignancy within the prior 5 years

- require high-dose steroids (≥20 mg prednisone)

Preoperative evaluation

Transplant candidates must undergo a thorough preoperative evaluation to exclude comorbid conditions that may affect outcomes. Cardiac screening typically consists of an echocardiogram and frequently left and right heart catheterization to assess for significant coronary disease and pulmonary hypertension. In addition to PFTs, the pulmonary evaluation is completed with a quantitative ventilation/perfusion scan and a chest CT. These studies can help guide which lung to transplant in single lung recipients and the order in which to transplant the lungs in bilateral transplants.

Organ allocation

Donor lungs are allocated to individual transplant candidates according to the Lung Allocation Score (LAS). Each candidate is assigned an LAS based on the probability of death on the waitlist as well as the probability of post-transplant survival.

Disease-specific guidelines

Obstructive airway disease
Given the limited 5-year survival after lung transplant, only patients with a high risk for COPD-related mortality who have failed maximal medical

therapy with oxygen supplementation and dilator therapy should be considered for transplantation. Lung volume reduction surgery should be considered before transplantation in patients who are suitable candidates. Although based on limited data, current guidelines recommend listing patients with COPD when their postbronchodilator FEV_1 is less than 20-25% predicted, $PaO_2 < 55$ mm Hg at rest, $PaCO_2 > 55$ mm Hg or with the onset of secondary pulmonary hypertension. In recent years there has been a trend toward bilateral lung transplants in patients with obstructive lung disease due to a small but statistically significant survival benefit.

Idiopathic pulmonary fibrosis

Patients with idiopathic pulmonary fibrosis (IPF) have the worst survival rate compared to all other lung disease while waiting on the transplant list. As such, IPF patients should be referred for transplantation evaluation very early in their course, even before significant symptoms arise. Those IPF patients who develop early severe lung restriction and hypoxemia appear to have the poorest prognosis and therefore should be considered for transplant.

Cystic fibrosis and bronchiectasis

Cystic fibrosis (CF) is the primary cause of end-stage obstructive pulmonary disease in the first 3 decades of life. Patients with septic lung disease such as cystic fibrosis and bronchiectasis must receive bilateral lung transplantation to prevent the spread of infection from a colonized native lung to a transplanted lung. Although controversial, most experts believe CF patients should be referred for transplant when their FEV_1 declines to 30% predicted as this is associated with a 50% 2-year mortality. The presence of hypoxemia, hypercapnea and weight loss should prompt consideration for transplant as well.

Pulmonary hypertension

With the advent of prostacyclins and other effective vasodilator therapies, patients with primary pulmonary hypertension are being transplanted less frequently. Nonetheless, patients with progression of their disease despite optimal medical therapy should be considered for transplant. Suggested criteria for transplantation include mean PAP > 50, RA pressure > 10 mm Hg, cardiac index < 2.5 $L/min/m^2$, NYHA class III or IV, and syncope.

Donor considerations

Aside from being ABO compatible, the ideal lung donor will be less than 55 years of age, have a $PaO_2 > 300$ mm Hg on 100% FiO_2 with a PEEP of 5 cm H_2O as well as a normal CXR and bronchoscopic exam.

Technical considerations

For single lung transplants, anterolateral or posterolateral thoracotomies can be used. For bilateral lung transplants, bilateral anterolateral or clamshell approaches are typically used. If the need for CPB is expected, central cannulation can be achieved with relative ease via a right thoracotomy. However, if only a left thoracotomy is used (i.e., for a left single lung transplant), femoral cannulation is generally favored.

Immunosuppression

Immunosuppression typically consists of corticosteroids, calcineurin inhibitors, and a cell-cycle inhibitor. Cyclosporine and tacrolimus are calcineurin inhibitors that block the expression of IL-2, resulting in the inhibition of T lymphocyte proliferation. Mycophenolate mofetil (MMF) and azathioprine both inhibit *de novo* purine synthesis, which results in the suppression of T and B lymphocyte proliferation.

Postoperative complications

Technical complications include stricture or dehiscence of the bronchial anastomoses. A bronchoscopy should be performed at the end of the procedure to assess the bronchial anastomosis. Strictures at the PA anastomosis occur less frequently but should be suspected when there is persistent pulmonary hypertension and unexplained hypoxemia. A nuclear perfusion scan will show unequal distribution of blood flow into the lungs. An angiogram will show a 15-20 mmHg gradient across the anastomosis. The anastomosis may need to be revised depending on the clinical status of the patient. Impairment of venous drainage across the atrial anastomosis will result in high PA pressures and ipsilateral pulmonary edema. TEE may be used to assess the anastomosis.

Infectious complications are caused by bacterial, viral, and fungal agents. Bacterial infections occur most commonly in the early postoperative period. CMV is the leading cause of postoperative infections in lung transplant recipients.

One quarter of lung transplant recipients will develop primary graft dysfunction (PGD), which carries a mortality rate as high as 30%. Ischemia-reperfusion injury underlies most cases of PGD.

Acute rejection develops in as many as 75% of recipients, usually within the first 3 months following lung transplantation. The signs and symptoms of acute rejection include low-grade fever, dyspnea, fatigue, hypoxemia, 10% or greater decrease in FEV_1 from baseline and the development of infiltrates on CXR. Acute rejection is a risk factor for the development of chronic rejection and its histologic counterpart, bronchiolitis obliterans. Histologic confirmation is not necessary for a diagnosis of chronic rejection. Bronchiolitis obliterans syndrome (BOS) is the term used for a decline in post-transplant FEV_1 once other causes have been excluded. BOS is generally not reversible, but modifications to the immunosuppression regimen can sometimes slow the progression of the disease.

Survival

According to the most recently published estimates of the International Society for Heart and Lung Transplantation, one-year survival after lung transplantation is 79% while five-year survival is only 52%. Patients with a preoperative diagnosis of primary pulmonary hypertension or IPF carry a worse prognosis than those with other diagnoses.

15. Thoracic infections and hemoptysis

Benjamin Wei, Matthew Hartwig

Mycobacterial infections

The indications for surgery for *Mycobacterium tuberculosis* (MTB) infections include: massive hemoptysis, bronchopleural fistula, bronchial stenosis, to rule out malignancy, entrapped parenchyma, failure of medical treatment, persistent cavitary disease, or a destroyed lung or lobe. Prior to surgery, the patient should be treated with combination drug therapy for 3 months and sputum cultures ideally should be negative. First-line therapy for MTB is 6 months of isoniazid and rifampin, with the addition of pyrazinamide and ethambutol for the initial 2 months. Multidrug resistant TB (MDR-TB) demonstrates resistance to both isoniazid and rifampin, and the need for surgery is increased in these patients.

MTB may also cause pericardial effusion or constrictive pericarditis. Pericardial biopsy is used to make the diagnosis though high levels of adenosine deaminase activity in the pericardial fluid are indicative of MTB. The treatment for MTB-related effusion is antibiotics and drainage. The treatment for constrictive pericarditis is antibiotics and pericardiectomy. MTB can also cause pleural TB, which results in a lymphocyte-rich effusion. Diagnosis is made by pleural biopsy, not by fluid culture, which results in no growth. Treatment is with antibiotics, thoracostomy tube placement for large effusions, and decortication for trapped lung or empyema. MTB can result in hemoptysis and predispose the patient to the formation of aspergillomas in areas of cavitary lung tissue. Uncommonly, MTB can cause endobronchial stenosis from scarring, but more likely results in extrinsic compression of the airway by infected lymph nodes. In the setting of endobronchial stenosis, treatment is inhaled corticosteroids, with the addition of incision and drainage of the lymph nodes – not excision – if steroids are unsuccessful.

Non-tuberculous mycobacterial (NTM) infections include *Mycobacterium avium* and *intracellulare*, which together represent the *M avium* complex and are the most common cause of NTM infections. *Mycobacterium chelonae*, *abscesssus*, and *fortuitum* are other, more virulent NTM species. NTM infections tend to occur in diseased lung, infect women more commonly than men, and predominantly occur in Caucasian patients. NTM infections are more resistant to drug therapy than MTB. Patients with localized disease may be amenable to surgical therapy, which should be considered earlier in the course of treatment.

Preoperative nutrition should be optimized, with enteral or parenteral feeding if necessary to raise the albumin >3 g/dL, as these patients are often cachectic. Mycobacterial infections can cause the formation of dense adhesions between parietal and visceral pleura; therefore an extrapleural dissection is preferentially performed. All grossly infected tissue should be resected; parenchyma containing only nodules may be spared. Tissue flaps should be used to reduce bronchial stump complications. Anti-tubercular medications should be continued postoperatively for 12-24 months. Operations for mycobacterial infections have a higher complication rate than resections for other disease processes, specifically a high rate of bronchopleural fistula.

Lung abscess

Patients with a lung abscess can present with pneumonia-like symptoms, including foul-smelling sputum if the abscess drains into the tracheobronchial tree. Rupture into the pleural space may result in pyopneumothorax, with the rapid onset of respiratory failure and septic shock.

Lung abscesses can be classified as primary or secondary, with aspiration being the most common etiology overall. An atypical bacteria, *Actinomyces*, classically causes multiple abscesses throughout the body, including the lungs. These infections are generally penicillin-sensitive.

A CT scan of the chest remains the most accurate method of diagnosis, which demonstrates a cavity with an air fluid level or areas of parenchymal necrosis. The first-line treatment for lung abscesses is prolonged antibiotic therapy directed by culture results. Sampling of the abscess is most accurately done via CT-guided or bronchoscopic needle aspiration. A lack of response to appropriate antibiotic therapy is justification for bronchoscopy, to rule out an obstructive process.

External drainage is used as an adjunct to antibiotics, and is reserved for treatment failure, giant abscesses (>8 cm in diameter), contralateral contamination, and rupture. Percutaneous drainage can be image-guided for multicentric abscesses and those that may be difficult to access with blind tube thoracostomy. Internal drainage via bronchoscope should not be performed. A pleural effusion in this setting is not unusual and if adequately drained can be managed with chest tube placement. Surgery is reserved for empyema, bronchopleural fistula, major hemoptysis, suspicion of cancer, or failure of non-operative therapy.

Mycotic infections

Histoplasmosis

Histoplasmosis is endemic to the Mississippi Valley, transmitted by contact with bat or bird feces, and usually self-limited. After the spores are inhaled, they germinate into yeast and are contained by macrophages. Acute pulmonary histoplasmosis is often asymptomatic, but may result in a self-limited flu-like illness. These patients do not require treatment. Disseminated histoplasmosis can occur in immunocompromised patients, who require treatment with amphotericin. Granulomas form as a reaction to the organisms, which eventually caseate and can calcify. These granulomas can compress or erode into structures such as the tracheobronchial tree (causing obstruction and/or hemoptysis) and the esophagus (causing esophageal leak). Histoplasmomas are healed areas of primary histoplasmosis that manifest as asymptomatic pulmonary coin-lesions, which may require surgical biopsy to differentiate from lung cancer. Rarely, fibrosing mediastinitis as a result of histoplasmosis can cause progressive compression of structures in the chest such as the SVC, esophagus, pulmonary vessels, and tracheobronchial tree. Chronic cavitary histoplasmosis occurs in patients with intrinsic lung disease and mimics TB. Definitive diagnosis of histoplasmosis relies on isolation of the organism in culture, as a positive serology may reflect a remote history of exposure to the organism.

Coccidiomycosis

Coccidiomycosis is a dimorphic fungus found in the southwest US, Mexico, and Central America. The spores are found in the soil and inhaled, and can result in primary pulmonary coccidiomycosis ("Valley fever"), which is usually self-resolved in the immunocompetent host. Erythema nodosum remains a positive prognostic sign of cell-mediated immunity. Diagnosis is made by serology and culture. Persistent symptoms justify treatment with antifungal therapy. Chronic infection may result in cavitation of lung or formation of granulomatous nodules. These cavities are often located peripherally and may rupture into the pleural space, resulting in effusion, pneumothorax, empyema, or bronchopleural fistula. Surgical intervention may be needed for these complications, and also to differentiate *Coccidioides* nodules from cancer.

Blastomycosis

Blastomycosis is found in the southeastern and central US, the spores of which are located in the soil and inhaled to cause disease. Like *Histoplasma* and *Coccidioides*, *Blastomyces* also induces a granulomatous reaction. It can result in pulmonary blastomycosis, cutaneous blastomycosis (multiple ulcerated skin nodules in disseminated cases), and disseminated blastomycosis. Diagnosis is made by microscopy (wide-based budding with double refractile walls) and DNA-based diagnosis, as culture can be time-consuming and serology not useful. Treatment is with antifungals. The role of surgery is to rule out malignancy.

Cryptococcus

Cryptococcus is an encapsulated yeast found in the soil worldwide. It can induce a granulomatous reaction that forms a nodule or mass mimicking lung cancer. It has a tendency to invade the meninges, especially in those with impaired immunity. Diagnosis is made by microscopy (organism with a capsule and narrow budding) and culture. If pathology shows the presence of *Cryptococcus* in a lung mass, the patient's CSF should be analyzed and the patient should be treated with amphotericin if there is evidence of meningitis.

Mucormycosis

Mucor is an omnipresent yeast found in the soil that thrives in acidic, hyperglycemic environments, making patients with diabetic ketoacidosis particularly susceptible. Other risk factors include corticosteroid use and neutropenia. The pulmonary form of disease presents as pneumonia refractory to antibacterial therapy. Pulmonary mucormycosis causes infarction of lung tissue, with possible PA rupture and hemoptysis, as well as invasion of adjacent chest wall and mediastinal structures. Diagnosis is made by microscopy (broad aseptate hyphae with right-angled finger-like projections). Treatment involves correction of diabetic ketoacidosis, reversal of immunosuppression, GM-CSF if the patient is neutropenic, amphotericin therapy, and rapid and aggressive surgical resection.

Aspergillosis

Aspergillus is a ubiquitous fungus found in the soil. In patients who are immunocompromised or have structural lung disease, *Aspergillus* can cause the formation of aspergillomas or result in invasive pulmonary aspergillosis. Certain patients, especially those with asthma and cystic fibrosis, have a hypersensitivity to the fungus that results in allergic bronchopulmonary aspergillosis (associated with eosinophilia and IgE elevation). Aspergillomas typically form in a pre-existing cavity. Cross-sectional imaging shows a fungus ball within a thick-walled cavity, sometimes surrounded partially by a crescent of air (Monod's sign). The combination of this radiologic finding with positive serology or culture is diagnostic. The organism is visualized using Gomori methenamine silver stain or Calcofluor. Birefringent calcium oxalate crystals can be visualized in the sputum with polarizing light microscopy. In addition, levels of galactomannan, a component of the cell wall, can be measured in serum or bronchoalveolar lavage fluid.

If asymptomatic, aspergillomas should not be treated, as some of them resolve spontaneously. If symptomatic and the patient can tolerate the surgery, they should be removed. Hemoptysis is the most common symptom and often responds well to bronchial artery embolization; however recurrence of bleeding and hemothorax occurs more than 50% of the time and resection of the mass should be undertaken if possible. Antifungal therapy is not helpful for the treatment of aspergilloma.

Invasive pulmonary aspergillosis can occur in immunocompromised patients, and results in a necrotizing bronchopneumonia that fails to respond to antibacterial treatment. CT scan may show multiple nodules, some of which may be surrounded by blood or air. Diagnosis is made by bronchoalveolar lavage culture. Invasive pulmonary aspergillosis is treated with antifungals, but the disease has a high mortality rate. Surgery is reserved for when the diagnosis is in question, or for the rare patient who has resectable disease.

Pneumocystis

The yeast-like fungus *Pneumocystis* serves as the causative agent in the formation of pneumocystis pneumonia (PCP). While the fungus is commonly found in the lungs of healthy individuals, opportunistic infection is usually limited to those with immunocompromised states. The most common treatment for PCP is Bactrim.

Hemoptysis

Massive hemoptysis may result in asphyxiation or exsanguination; the most common causes of which are bronchiectasis, cancer, TB, and mycetoma. Initial priorities include stabilization of the airway, with intubation if necessary, and resuscitation of the patient. The patient should be placed in lateral decubitus position with the suspected origin of hemoptysis on the dependent side. Nasopharyngeal and GI sources of bleeding should be ruled out. Antitussives should be given and bronchodilators should be avoided because they can cause vasodilation and exacerbation of bleeding. Bronchoscopy should be performed to evacuate blood, visualize the airway, and obtain selective intubation of the non-bleeding side. Balloon occlusion of the affected side can also be performed. Bronchoscopic measures to control bleeding include lavage with ice-cold saline or epinephrine, directed cautery, application of pro-coagulants such as fibrin or thrombin, and balloon tamponade.

The source of hemoptysis is the bronchial arteries in over 95% of cases; therefore bronchial artery embolization (BAE) should be attempted. PA angiography with vaso-occlusion or endovascular stenting can be performed if a PA source is suspected or if BAE is unsuccessful. A pre-procedure CT scan can help define the etiology of the hemoptysis in patients with a stable airway and hemodynamics. Because the early risk of re-bleeding after BAE may be as much as 30%, the patient for whom BAE is successful may benefit from a semi-elective lung resection under more controlled conditions, a decision which depends on the etiology of the bleed and the angiographic characteristics of the lesion. If angiographic measures fail, or if the patient is too unstable, emergent surgical intervention is necessary. Surgical resection of the relevant lobe is performed with the attendant higher morbidity and mortality rates compared to elective or semi-elective resection.

16. Benign pleural disease

Robroy H. MacIver

Pneumothorax

The most common cause of primary spontaneous pneumothorax is the rupture of an apical subpleural bleb. Spontaneous pneumothorax is seen in men more commonly than women by a ratio of 6:1. A typical presentation is of sudden onset of chest pain with shortness of breath. Often the presentation is after heavy exertion. Spontaneous pneumothorax is rarely seen before puberty. Other conditions such as cystic fibrosis and COPD can also make patients more prone to pneumothoraces. Tension pneumothorax from spontaneous pneumothorax is rare secondary to the collapsed segment normally closing off the leaking lung.

Secondary causes of pneumothorax such as central line placement, bronchoscopy, thoracentesis and lung biopsy are also frequent etiologies. More rare causes include catamenial pneumothorax (from pleural endometriosis), lung cancer, metastatic tumors, and lymphangiomatosis (proliferation of spindle cells along bronchioles leading to air trapping and thin-walled cysts).

Diagnosis

The diagnosis of pneumothorax can vary depending on clinical severity. If the patient is not *in extremis,* a standard CXR is sufficient in addition to the physical exam revealing decreased breath sounds and possible crepitus. Various grading scales exist, but in general, collapse is graded as minimal or small if only a rim of air surrounds the lung and moderate if the lung is collapsed half way to the heart border.

Treatment

Early treatment options for spontaneous pneumothorax vary from observation, aspiration, tube thoracostomy with either water seal or Heimlich valve, or percutaneous catheter placement, depending on severity and clinical presentation. Operative intervention is indicated for a persistent air leak lasting one week, a second recurrence, patients with only one lung, and patients with high risk of recurrence and for which recurrence is dangerous (e.g., pilots and divers). The chance of recurrence is 20-50%. Either talc or doxycycline pleurodesis is acceptable. Most centers now complete this procedure via VATS. Complications of pleurodesis include fever and pleuritic chest pain. Blebs should be resected; some groups advocate apical resection even in the absence of blebs.

Fibrothorax

The best treatment of fibrothorax is prevention. Failure to adequately recognize and treat hemothorax, empyema, or large pleural effusions occurs frequently and is the most common cause of fibrothorax. Regardless of the undrained fluids' nature, the resultant inflammatory response eventually leads to a dense, avascular collagen matrix that does not affect the underlying pleura.

Diagnosis

Physical exam may reveal collapsed intercostal spaces and decreased size of the thorax. CXR reveals radiodensities in the dependent portions of the lung. CT scans are helpful in determining underlying lung disease. PFTs will reveal a restrictive ventilatory defect with reduction of total lung capacity, vital capacity, and FEV_1. DLCO will be normal. Fibrothorax can sometimes be confused with mesothelioma and malignant metastatic spread to the pleural space. Biopsy by percutaneous, open, or VATS should be performed prior to any definitive treatment if cancer is a consideration.

Treatment

Decortication remains the main treatment for fibrothorax. Decortication occurs in three main steps. The first is blunt dissection of the parietal peel. The plane should be between the endothoracic fascia and the parietal pleura. Next the pleural cavity is entered and any fluid or debris is evacuated. Finally, the visceral pleura is dissected. The plane lies between the visceral pleura and the fibrous peel. Expansion of the lung can facilitate this step. Care must be taken to avoid damage to the phrenic nerve and diaphragm.

Empyema

Empyema is defined as a pleural effusion with positive bacteriologic cultures. Findings in analysis of pleural fluid include a pH <7, glucose <50 mg/dL, and an LDH >1000 IU/L. The etiology is diverse and includes pneumonia, trauma, instrumentation, and spread from other primary sites of infection. Bronchopleural fistulas can either be an etiology or a complication of an empyema.

Classically, the stages of empyema are broken down into three stages:

- *Stage I:* parapneumonic effusion (exudative)

- *Stage II:* fibrinopurulent phase; often includes bacterial invasion

- *Stage III:* chronic phase (organizing phase); includes in-growth of fibroblasts and capillaries

The most common organisms are *S. aureus*, gram negative bacteria, and anaerobes. Approximately half are polymicrobial.

Treatment

Prompt drainage remains the mainstay of treatment. Often, simple tube thoracostomy is not sufficient and either VATS or open drainage is necessary. Full lung re-expansion is needed to close off the potential space where infection can collect. In cases of chronic empyema leading to an entrapped lung, decortication is indicated to allow expansion of the lung.

Bronchopleural fistulas or severe empyema often require more aggressive treatment such as with a Clagett window or an Eloesser flap. Both of these procedures allow for continued drainage, irrigation, and frequent dressing changes. The Eloesser flap is considered more permanent as the skin is sutured to the pleura to epithelialize the tract to facilitate keeping it open. Other options of obliterating the space lost to infection include muscle flap coverage. The latissimus is the most commonly used muscle flap for this purpose.

17. Malignant pleural effusions and malignant pleural mesothelioma

Bryan M. Burt, Ravi K. Ghanta

Malignant pleural effusions

Malignant pleural effusions (MPE) cause significant morbidity for patients with cancer. Lung cancer is the leading cause of MPE (40% of cases), followed by metastatic breast cancer (25%), lymphoma-induced effusions (10%), ovarian cancer (5%), and gastric cancer (5%). Pleural seeding, either by direct tumor extension, hematogenous or lymphangitic spread is accompanied by accumulation of pleural fluid. This is often secondary to the production of angiogenic factors that increase vascular permeability, lymphatic obstruction that perturbs the normal absorption of 2-3 L of pleural fluid per day, and direct production of fluid by the tumor. After diagnosis, patients with MPE experience a median survival of only 4 to 6 months. Dyspnea is the principal symptom and it is progressive, leading to symptoms at rest, and underscoring the need for palliation.

Systemic therapy

Small effusions usually can be treated by malignancy-specific chemotherapy and RT to the primary lung lesion. However, neither of these treatments is effective for moderate to large effusions, and treatment should proceed to local therapies focused on symptom control.

Thoracentesis

All cancer patients with an effusion should undergo thoracentesis for diagnosis and to weigh the contribution of the effusion to the patient's symptoms. Thoracentesis is performed with US-guided aspiration for small to moderate effusions to prevent complications such as pneumothorax or hemothorax. Large effusions usually do not need image guidance. Radiologic assessment with CXR or chest CT after thoracentesis is helpful in determining the extent of disease and the degree of lung entrapment. Patients with recurrent MPE after thoracentesis can be managed in several ways. Repeat thoracentesis is an option for patients with an extremely short life expectancy (<2 months). For patients whose symptoms improve after initial thoracentesis and then develop recurrent effusions, the surgical option of pleurodesis or indwelling pleural catheter placement should be considered. The optimal surgical therapy is dependent on the degree of lung entrapment and the preference of the patient.

Pleurodesis

Pleurodesis eliminates the pleural space, but is only possible when there is pleural apposition. If the lung fully expands following thoracentesis, the patient may undergo pleurodesis with a chemical sclerosant such as talc, doxycycline, or bleomycin. Patients must be medically fit enough to tolerate the systemic inflammatory response that occurs after chemical pleurodesis, especially with talc. Talc pleurodesis has high success rates of 80-95% at 90 days but has been associated with acute respiratory distress syndrome and death in a minority of patients and warrants extreme caution in the medically compromised and elderly population. As a result, one of the most frequent and effective uses remains in the treatment of metastatic breast cancer. Options for pleurodesis include:

- VATS drainage of effusion and installation of sclerosant

- Chest tube placement followed by sclerosant instillation

- Indwelling pleural catheter placement followed by sclerosant instillation

Indwelling pleural catheters

Following thoracentesis, patients with trapped lung secondary to long-standing fibropurulent effusion and fibrin peels are not candidates for pleurodesis. Pleural apposition is not possible in this group and the pleural space cannot be obliterated. These patients are best managed with a long-term indwelling pleural catheter such as the Pleur-X catheter draining system. These catheters can be placed in the operating room with VATS or at the bedside either via open or Seldinger techniques.

Malignant pleural mesothelioma

Primary pleural tumors are rare malignancies. Malignant pleural mesothelioma (MPM) is the most common primary pleural tumor, accounting for 2000 to 3000 cases per year in the United States. The peak incidence of MPM is in the sixth decade of life and males are affected more often than females (5:1). Exposure to asbestos is the causative factor in 85% of cases and the latency period from exposure to development of the disease is 15 to 50 years. Conversely, the benign variant of mesothelioma is not associated with asbestos exposure. Non-asbestos causes of MPM include RT, non-asbestos mineral fibers, and exposure to simian virus 40.

Presentation and diagnosis

Dyspnea is the most common symptom. Chest pain is the second most common symptom and is a poor prognostic indicator as it often represents chest wall invasion. Decreased breath sounds, dullness to percussion and limited chest wall excursion may be present. Chest wall masses may be found at previous biopsy sites. PET-CT scanning with IV contrast is the primary imaging modality for diagnosis and staging, providing insight into nodal involvement and occult metastases. MRI is useful to determine invasion into the chest wall and transdiaphragmatic extension. MPM may appear as pleural effusion, subtle pleural thickening, discrete pleural-based masses or a thick confluent pleural rind with encasement of the entire lung. Pleural fluid cytology is diagnostic in only 30-50% of cases. The presence of high levels of pleural fluid hyaluronic acid is suggestive of the disease. Thoracoscopic pleural biopsy is more accurate than percutaneous needle biopsy and is the preferred approach for obtaining tissue for definitive diagnosis. The location of the incision needs to be carefully planned to permit subsequent resection based on the high rate of port site seeding.

Pathology and staging

MPM may be classified into three major subcategories: epithelioid, sarcomatoid, and biphasic (mixed). Epithelioid MPM accounts for about two-thirds of cases and is associated with a better prognosis than is sarcomatoid and biphasic MPM. To be classified as biphasic MPM, the tissue must be composed of at least 10% epithelioid and sarcomatoid components. There is a lack of a uniformly accepted staging system for MPM and the two most commonly used systems are the International Mesothelioma Interest Group TNM staging system and Brigham & Women's Hospital (BWH) staging system. The BWH staging system is a surgical staging system that considers resectability, tumor histology, and nodal status. The TNM system has been endorsed by the American Joint Commission on Cancer. Table 17-1 depicts the TNM system with staging classification.

Treatment

MPM is a locally aggressive cancer that is difficult to treat. Palliative treatments such as pleurodesis were found to improve quality of life, and results in a median survival of 6 to 9 months. The best result of chemotherapy was shown in a large randomized clinical trial that demonstrated a benefit of combination cisplatin and premetrexed (12 month median survival) over cisplatin alone (9 month median survival).

The surgical approaches to this disease include extrapleural pneumonectomy (EPP) and pleurectomy/decortication (P/D). EPP involves the *en bloc* resection of the lung, parietal and visceral pleura, pericardium, and ipsilateral hemidiaphragm and is associated with 3-4% mortality in large centers. P/D entails resection of the parietal and visceral pleura with or without resection of the pericardium and diaphragm and is associated with 1-2% mortality. Many have suggested that one approach is superior to the other, but no prospective, randomized trial, has ever been carried out. Typically, P/D is reserved for high risk or advanced disease. Regardless of the approach, results of surgical treatment alone were disappointing. This lead to the use of multimodality therapy using surgery combined with chemotherapy and/or RT. This is generally advocated for clinical stage I-III epithelial and mixed malignant mesothelioma, while stage IV and sarcomatoid histology are generally palliated with chemotherapy alone. Some centers utilize intrapleural chemotherapy at the time of operation. Median survivals with various combinations of multimodality therapy have ranged from 9 to 26 months, with certain subsets such as the patients with epithelial histology, having median survivals of 26 months.

Table 17-1. International staging of pleural mesothelioma *(Adapted with permission from Sobin L, Gospodarowicz M, Wittekind C. TNM Classification of Malignant Tumours. 7th edition. Oxford: Wiley-Blackwell; 2009).*

TNM descriptors	
T – Primary Tumor	
Tx	Primary tumor cannot be assessed
T0	No evidence of primary tumor
Tis	Carcinoma in situ
T1	Tumor involves ipsilateral parietal pleura, with or without focal involvement of visceral pleura
T1a	Tumor involves ipsilateral parietal pleura. No involvement of visceral pleura.
T1b	Tumor involves ipsilateral parietal pleura with focal involvement of visceral pleura
T2	Tumor involves any of the ipsilateral pleural surfaces with at least one of the following: - Confluent visceral pleura tumor (including the fissure) - Invasion of diaphragmatic muscle - Invasion of lung parenchyma
T3	Tumor involves any ipsilateral pleural surfaces with at least one of the following: - Invasion of endothoracic fascia - Invasion into mediastinal fat - Solitary focus of tumor invading soft tissues of the chest wall - Non-transmural involvement of the pericardium

T4	Tumor involves any ipsilateral pleural surfaces with at least one of the following:
	- Diffuse or multifocal invasion of soft tissues of chest wall
	- Any involvement of rib
	- Invasion through diaphragm to peritoneum
	- Direct extension to contralateral pleura
	- Invasion into the spine
	- Extension to internal surface of pericardium
	- Pericardial effusion with positive cytology
	- Invasion of myocardium
	- Invasion of brachial plexus

N – Regional Lymph Nodes	
NX	Regional lymph nodes cannot be assessed
N0	No regional lymph node metastasis
N1	Metastasis in ipsilateral bronchopulmonary and/or hilar lymph nodes
N2	Metastasis in subcarinal lymph nodes and/or ipsilateral internal mammary or mediastinal lymph nodes
N3	Metastasis in contralateral mediastinal, internal mammary, or hilar nodes and/or ipsilateral or contralateral supraclavicular or scalene lymph nodes

M – Distant Metastasis	
M0	No distant metastasis
M1	Distant metastasis

Stage	T	N	M
IA	1a	0	0
IB	1b	0	0
II	2	0	0
III	1, 2	1	0
	1, 2	2	0
	3	0 – 2	0
IV	4	Any	0
	Any	3	0
	Any	Any	1

18. Chylothorax
Samuel J. Youssef

The thoracic duct is a channel draining lymphatic fluid from the body to the venous system. During development, the *cisterna chyli* joins the bilateral jugular lymphatic sacs forming the thoracic duct. It is originally a bilateral conduit that merges into a single system. This configuration is highly variable, seen only 60% of the time.

The thoracic duct originates with the *cisterna chyli* between T10 and L3 and enters the chest through the aortic hiatus to the right of the aorta. It courses anterior to the vertebral bodies between the aorta and azygos vein and posterior to the esophagus. At T5, it crosses to the left as it passes posterior to the aortic arch and lies on the left side of the esophagus. In the neck, it arches laterally at C7 and lies anterior to the subclavian artery, superficial to the phrenic nerve and anterior scalene muscle. It then passes behind the carotid sheath and terminates as single (80%) or multiple (20%) branches into the left jugulo-subclavian junction.

Lymph from the right side of the head, neck, and chest wall as well as from the right lung, heart, dome of liver, and right diaphragm drains into a right lymphatic duct which then drains into the posterior junction of the right subclavian and jugular veins.

Chyle

The primary physiologic role of the thoracic duct is to deliver digestive fat (60% of ingested fat) to the venous system. Concentrations of fat, protein, and lymphocytes vary depending on the timing, composition, and amount of food ingested. Fatty acids <10 carbon atoms bypass the lymphatic circulation and enter directly into the portal system. Hence, a diet consisting of medium chain triglycerides reduces thoracic duct flow. T-lymphocytes are the main cellular components of thoracic duct lymph. Chyle is bacteriostatic, and its alkaline pH results in little pleural reaction.

The lymph flow varies between 30 and 190mL/hr. It is driven by the absorption of intestinal food/liquid and augmented by intestinal contractions. The negative transdiaphragmatic pressure gradient as well as the duct's valves help the upward flow. The normal intraductal pressure ranges from 10-25 cmH$_2$O.

Chylothorax

Congenital chylothorax is the most common cause of pleural effusion in the neonatal period. It presents as respiratory distress at birth or in first weeks of life. It is associated with syndromes of abnormal lymphatic development. The thoracic duct may be atretic or have multiple dilated lymphatic channels or fistulas. Treatment is conservative, with expected resolution in 4-5 weeks. Continued breastfeeding does not prevent resolution. Thoracentesis is appropriate for initial relief. In the absence of ascites, pleuro-peritoneal shunting is used for persistent chylothorax.

Traumatic chylothorax may occur after blunt or penetrating trauma. The most common non-penetrating method is by hyperextension of the spine with rupture just above the diaphragm. Often, the duct has been fixed as a result of prior disease or malignancy.

Surgical injuries occur during esophagectomy, aortic operations, coarctation repair, ligation of PDA, left pneumonectomy, removal of posterior mediastinal tumors, and sympathectomy. Injuries are not recognized intraoperatively because patients have had no oral intake for hours prior. Duct injuries below T6 level tend to present on the right while injuries above T6 present on the left. The incidence of chylothorax after esophagectomy varies between 0.5-3.4% and does not depend on approach.

Neoplastic chylothorax occurs by invasion, compression, or tumor embolism of the thoracic duct. Lymphoma is the most common malignancy (50% of cases) followed by lung cancer and retroperitoneal sarcoma.

Presentation and diagnosis

Presenting signs may be widened mediastinum, pleural effusion, or rarely pericardial effusion. Drainage is necessary to relieve symptoms. Ongoing external drainage may rapidly deplete nutritional, fluid, electrolyte, and lymph reserves. Most postoperative cases drain in excess of 1 L/day. If this persists for more than 1 week, mortality and morbidity rises. Spontaneous healing of a nonsurgical fistula may occur in less than half of patients. Death ensues unless the fistula is surgically closed.

Diagnosis is suggested by the presence of non-clotting milky fluid in the pleural space. Triglyceride levels >110 mg/dL are 99% diagnostic. Levels < 50 mg/dL exclude chylothorax with 95% probability. For levels 50-110 mg/dL other studies such as inspection for chylomicrons are warranted. The presence of chylomicrons is a very specific finding. Fat globules stain with Sudan-3 and can be seen in the setting of chylothorax. Chylothorax should be distinguished from pseudochylothorax, which results from accumulation of cholesterol in long-standing pleural effusions. Pseudochylothorax was seen with TB in the past, but now the most common cause is rheumatoid pleurisy. Pseudochylothorax has cholesterol

>200 mg/dL with cholesterol crystals and no chylomicrons. Chylothorax usually has a cholesterol-to-triglyceride ratio < 1.

Management

Medical management is an appropriate initial strategy. This entails drainage of the pleural space, reduction of chyle flow, hydration, and nutrition. Approximately 25-50% of leaks close spontaneously. Infection is uncommon since chyle is bacteriostatic. A reduction in dietary intake and reduction in long chain fatty acids reduces lymph flow. Medium-chain triglycerides are administered as they are preferentially taken up by the portal circulation. TPN may often be preferred. Fistula healing most often occurs due to obliteration of the pleural space rather than vessel closure. Chemical pleurodesis may be used, especially in malignant fistulas. Lymphatic obstruction by tumor should undergo chemo/radiotherapy to relieve obstruction or promote fibrosis. Pleuroperitoneal shunting may be used with malignant chylothorax or when thoracotomy is contraindicated and the lung entrapped. Occlusion of the shunt occurs in 10% and ascites is a contraindication. Somatostatin can be used to decrease foregut secretions and lymph volume.

Percutaneous transabdominal duct catheterization and embolization can be effective in patients too frail to undergo duct ligation. Patients with previous abdominal surgery involving retroperitoneal organs may not be suitable for this intervention.

Thoracic duct ligation has reduced the mortality from over 50% to 10%. Idiopathic chylothorax in neonates and non-traumatic chylothorax should be managed non-operatively.

Indications for duct ligation include:

- Average daily loss of >1500 cc/day in adults or >100cc/day in children over a five day period despite conservative management

- Persistent leak for over two weeks

- Nutritional or metabolic complications

- Entrapped lung with inability to adequately drain the collection with a chest tube

- Post-esophagectomy chylothorax (given the high morbidity and mortality in these patients from immunological and metabolic imbalances)

Surgical techniques include direct ligation of the thoracic duct, mass ligation, thoracoscopic ligation, pleurectomy, fibrin glue, and placement of a pleuroperitoneal shunt. Mass ligation of all tissue between the aorta, spine, esophagus, azygos vein, and pericardium is performed above the diaphragmatic hiatus via the right pleural space and is the best way to ligate the thoracic duct. Visualization of a leak can be aided by ingestion of 6 to 8 ounces of cream or olive oil 2-3 hours prior to surgery. Prophylactic ligation of the thoracic duct during esophagectomy has been advocated.

19. Chest wall deformities

Jeremiah T. Martin

Classification

Chest wall deformities can be broadly classified into *pectus excavatum*, *pectus carinatum*, Poland's Syndrome, sternal defects (including cleft sternum, *ectopia cordis* and Cantrell's pentalogy), and miscellaneous conditions (including Jeune's disease and Jarcho-Levin syndrome).

Pectus excavatum

Occurring in up to 1 in 300 live births, *pectus excavatum* is the most common of the congenital chest wall deformities. It is characterized by sternal depression and flaring of the costal margins.

The etiology of *pectus excavatum*, similar to the other deformities, is poorly understood; however there appear to be hereditary patterns in addition to association with other musculoskeletal conditions such as Marfan's syndrome. It appears that excessive growth of the lower costal cartilages is responsible. The manubrium and first and second ribs are usually spared. While it may be symmetric, there is frequently a greater depression towards the right. In addition, the deformity is progressive, with the potential for significant worsening during the adolescent growth spurt.

The physiologic impact of the deformity is difficult to consistently demonstrate, however, patients with *pectus excavatum* can demonstrate reduced vital capacity, and exercise tolerance is generally improved after repair. *Pectus excavatum* may cause depression of the RV with reduction in cardiac performance, and specifically mitral valve prolapse due to sternal pressure on the annulus. However, esthetic concerns remain the most common reason for repair.

Patients with *pectus excavatum* are generally asymptomatic, but may present with decreased exercise tolerance. Psychosocial factors and cosmetic concerns are the most common reason for presentation. Pain may also be a presenting feature at the site of deformity.

Up to 25% of patients will have associated scoliosis, and therefore a complete examination and workup for associated musculoskeletal conditions must be undertaken. The most common score, the Haller index, is calculated as the ratio of the lateral diameter of the chest to the minimum distance between the sternum and the spine. A normal chest has an index of 2.5 with larger numbers indicating more severe disease.

EKG abnormalities are common and caused by the configuration of the chest wall. Normal pulmonary function testing does not correlate well with degree of exercise limitation. Echocardiography may be helpful if mitral prolapse is suspected.

Surgical correction is the standard of care. Cosmetic results are generally excellent, with variable improvement seen in exercise tolerance. Three approaches should be mentioned:

- The *Ravitch repair* is an open repair involving subperichondrial resection of all deformed costal segments, creation of a wedge sternal osteotomy to allow sternal elevation, and sternal fixation usually with a retrosternal bar or other support. The procedure is conducted through either a midline or a transverse inframammary incision.

- *Sternal eversion* has also been described with creation of what is essentially a free graft of sternum. This is less commonly practiced due to the potential for devastating complications.

- Minimally invasive repair utilizing the *Nuss procedure*, originally described in 1998, is now practiced with increasing frequency. Under thoracoscopic guidance, a convex bar is passed behind the sternum through the anterior mediastinum, and subsequently rotated to push the sternum and deformed cartilages forward. It is fixed laterally to the chest wall. Although the promise of a minimally invasive approach seems appealing, limitations include the need to perform the procedure before the growth spurt. It also appears to be associated with greater pain than the open approach. The bar generally needs to remain in place for 3 years. Risk of recurrence is not well established but is up to 7%.

Pectus carinatum

Pectus carinatum, much less common than *excavatum*, accounts for approximately 10% of the chest wall deformities, and is much more likely to occur in boys. Unlike *excavatum*, *carinatum* presents much later in childhood, and in addition to the cosmetic concerns, is more likely to present with pain. The defect may be a site of recurrent trauma and may be painful for the child to sleep prone. In these cases the Haller index is generally less than 2. Orthotopic bracing may be used with limited success, and again surgical repair is indicated for severe cases. Similar to the repair of *pectus excavatum*, subperichondrial excision of the affected costal elements with one or more sternal osteotomies are required.

Poland's syndrome

The original description of this deformity included unilateral absence of the pectoralis major and minor muscles associated with syndactily. Occurring in approximately 1 in 30,000 live births, the pathophysiology is poorly understood but may involve an in-utero vascular event of the affected subclavian supply. Patients with Poland's are also likely to have breast involvement, which may include amastia, and absence of axillary hair. Chest wall deformities, when they occur in this setting, may be profound due to rib aplasia. Surgical repair depends on the extent of chest wall involvement and may require rib grafts from the contralateral side and the use of patch material.

Sternal defects

Sternal defects range from a simple cleft to complete absence of the sternum and chest wall. Failure of fusion of the embryonic sternum is felt to be the developmental cause.

- *Sternal cleft.* Involves usually the upper portion of the sternum and is usually noted initially when the infant cries and a protrusion is noted. The heart, lungs, and overlying skin are generally normal. Repair is indicated to protect the mediastinal structures.

- *Ectopia cordis.* Results in complete failure of midline covering of the heart (skin, sternum, pericardium), and part or all of the heart may be positioned outside of the body. The heart is usually rotated anteriorly and in almost all cases underlying congenital cardiac defects are noted.

- *Thoracoabdominal ectopia cordis / Cantrell's pentalogy.* Distinct in that the heart is covered by a thin membrane and not rotated. The abdominal wall and diaphragm also have developmental defects. It is also associated with the development of a diverticulum of the LV of unclear significance. The five findings are omphalocele, anterior diaphragmatic hernia, sternal cleft, ectopia cordis, and an intracardiac defect: either VSD or ventricular diverticulum.

Miscellaneous conditions

- *Jeune's Syndrome (asphyxiating thoracic dystrophy).* Narrow bell-shaped chest, which is severely restrictive. The ribs are oriented horizontally and are foreshortened. Pulmonary development is limited as is respiration due to extremely poor respiratory mechanics.

- *Jarcho-Levin syndrome (spondylothoracic dysplasia).* Characterized by the presence of alternating hemivertebrae, which are short in height, resulting in very close approximation of the ribs. Very poor respiratory mechanics are noted.

Both of these conditions are associated with poor outcomes due to difficulty with pulmonary development and the frequent occurrence of pulmonary complications.

20. Chest wall tumors

Robert A. Meguid

Tumors of the chest wall are rare, accounting for less than 1% of all tumors. They can be divided into benign and malignant lesions and stratified by histopathology. Primary malignant chest wall tumors include chondrosarcomas (35%), plasmacytomas (25%), Ewing's sarcomas (15%), osteosarcomas (15%), lymphoma (10%), plus other rare tumors. In addition, several neoplasms metastasize to the chest wall, including melanoma, breast carcinoma, lung carcinoma, mesothelioma, and renal cell carcinoma.

Benign tumors of the chest wall include fibrous dysplasia (40%), chondromas (30%), osteochondromas, desmoids, lipomas, neurofibromas, and giant cell tumors, among others. In general, benign tumors of the chest wall are characterized by slow growth.

Presentation

Approximately 80% of chest wall tumors present as painful, enlarging lesions. Depending on tumor histopathology, they vary in rapidity of growth with benign chest wall tumors growing slower than malignant. Presenting pain may be due to displacement or invasion of adjacent structures, and pathologic fracture of ribs. The remaining 20% are incidentally-found asymptomatic masses. Patients may also present with dyspnea, night sweats, fevers, or generalized malaise.

Workup

Following careful history and physical examination, imaging should be obtained. While tumors have different appearances on imaging due to differing histopathology, chest CT and MRI with or without contrast-enhancement are useful. Staging is dependent on the primary tumor type, and PET-CT can aid in this, especially for bone and soft-tissue sarcomas.

Tissue diagnosis should be made prior to surgical resection to guide neo-adjuvant therapy. Core needle biopsy or incisional biopsy should be pursued, with excisional biopsy of lesions less than 5cm.

Primary malignant chest wall tumors

- *Chondrosarcomas.* The most commonly occurring malignant primary tumors of the chest wall. 80% develop from the costochondral arches of the ribs and 20% from sternum. They may develop from benign tumors of the cartilage, or may be associated with trauma.

They occur most commonly in males less than 20 or greater than 50 years of age. Patients present with a slowly enlarging mass, associated with pain. CXR shows a lobulated mass arising in the medullary portion of the rib or sternum. Treatment is wide resection.

- *Plasmacytomas* (or solitary plasma cell tumor myeloma). Account for 20-30% of primary tumors of the chest wall and occur later in life. They tend to occur in the ribs and sternum and progress to multiple myeloma with greater frequency than extraosseous plasmacytomas. They present as painless masses with an osteolytic appearance on CXR. Workup should rule out extrathoracic lesions. Treatment of solitary plasmacytomas is RT. Surgical resection can be used for refractory cases. Chemotherapy is only used for disease progression.

- *Ewing's sarcomas.* The most common malignant lesion of the ribs in children, they develop from neural crest cells. These aggressive tumors invade and displace adjacent structures, and may present as solitary or multiple masses. Patients present with a painful mass and commonly, fever and malaise. Some patients may also have leukocytosis and an elevated erythrocyte sedimentation rate. On CXR, these tumors appear as lytic lesions with surrounding destruction (small holes or mottled appearance) and tend to have a characteristic onion-peel appearance from new bone formation. Treatment is surgery plus RT. Chemotherapy may be used preoperatively to shrink the tumor.

- *Osteosarcomas.* Occur most frequently in the ribs, scapulae, or clavicles of young adults. They are more prone to recurrence and metastasis than osteosarcomas of the extremities. They present as painful masses with elevated alkaline phosphatase levels. On CXR, they have a classic "sunburst" pattern and elevation of the periosteum (Codman's triangle sign) secondary to new bone formation. They are treated with chemotherapy followed by resection, with prognosis predicted by response to chemotherapy. RT is usually ineffective.

- *Lymphomas.* The most common type of chest wall lymphoma is extranodal diffuse large B-cell lymphoma. Lymphoma occurs in immunocompromised patients (transplant patients, HIV positive patients). Treatment is RT and chemotherapy (CHOP: cytoxan, adriamycin, vincristin, & prednisone).

- *Soft tissue sarcomas.* Workup includes MRI to identify infiltration and relation to adjacent vital structures, and chest CT to rule out pulmonary metastases. Treatment is wide local resection with 1 cm margins, including excision of biopsy sites. RT is indicated for residual disease, inadequate margins, tumors greater than 5 cm, and highly invasive tumors. Local recurrence is treated like the initial occurrence, and solitary pulmonary lesions can be resected. RT-induced sarcomas, which tend to be very aggressive, are treated similarly.

- *Malignant fibrous histiocytoma.* Painless, slowly enlarging violaceous chest wall mass, associated with history of RT. Most common in patients 50-70 years of age. Treatment is wide resection.

- *Other tumors.* Other malignant chest wall tumors include neuroblastomas, ganglioneuroblastomas, malignant schwannomas.

- *Metastases.* In general, solitary tumor metastases to the chest, most commonly from melanoma, breast carcinoma, lung carcinoma, mesothelioma, and renal cell carcinoma, are treated with resection and sometimes RT.

Benign chest wall tumors

- *Fibrous dysplasia of the bone.* The most common benign rib lesion in children, represents a maturation defect and can be associated with trauma. It presents as a painless mass. CXR shows as a fusiform mass with thinning of the cortex and no calcifications. Treatment is resection where deformity has occurred.

- *Chondromas.* The most common benign tumor of cartilage. They appear similar to malignant chondrosarcomas, necessitating surgical biopsy or resection to rule out malignancy.

- *Osteochondromas.* Typically present as masses associated with rib fractures and are resected to prevent further tissue displacement.

- *Desmoid tumors.* Histologically benign tumors developing from the muscular aponeurosis; locally aggressive. They occur more commonly in females, people with familial adenomatous polyposis (FAP) and at sites of prior trauma or scarring. Histologically, they contain sheets of fibroblasts with abundant collagen. They present as a painful mass, fixed to deep tissues but not to skin. Treatment is wide resection with 2-4 cm microscopically negative margins. Between one quarter and one half recur locally. RT is used following margin-positive resections, but the use of chemotherapy is not supported by trials.

- *Other benign chest wall tumors.* Lipomas, fibromas, neurofibromas, ganglioneuromas, schwannomas, and giant cell tumors.

Treatment

A multidisciplinary approach should be utilized for management of chest wall tumors, due to the infrequency with which they are encountered by most practitioners. While most lesions are treated with resection, including benign lesions, specific treatment nuances exist, as discussed above.

Post-resection defects less than 5cm or those covered by the scapula do not warrant reconstruction beyond coverage with local tissue advancement. Reconstruction is warranted for defects greater than 5cm or involving two or more adjacent ribs. This usually entails coverage with a methyl methacrylate and non-absorbable mesh "sandwich". In addition, tissue transfer can be used to cover defects; tissue includes latissimus dorsi, rectus abdominus, and pectoralis muscle and myocutaneous flaps. These are particularly useful in irradiated tissue beds. Use of such flaps, or more complex tissue rearrangement, may necessitate the assistance from plastic/ reconstructive surgeons.

Aside from local recurrence, malignant chest wall tumors can metastasize to the lungs or liver. Therefore, long-term surveillance is warranted, and accomplished by serial chest CT at progressive intervals, based on initial tumor aggressiveness.

21. Thoracic outlet syndrome
Matthew D. Taylor

Thoracic outlet syndrome (TOS) is defined as a constellation of symptoms related to compression of the neurovascular elements found in the thoracic outlet including the brachial plexus, subclavian artery, and subclavian vein.

Classification

There are three classifications of TOS based upon the site of anatomic compression. Neurogenic TOS is the most common form of TOS, representing 90-95% of all cases. Arterial and venous TOS account for the remaining 5-10%. Venous TOS may progress to Paget-Schroetter syndrome (axillosubclavian vein thrombosis), otherwise known as effort thrombosis, which occurs in individuals performing persistent repetitive motion of the arm.

Etiology

Causes of TOS include:

- Anterior scalene muscle hypertrophy causing brachial plexus compression and/or subclavian artery compression

- Costoclavicular syndrome resulting in narrowing of the space between the clavicle and first rib

- Presence of a cervical rib

- Trauma

Presentation

TOS is more common in patients age 20-40 years and in women compared to men (4:1 ratio). Symptoms may include pain, numbness, and tingling of the arm and hand. In the case of venous TOS, patients may develop significant arm swelling if occlusive thrombus is present. Patients with arterial TOS may develop distal embolism due to arterial stenosis.

Four clinical examination maneuvers may be performed to elicit signs/symptoms of TOS:

- *Costoclavicular test.* Patient holds the shoulders down and backward to narrow the costoclavicular space.

- *Adson test.* Patient takes a deep breath while extending the neck and turning the head toward the side. Causes narrowing of the interscalene triangle.

- *Roos test.* Patient holds both arms at 90 degrees of abduction and external rotation with the shoulders drawn back. Hands are opened and closed for 3 minutes.

- *Wright test.* Patient hyperabducts and externally rotates arm.

Diagnosis

In addition to the H&P, X-ray of the cervical spine and chest should be performed to exclude cervical vertebral anomalies or a cervical rib. CT scan with IV contrast or MRI should be performed in the neutral position and with arms above the head. Obtaining imaging in both positions may better define the anatomic abnormality. Because the majority of patients have neurogenic TOS, arteriogram or venogram is not routinely performed unless symptoms such as arm swelling or digit ischemia are present.

Treatment

Initial treatment should be focused on physical therapy maneuvers to strengthen the structures of the shoulder girdle and correcting posture. Surgical therapy is reserved for patients who have not responded to conservative therapy after several months. Surgical decompression is accomplished by performing a first rib resection with scalenectomy approached by a transaxillary or supraclavicular approach. For venous TOS, combined supraclavicular and infraclavicular incisions may be necessary for adequate exposure. With symptomatic arterial stenosis, first rib resection and scalenectomy are combined with arterial reconstruction. Venous TOS is treated with thrombolysis followed by decompression (first rib resection and/or scalenectomy) and venous angioplasty or reconstruction.

22. Diseases of the diaphragm

Daniela Molena

The diaphragm is a muscular-fibrous structure that divides the chest from the abdomen and it represents the fulcrum of ventilatory mechanics. Normal function of both hemidiaphragms is necessary for optimal respiratory dynamics. When the diaphragm contracts, the rib cage expands, negative intra-thoracic pressure is created, and ventilation is initiated.

Anatomically, the diaphragm has a peripheral muscular and a central fibrous component. The muscular fibers originate from the circumference of the thoracic outlet (xiphoid process, lower bilateral 6 ribs, arcuate ligaments, and lumbar vertebrae) and converge into a central tendon creating a half-dome shape. There are 3 main openings in the diaphragm which allow for the passage of major structures from the chest to the abdomen: the caval opening for the IVC, the esophageal hiatus for the esophagus and vagus nerves, and the aortic hiatus for the aorta, thoracic duct, and azygos vein. The diaphragm is innervated solely by the phrenic nerves, which originate from the third, fourth and fifth cervical nerves and provide both sensory and motor functions.

Congenital diaphragmatic hernias

Congenital diaphragmatic hernias (CDH) occur as a result of embryologic developmental defects during gestation. The diaphragm develops between the 7th and 10th weeks of gestation from four embryologic components: the septum transversum, the right and left pleuroperitoneal membranes, and the dorsal mesentery of the esophagus. Muscle fibers then migrate from the third, fourth, and fifth cervical myotomes to complete the structure of the diaphragm. Failure of growth and fusion of these precursors lead to diaphragmatic defects. CDH are rare disorders occurring in about 1 every 2000-3000 live births but are associated with high morbidity and mortality. Decreased survival is mainly due to associated congenital abnormalities, prematurity, and low birth weight.

The cause of CHD is not well known. Familiar association is present in less than 2% of cases; different patterns of inheritance have been reported and chromosome abnormalities are present in one third of cases. The diagnosis can be made *in utero* with a prenatal US. Occasionally, CDH are incidentally discovered in adulthood during radiological testing for other reasons.

The posterolateral defect, also known as *Bochdalek's hernia*, is the most common and constitutes 90% of all CDH. It occurs more frequently in men than women with 3:2 ratio, it is left-sided in 80-90% of cases and it is associated with other congenital abnormalities including cardiac, renal, neural and GI defects.

Pulmonary hypoplasia and pulmonary hypertension are due to early herniation and entrapment of the abdominal organs into the chest causing compression of the lung parenchyma, directly on the ipsilateral side, and indirectly on the contralateral by means of mediastinal shifting. Respiratory impairment is thus the main symptom with severity ranging from life-threatening respiratory distress requiring mechanical ventilation or occasionally ECMO to only minor respiratory difficulty. Feeding problems and growth retardation may be present as well.

CXR of the neonate is diagnostic by showing intestinal loops or the tip of an orogastric tube in the chest. Despite improvement in early diagnosis and aggressive intensive care management, Bochdalek's hernia carries a mortality rate that approaches 50%. Surgical repair is typically approached from the abdomen and it entails reduction of the hernia content into the abdomen, resection of the hernia sac if present (20% of cases), and closure of the diaphragmatic defect either primarily of with a nonabsorbable patch. Extralobar pulmonary sequestrations and associated abdominal abnormalities, when present, are resected or corrected at the time of the hernia repair if the neonate is on stable condition. Prenatal tracheal occlusion has been shown to reverse lung hypoplasia in animal models.

Morgagni's hernia is an anterior defect that occurs between the xiphoid process and the costochondral attachments of the diaphragm. It constitutes less than 2% of all CDH, it is usually asymptomatic, and it is often diagnosed incidentally. Surgical correction is advised even in the absence of symptoms in order to avoid life-threatening complications like incarceration or strangulation. Repair is approached through the abdomen, and the defect is closed either primarily or with mesh. The outcome and prognosis are excellent. Minimally invasive approaches have been described with good results in adults.

Acquired diaphragmatic hernias

Acquired diaphragmatic hernias are mostly due to trauma. Diaphragmatic rupture occurs in about 3-5% of all patients admitted for trauma. It is usually associated with severe injury and high mortality rate, and it is mostly due to blunt trauma. Patients are either asymptomatic or critically ill due to other injuries. The diagnosis is often missed or delayed. Visualization of herniated abdominal organs in the chest or the presence of an orogastric tube above the level of the diaphragm are suggestive signs of diaphragmatic injury. MRI and CT imaging show high sensitivity and specificity. Surgical repair is advised in order to avoid complications such as strangulation and obstruction. Prognosis is highly influenced by the severity of associated abdominal and overall injury scores.

Eventration and paralysis

Eventration of the diaphragm is a rare congenital developmental defect in which myoblasts fail to migrate to the muscular portion of the diaphragm impairing its ability to contract. It is frequently associated with other congenital abnormalities like spine and skeletal defects, hypoplastic lungs, sequestrations, and transposition of the viscera.

Diaphragmatic paresis or paralysis is an acquired condition, usually involving one hemidiaphragm, which results from an interruption in the conduction of the phrenic nerve impulse. The most common cause is the injury to the phrenic nerve due to surgery to the chest or neck, or direct invasion by a neoplasm. Idiopathic paralysis or phrenic nerve injury due to central line placement, spinal cord injury, or brachial plexus neuropathy (Parsonage-Turner syndrome) have been described. Neurologic diseases such as myelitis, encephalitis, poliomyelitis, or herpes zoster can impair the function of both hemidiaphragms.

The main symptom of diaphragm paralysis or eventration is dyspnea due to ventilation impairment and ventilation/perfusion mismatch of the basal portion of the lungs. Orthopnea is more typical of diaphragmatic paralysis due to shifting of the abdominal organs towards the chest and reduction of lung volume. Most adult patients are however asymptomatic and the elevated hemidiaphragm is incidentally found on a chest radiograph. PFTs will show a restrictive pattern and when done in a supine position, a 20-50% reduction of the total lung volumes. The sniff test has been classically described as the test of choice to distinguish paralysis from eventration (paradoxical upward motion of the paralyzed diaphragm greater than 2 cm during sniffing under fluoroscopy). However, this is not very specific and at times difficult to interpret. US and MRI have been used as valuable alternatives to fluoroscopy in the evaluation of diaphragmatic motion. CT and MRI can be useful to assess the content of a partial eventration. Definitive diagnosis of phrenic nerve paralysis can be made by phrenic nerve stimulation with electromyography.

Surgical plication is the preferred treatment for both conditions and it is indicated to relieve symptoms. The goal of plication is to reduce the paradoxical excursion of the diaphragm during inspiration, hence increasing both end-inspiratory and end-expiratory lung volumes. If paresis is suspected, a 1- to 2-year observation time might be warranted unless symptoms are so severe to impair quality of life or effective rehabilitation.

Plication can be done through a laparotomy or thoracotomy with good results, and mostly involves placing imbricating stitches in the central tendon of the diaphragm. Minimally invasive techniques have been shown to have equivalent success perhaps with less morbidity.

Diaphragmatic pacing

Diaphragmatic pacing is a rarely used technique that uses the application of electrical impulses to the phrenic nerve or diaphragm in order to stimulate diaphragmatic contraction. The main goal is to improve respiration in patients who would otherwise be dependent on a mechanical ventilator. The fundamental requirements for its successful application are the presence of intact phrenic nerves and a normal diaphragm. There are few indications for diaphragmatic pacing: central alveolar hypoventilation (Ondine's curse) and high cervical cord injury (above C3). Recently, it has been used in patients with amyotrophic lateral sclerosis with the goal to delay the need for mechanical ventilation by keeping diaphragmatic strength with electrical stimulation. The phrenic nerve can be stimulated by contact with an electrode placed either in the neck or in the chest. Direct stimulation of the diaphragm with electrodes implanted on areas of phrenic nerve entry has been reported and can be achieved through a laparoscopic approach.

Tumors of the diaphragm

Primary tumors of the diaphragm are very rare, and for the most part benign. The most common are congenital cysts (bronchogenic, mesothelial, or teratoid) and lipomas. Other benign tumors arise either from mesothelial cells (fibromas, angiomas, chondromas, hemangiomas, leiomyomas, hamartomas, desmoids, and solitary fibrous tumors) or neurogenic cells (neurilemmomas and neurofibromas). Primary malignant tumors are rare and mostly of mesenchymal origin (rhabdomyosarcomas and leiomyosarcomas).

Clinically silent, tumors are usually incidentally discovered on CXR or autopsy. Neurogenic tumors can be associated with hypertrophic pulmonary osteoarthropathy. Large masses can cause symptoms by compression of surrounding structures. On CXR, diaphragmatic tumors present as smooth or lobulated masses protruding into the base of the lung and they are difficult to differentiate from effusion, eventration, hernias, or lung or abdominal masses. CT or MRI can usually confirm the presence of a mass in the diaphragm even though it is challenging to determine whether a large tumor arises from the diaphragm, the lung, the pleura, or abdominal organs.

Surgical resection is the definitive treatment and the diaphragmatic defect can be closed primarily or with a prosthetic mesh. The prognosis reported for malignant tumors is dismal.

The diaphragm can be involved by thoracic or abdominal tumors by direct extension, commonly by lung cancer, mesothelioma, and hepatic carcinoma. In some instances en-bloc resection of the diaphragm and reconstruction with prosthetic material is necessary.

Other rare diaphragmatic conditions

Porous diaphragmatic syndromes

Variety of clinical conditions characterized by the passage of fluids, gases, tissues, secretions, or intestinal content through diaphragmatic pores from the abdominal to the chest cavity. When these pores are identified, then primary closure is curative.

Catamenial pneumothorax

It is defined as a spontaneous pneumothorax that occurs in women in relation to their menses. It can be considered part of the porous diaphragmatic syndromes since diaphragmatic defects have been reported in up to 60% of cases and it is hypothesized that these pores allow passage of air from the abdomen into the chest causing pneumothorax. Endometrial implants in the visceral pleura can be found as well, and pelvic endometriosis has been reported in 20-70% of cases. Combined medical hormonal therapy and surgery seem to offer the best results. Surgical treatment involves correction of the diaphragmatic defect, resection of the endometrial implants, and pleurodesis or pleurectomy.

Agenesis of the diaphragm

Isolated diaphragmatic agenesis is extremely rare and only few cases are reported in the literature. It is usually diagnosed early after birth and it is associated with high mortality. Rare adult cases have been reported as well. In contrast with other congenital diaphragmatic hernias, a familial inheritance with multifactorial genetic etiology has been shown.

Cantrell's pentalogy

The full spectrum of this syndrome consist of deficiency of the anterior diaphragm, a supraumbilical abdominal wall defect, defect of the diaphragmatic pericardium, congenital intracardiac abnormalities, and a defect of the lower sternum. These defects cause omphalocele with associated *ectopia cordis*. It is a rare condition, often incomplete, due to developmental failure of the lateral mesoderm during the third week of gestation. The prognosis depends on the severity of the defects and the treatment consists of correction of the ventral hernia, diaphragmatic defects, sternal defects, and cardiovascular associated anomalies.

23. Anatomy and physiology of the esophagus
Ryan A. Macke

Anatomy

The esophagus is a tubular structure made up of 4 layers: mucosa, sub-mucosa, muscularis propria, and adventitia. The mucosa is broken down into 3 additional layers: the mucous membrane, made up of non-keratinized squamous epithelium; the lamina propria, a thin layer of connective tissue; and the mucosa muscularis, a thin layer of smooth muscle. The submucosa contains vascular, lymphatic, and nervous plexuses, as well as connective tissue and glands. The muscularis propria is comprised of an outer longitudinal and inner circular muscle layer. The adventitial layer is made up of loose connective tissue that approximates the esophagus to adjacent structures and contains additional vascular, lymphatic, and nervous networks. The esophagus does not have a serosa, as seen in the remainder of the GI tract.

As noted above, the muscularis propria transitions from striated muscle in the proximal esophagus to smooth muscle distally. The longitudinal muscle layer originates from the posterior aspect of the cricoid cartilage, with two muscle bundles wrapping around laterally and meeting on the dorsal aspect of the esophagus roughly 3 cm below the cricoid. This orientation leaves a V-shaped area of weakness, known as Laimer's triangle, on the dorsal esophagus just distal to the cricopharyngeus muscle that is covered only with the circular muscle layer. In contrast, Killian's triangle is an area of weakness proximal to the cricopharyngeus muscle. The inner circular layer is in continuity with the inferior constrictor muscles and is thicker than the outer layer. Circular fibers have a transverse orientation in the proximal and distal esophagus, while the remaining fibers have an oblique spiraling orientation that aids in peristalsis.

The esophagus has a segmental blood supply. The inferior thyroid arteries are the main arterial inflow to the cervical esophagus. The thoracic esophagus is supplied by bronchial arteries, typically one right and two left-sided branches, as well as direct branches from the descending aorta. The left gastric and inferior phrenic arteries supply the abdominal esophagus. Longitudinal anastomoses are formed within the muscle and submucosa, providing collaterals that allow the esophagus to be mobilized without significant risk of ischemia.

Venous drainage is also segmental. The submucosal venous plexus drains into a periesophageal venous plexus. Inferior thyroid veins then drain the cervical esophagus, while the bronchial, azygos, and hemiazygos veins drain the thoracic esophagus. These veins then empty into the SVC. The abdominal esophagus drains into the coronary vein of the portal system. The submucosal venous plexus of the stomach and esophagus are connected, thus permitting the coronary-azygos vein portosystemic shunt seen in portal hypertension.

Esophageal lymphatic drainage is not segmental, but rather intramural and longitudinal. Networks of lymphatics are found in the submucosa (most extensive), muscularis propria, and adventitia. Submucosal lymphatics drain into collecting trunks, which then pierce the muscularis propria and enter the periesophageal regional lymph nodes. These trunks may also drain directly into the thoracic duct. Because of the extensive intramural longitudinal lymphatic connections, lymph can spread in varying directions. In theory, lymph from the proximal esophagus drains into the deep cervical nodes, the middle third drains into the superior and posterior mediastinal nodes, and the distal third drains into the gastric and celiac nodes. However, obstruction of the ducts by tumor or inflammation may alter this flow, possibly explaining the unpredictable lymphatic spread seen in esophageal cancer.

The majority of the innervation of the esophagus occurs either directly by the vagus nerves (including the recurrent laryngeal branches) or indirectly through its fibers. This includes motor, sensory, parasympathetic, and sympathetic pathways. The recurrent laryngeal nerves supply the cricopharyngeus muscle and cervical esophagus and therefore injury to these nerves can lead to aspiration and dysmotility. The mid-esophagus is supplied predominantly by direct branches of the vagus nerves. The distal thoracic esophagus is innervated by the anterior and posterior esophageal plexuses, which are comprised of fibers from both vagus nerves after each nerve passes posterior to the hilum. The fibers of each plexus then converge to reform the left vagus anteriorly and the right vagus posteriorly, with both nerves having fibers from the original contralateral vagus. The intrinsic innervation of the esophagus is provided by the myoenteric (Auerbach's) plexus, which lies between the outer muscle layers, and the submucosal (Meissner's) plexus, which lies in the submucosa.

Anatomic points of narrowing provide landmarks for endoscopic examination and can aid in localizing pathology. These points and average measurements are listed in Table 23-1.

Table 23-1. Endoscopic points of narrowing and average measurements.

Anatomic point	Distance from incisors	
	Men	Women
Upper esophageal sphincter	14 cm	15 cm
Crossing of left mainstem bronchus and aortic arch	22-24 cm	24-26 cm
Lower esophageal sphincter	36-38 cm	38-40 cm

Physiology

Swallowing is a complex series of events that can be divided into three phases: oral, pharyngeal, and esophageal. The oral phase is voluntary, whereas the final two phases are not. The purpose of the esophageal phase is to transport a bolus through an opened UES, down the esophagus, and through an opened LES. The UES is a high-pressure area approximately 2-3 cm in length that separates the pharynx from the esophagus. The cricopharyngeus is the key muscle involved in UES function. At rest, the UES is tonically contracted, preventing reflux into the pharynx and aspiration. Relaxation is triggered by a voluntary swallow, allowing a bolus to pass through. Contraction with pressures twice the resting pressure then occurs, followed by a return to baseline. In contrast, the esophageal body is not tonically contracted. The longitudinal and circular muscle layers combine to create peristaltic contractions that occlude the lumen and push the bolus distally to the LES. The LES is both a physiologic and anatomic area whose main purpose is preventing esophageal reflux by remaining tonically contracted. Relaxation occurs in response to peristalsis in the esophageal body or gastric distension. Transient relaxation of the LES also occurs, spanning 5 to 30 seconds, and can lead to normal, brief periods of physiologic reflux. The following substances are known to cause LES relaxation: secretin, cholecystokinin (CCK), glucagon, gastric inhibitory peptide (GIP), vasoactive intestinal peptide (VIP), and neurotensin. Extrinsic factors that can cause increased LES pressure include increased intra-abdominal pressure, acting on the abdominal portion of the LES, and contraction of the diaphragm at the level of the crus during a Valsalva maneuver. Additionally, gastrin causes LES contraction.

Esophageal contractions can be categorized as primary, secondary, and tertiary waves. Primary waves are normal peristaltic contractions triggered by voluntary swallowing. Peristaltic contractions occurring in response to esophageal distention or irritation are referred to as secondary waves, which carry out a "housekeeping" function. Tertiary waves are not coordinated and do not produce effective peristalsis. Tertiary waves are seen in normal patients and can occur spontaneously or in response to a swallow. However, a greater frequency of tertiary contractions may be seen in patients with dysmotility disorders.

24. Esophageal cancer

Carlos J. Anciano

Epidemiology

Esophageal cancer is among the 10 most common malignancies world-wide. In the US, 15,000 new cases are diagnosed every year.

Squamous cell is the most common type of esophageal cancer worldwide. Risk factors include alcohol and tobacco consumption (x100 risk when combined), dietary factors (nitrosamines and high-cholesterol consumption), achalasia, Plummer-Vinson syndrome, HIV, and Epstein-Barr viruses. It has a male predominance of 2-3:1. Most tumors present in the middle third of the esophagus.

Adenocarcinoma is now the most common type in the US, representing the fastest growing solid malignancy in the country. Most adenocarcinomas are thought to develop following the metaplasia-dysplasia-carcinoma sequence in Barrett's epithelium related to GERD, particularly in long-segment disease. Other potential risk factors include nitrates, obesity, smoking, LES relaxing drugs, mixed acid-bile reflux, TP53 gene mutations, and chronic esophageal inflammation. The great majority of these tumors involve the distal esophagus.

Diagnosis

The classic presentation of esophageal cancer is dysphagia to solids. The typical patient with esophageal adenocarcinoma is a middle aged male, of middle or high socioeconomic status, with a long history of GERD and known hiatal hernia, without any weight loss or palpable node metastases at the time of presentation. On the contrary, patients with squamous cell cancer tend to present with a few months of dysphagia and weight loss, are heavy tobacco and alcohol consumers, from endemic areas, and lower socioeconomic class. Odynophagia, hemoptysis, and hoarseness may be present. Vocal chord palsy is usually related to more proximal tumors or metastatic disease.

The first study for workup of dysphagia is barium swallow esophagography. Flexible endoscopy with brushings and multiple biopsies is the procedure of choice for tissue diagnosis. EUS with FNA can be useful in the evaluation of malignant strictures.

Staging

The TNM staging of the American Joint Committee on Cancer (AJCC) and the International Union Against Cancer (UICC) was modified in

2009 to include separate stage groupings based on histology (Table 24-1). Clinical staging (cTNM) is achieved using CXR, barium contrast studies, bronchoscopy, CT, EUS or US with FNA, FDG-PET, thoracoscopy, and laparoscopy.

T stage is determined by EUS. The layers of the esophagus by EUS are:

- *First layer (hyperechoic):* Interface between lumen and mucosa

- *Second layer (hypoechoic):* Deep mucosa including muscularis mucosa

- *Third layer (hyperechoic):* Submucosa

- *Fourth layer (hypoechoic):* Muscularis propria

- *Fifth layer (hyperechoic):* Adventitia

Therefore, T staging is determined the following way: T1 (not beyond submucosa - 1st to 3rd EUS layers), T2 (confined to muscularis propria - 4th EUS layer), T3 (beyond muscularis propria - 5th EUS layer). T4 is determined by CT showing obliteration of fat planes surrounding the esophagus.

N and M staging is determined with a combination of diagnostic techniques. Intrathoracic or abdominal nodes > 1cm or supraclavicular nodes > 0.5 cm are suggestive of malignancy. Cervical and celiac nodes are considered M disease. PET is useful determining N and M stages, generally requiring tissue confirmation of the enhanced areas.

Metastases may be found in liver (35%), lung (20%), bone (9%), adrenals (2%), brain (2%), and pericardium, pleura, soft tissues, stomach, pancreas, and spleen. Thoracoscopy and laparoscopy are used selectively for nodal sampling, ascites/pleural cytology, conduit conditioning, and T stage resectability assessment.

Treatment

Early stage I (T1) tumors may undergo endoscopic treatment. Endoscopic mucosal resection (EMR), photodynamic therapy (PDT), and laser ablation are options. Nodal involvement must be excluded. T1a (mucosal) lesions carry a 0-12% node positive rate while T1b a 25-40% rate. Multifocal neoplasia, skip lesions, and lymphovascular invasion must be considered. Endoscopic treatment must be tailored to very early stages and poor surgical candidates.

Surgical resection offers the best curative chance. It is indicated for tumors without regional (N) or distant (M) disease as a single modality therapy, and as part of multimodality therapy for advanced stages in the setting of neoadjuvant treatment or as part of palliation.

There are different surgical approaches used, each with its own advantages and disadvantages:

- *Transhiatal esophagectomy.* The intrathoracic esophagus is excised without a thoracotomy. The conduit (usually stomach) is advanced and a cervical anastomosis is constructed. It avoids the pulmonary morbidity associated with a thoracotomy. It has a higher risk of recurrent laryngeal nerve injury (11%), strictures (28%), and leak rates (12-16%), although leaks are easier to control. It has comparable 5-year survival rates (20-25%) with a 5% perioperative mortality. It is preferred for mid to low tumors, non-bulky, early stage disease, in patients with pulmonary comorbidities. Some people argue that it compromises nodal tissue removal.

- *Transthoracic esophagectomy (Ivor-Lewis).* It is the most commonly performed technique. A right thoracotomy is performed (a left thoracotomy or thoracoabdominal incision can be used for distal tumors requiring phrenotomy) as well as a laparoscopy or laparotomy for intra-abdominal mobilization. It allows for a 2-field node dissection. The anastomosis is created in the chest. It has similar survival rates, and lower leak (10%), stricture (16%), and recurrent laryngeal nerve injury (5%) rates.

- *Three-incision esophagectomy.* This technique can be employed for tumors at any level and involves a right thoracotomy with dissection of the esophagus, an upper midline laparotomy with mobilization of the conduit, and a neck incision for the anastomosis. Advantages include the direct visualization of the dissection in the chest and a cervical anastomosis. Leak rates and risk of injury to the recurrent laryngeal nerve are equivalent to the transhiatal technique.

Minimally invasive approaches with combinations of robotic assistance or thoracoscopic surgery with laparoscopy are performed in some centers. They are technically demanding with long learning curves. They offer an oncologically sound procedure with a long-term survival benefit yet to be determined.

Different conduits can be used for reconstruction:

- *Stomach.* Stomach is the preferred substitute for conduit due to its robust blood supply and isoperistaltic arrangement. Disadvantages include the risk of delayed gastric emptying, reflux burden, and the possibility of Barrett's disease recurrence in the esophageal remnant. Most surgeons use a pyloromyotomy/plasty to improve drainage.

- *Colon.* Colon is the preferred conduit for young patients with benign disease or gastric compromise (lye ingestion). The left colon is preferred over the right colon as it has a longer length, less vascular anatomic variation, and a smaller caliber. It has long-term functional benefits but requires colonoscopy, preoperative blood supply studies, three anastomoses, longer operative time, and more blood loss. Preservation of adequate arterial and venous supply is key. The mesentery is preserved when possible in order to allow adequate venous drainage and avoid outflow obstruction and thrombosis that can lead to graft necrosis. If graft necrosis is suspected, immediate endoscopy is indicated. If confirmed, the graft should be emergently excised and an esophagostomy performed.

- *Jejunum.* Jejunum is preferred in Roux-en-Y form when a gastrectomy is required for distal tumors. Merendino interposition (interposing a jejunal loop between the esophagus and proximal stomach), long jejunal loop (requires pedicle preparation), and free graft (cervical reconstruction) are less frequent.

The most frequent placement of the conduit is orthotopic (anatomic). The subcutaneous placement is rarely used due to cosmetics. A retrosternal placement is used when there is a fear for tumor involvement of the conduit in the posterior mediastinum (e.g., palliative surgery) or in delayed reconstructions with inflammatory scarring of the mediastinal pathway.

Neoadjuvant regimes are used with advanced locoregional disease as they can downstage tumors in up to 50% patients with a 10% complete response seen at the time of the resection. Complete response is the most important predictor of improved survival from these therapies. Patients that receive neoadjuvant therapies are more likely to complete the full course of chemoradiation when compared to those undergoing adjuvant treatment. In addition, using chemoradiation in a neoadjuvant way avoids radiation of the conduit and allows to assess the response of the tumor to therapy.

Adjuvant RT may be used to sterilize microscopic or gross residual local tumor, at the expense of damage to the conduit. There is no role for adjuvant chemotherapy in the absence of metastatic disease; nonetheless, aggressive histology and lymphovascular invasion should be considered.

Advanced stage confers a dismal prognosis. Chemoradiation is superior to either chemotherapy or RT alone. The most common regimen is cisplatin and 5-fluorouracil with a third agent (epirubicin or docetaxel), combined with 40-50 Gy of fractionated RT. Additive resection of squamous cell cancer reduces local recurrence without improved survival. Adenocarcinoma has a less significant response to chemoradiation, therefore surgery is performed more frequently.

Palliation includes all previous modalities as well as endoscopic dilations and stent placements. They aim for improvement in quality of life controlling dysphagia, odynophagia, blood loss, fistula-related morbidity, and nutrition.

Tracheoesophageal fistula presents in approximately 15% of patients with locally advanced esophageal cancer and is a devastating complication. The goal of treatment for these patients is palliation with control of the fistula to limit respiratory complications. The best treatment method depends on patient and tumor characteristics. Most fistulas are treated with stents with closure rates of 75-100%. Chemoradiation may be useful alone (for small fistulas with minimal spillage) or in combination with other strategies. Bypass and diversion may be reasonable in patients with good functional status and no regional or metastatic disease. Nutritional and supportive management is important, regardless of the main treatment strategy chosen.

Outcomes

Overall, esophageal cancer confers a 5-12% 5-yr survival (median survival 23 months). 5-year survival is 80% for early stage, 24% for local, 12% for locoregional, and 2% for distant disease. Poor prognostic factors are advanced age, African/American race, lower esophageal tumors, increased depth, > 5 nodes involved, and a high ratio of positive to negative nodes. Good prognostic factors are complete pathological response, minimal residual disease, high hospital volume (for stage I-II, >20 procedures/year).

Table 24-1. International staging of esophageal carcinoma *(Adapted with permission from Sobin L, Gospodarowicz M, Wittekind C. TNM Classification of Malignant Tumours. 7th edition. Oxford: Wiley-Blackwell; 2009).*

TNM Descriptors	
T – Primary Tumor	
Tx	Primary tumor cannot be assessed
T0	No evidence of primary tumor
Tis	Carcinoma in situ / high-grade dysplasia
T1	Tumor invades lamina propria, muscularis mucosae, or submucosa
T1a	Tumor invades lamina propria or muscularis mucosae
T1b	Tumor invades submucosa
T2	Tumor invades muscularis propria
T3	Tumor invades adventitia
T4	Tumor invades adjacent structures
T4a	Tumor invades pleura, pericardium, or diaphragm
T4b	Tumor invades other adjacent structures such as aorta, vertebral body, or trachea
N – Regional Lymph Nodes	
NX	Regional lymph nodes cannot be assessed
N0	No regional lymph node metastasis
N1	Metastasis in 1-2 regional lymph nodes
N2	Metastasis in 3-6 regional lymph nodes
N3	Metastasis in 7 or more regional lymph nodes
M – Distant Metastasis	
M0	No distant metastasis
M1	Distant metastasis

Nonanatomic cancer characteristics	
Histologic grade	
G1	Well differentiated
G2	Moderately differentiated
G3	Poorly differentiated
G4	Undifferentiated
Cancer location (based on proximal edge of tumor)	
Upper thoracic	From thoracic inlet to tracheal bifurcation (20-25 cm from incisors)
Middle thoracic	Proximal half of esophagus between tracheal bifurcation and GE junction (25-30 cm from incisors)
Lower thoracic	Distal half of esophagus between tracheal bifurcation and GE junction (30-40 cm from incisors)
GE junction	Distal thoracic esophagus, GE junction, or within the proximal 5 cm of the stomach (cardia) that extend into the GE junction or esophagus (40-45 cm from incisors)

Stage grouping: Adenocarcinoma				
Stage	T	N	M	G
0	Tis	0	0	1
IA	1	0	0	1–2
IB	1	0	0	3
	2	0	0	1–2
IIA	2	0	0	3
IIB	3	0	0	Any
	1–2	1	0	Any
IIIA	1–2	2	0	Any
	3	1	0	Any
	4a	0	0	Any
IIIB	3	2	0	Any
IIIC	4a	1–2	0	Any
	4b	Any	0	Any
	Any	3	0	Any
IV	Any	Any	1	Any

Stage grouping: Squamous cell carcinoma					
Stage	T	N	M	G	Location
0	Tis	0	0	1	Any
IA	1	0	0	1	Any
IB	1	0	0	2–3	Any
	2–3	0	0	1	Lower
IIA	2–3	0	0	1	Upper, middle
	2–3	0	0	2–3	Lower
IIB	2–3	0	0	2–3	Upper, middle
	1–2	1	0	Any	Any
IIIA	1–2	2	0	Any	Any
	3	1	0	Any	Any
	4a	0	0	Any	Any
IIIB	3	2	0	Any	Any
IIIC	4a	1–2	0	Any	Any
	4b	Any	0	Any	Any
	Any	3	0	Any	Any
IV	Any	Any	1	Any	Any

GE: Esophagogastric

25. Other esophageal tumors
Carlos M. Mery

Malignant esophageal tumors

Approximately 2% of esophageal malignant tumors are not adenocarcinomas or squamous cell carcinomas. Some of these tumors include:

- *Small cell tumors.* Neuroendocrine tumors found primarily in the distal third of the esophagus. Prognosis is poor. Treatment is by esophageal resection if the tumor is confined to the esophagus, followed by adjuvant chemotherapy. Some people advocate RT rather than surgical resection due to the poor outcomes.

- *Carcinosarcomas.* Polypoid lesions in the lower two thirds of the esophagus. They are composed by carcinomatous and sarcomatous elements.

- *Melanomas.* Usually present as polypoid, ulcerated masses in the lower two thirds of the esophagus. Most patients present with metastatic disease.

- *Leiomyosarcomas.* Found throughout the esophagus. Sometimes difficult to differentiate from leiomyomas. Treatment is by resection. Patients with low grade tumors may benefit from resection even if there is evidence of metastatic disease.

- *GI stromal tumors (GIST).* Mesenchymal submucosal tumors associated with mutations of *c-kit* gene that encodes a receptor tyrosine kinase (RTK). Size of tumor and number of mitoses define the aggressiveness of the tumor. Surgical resection is the treatment of choice. Patients with intermediate or high-risk tumors should be treated with adjuvant imatinib (Gleevec). Patients with bulky but resectable disease may benefit from neoadjuvant therapy with imatinib followed by resection. Advanced disease should be treated with imatinib. Surgical debulking may follow in selected patients with an adequate response to medical treatment.

Benign esophageal tumors

Benign esophageal tumors are rare. The most common benign tumors are leiomyomas, followed by esophageal cysts and polyps. These tumors are usually asymptomatic but may be associated with obstructive symptoms when larger than 5 cm. Workup includes barium esophagogram, CT, endoscopy, and EUS. Intramural tumors (e.g., leiomyomas) should not be biopsied endoscopically. Some of the most common benign tumors are:

- *Leiomyoma.* Most common benign tumor of the esophagus, more common in the lower third. It usually originates from the muscularis propria layer of the esophagus. Histologically, it appears as whorls of spindle cells with eosinophilic neoplasm within connective tissue. Surgical treatment is indicated for symptomatic patients, tumors increasing in size, or when the diagnosis is in doubt. Enucleation is the treatment of choice.

- *Esophageal cysts.* Congenital cysts are developed from persistent vacuoles in the wall of the foregut during development. They occur in close proximity or within the wall of the esophagus. Most cysts present in childhood with symptoms of esophageal or airway obstruction. Sometimes, they are found incidentally in the adult patient. Cysts should be surgically enucleated, even if asymptomatic, to prevent growth and obstruction.

- *Fibrovascular polyp.* Most common intraluminal benign tumor, mostly found in the upper esophagus and usually very large. Resection is indicated to avoid airway obstruction. Small tumors are excised endoscopically; larger tumors are excised surgically via an esophagotomy.

- *Squamous cell papilloma.* Very rare, mainly in older patients, in the distal third of the esophagus, associated with human papilloma virus. Indications for resection include obstruction and inability to differentiate from squamous cell carcinoma.

- *Granular cell tumor.* Submucosal tumors in the distal third of the esophagus, originating from Schwann cells. Large symptomatic tumors and those in which malignancy cannot be excluded should be resected.

- *Hemangioma.* Submucosal nodular tumors, blue in appearance, in the distal third of the esophagus. They can be associated with Osler-Weber-Rendu syndrome. They are usually asymptomatic but may present with bleeding and dysphagia. Biopsy is contraindicated due to the risk of bleeding. Diagnosis may be confirmed with CT and radionuclide angiography. Asymptomatic lesions are managed expectantly.

- *Inflammatory pseudotumor.* Mucosal inflammatory tumors, most common in the lower third of the esophagus. It is difficult to differentiate these tumors from cancer. Multiple biopsies are usually required. No particular treatment is needed.

- *Adenoma.* Polyps arising from columnar epithelium in the distal esophagus. Sampling is required to rule out dysplasia.

26. Congenital diseases of the esophagus

Jeremiah T. Martin

Embryology

Development of the foregut begins in the 4th week of life. The embryo folds upon itself laterally and cephalocaudad such that an endodermal lined cavity is formed, which will give rise to the epithelium and glands of the digestive tract. Foregut derivatives include the pharynx and respiratory system, which form as a single entity, but later the laryngotracheal bud grows and forms a septum, which develops from the lateral wall. Meanwhile, as the esophagus rapidly elongates, its lumen is quickly occluded by proliferating endothelium. This later recanalizes as a series of separate vacuoles, which grow and coalesce to form the final esophageal lumen. It is this complex process which gives rise to the variety of developmental anomalies that can occur.

Tracheoesophageal fistula / esophageal atresia (TEF/EA)

TEF/EA is caused by failure of lateral septation of the embryonic foregut into esophagus and trachea with the fistula tract presumed to arise from a defect in the branching lung bud. TEF most commonly presents with esophageal atresia and distal fistula (Type C, 84%). Following this, isolated EA is next most common (Type A, 8%).

The presence or absence of EA determines the mode of presentation. EA in utero may manifest as polyhydramnios. However, in those cases not diagnosed prenatally, symptoms generally develop soon after birth. The infant will suffer from excessive secretions, and inability to feed. The presence of distal fistula (most common) will cause gastric distention from the respiratory tract, and reflux of gastric contents to the trachea leads to respiratory morbidity. It is important to be aware of associated anomalies found in up to 50% of infants. Two important associations are:

- *VATER association:* vertebral defects, anal atresia, TEF, radial and renal dysplasia

- *CHARGE association:* coloboma, heart defects, atresia of nasal choanae, retardation of growth/development, genital anomalies, ear anomalies

The first test for diagnosis is the inability to pass a NGT into the stomach, which can be demonstrated coiled in the proximal esophagus on a lateral CXR. Careful administration of a small amount of contrast can further help characterize the presence of fistula; however the risk exists in proximal fistulae of passage of contrast into the airway. CT with reconstruction and MRI are also useful imaging modalities.

Surgical management will be required to restore GI continuity following proper resuscitation and treatment of any pulmonary complications in addition to workup for associated abnormalities. The infant should be managed with a NGT in the semi-sitting position and treated with antibiotics as necessary prior to surgery. If ventilation is required, care must be taken to watch for abdominal distention in the setting of distal TEF.

The surgical approach is through a right thoracotomy with division of the azygos vein, localization of the fistula and ligation/division of the tract. The esophagus should ideally be reconstructed primarily unless there is a significant distance which cannot be bridged. In this event, elongation of the esophagus may be performed by myotomies, but a staged procedure is likely to be required with interposition of conduit (gastric or colon). In this case, as in the case of isolated esophageal atresia where the atretic segment is more likely to be long, a gastrostomy will be required at the first procedure. Complications include pneumonia, anastomotic leak, stricture formation, and gastroesophageal reflux.

Esophageal cysts / duplication

Esophageal cysts are the second most common benign esophageal lesion after leiomyoma. Yet their occurrence is rare and represents a spectrum of pathology, which includes true esophageal duplication cysts, bronchogenic cysts, and enteric cysts. They are frequently asymptomatic until progressive enlargement leads to symptoms of obstruction. They may also present with complications, including ulceration (many contain ectopic gastric mucosa), hemorrhage, and infection. It is generally accepted that even incidental discovery is an indication for surgical excision.

Esophageal duplication cysts occur in approximately 1/8000 live births. They are defined by their presence within the esophageal wall, covered by two muscle layers, and contain an embryonic lining similar to that of the esophagus. Most commonly, they do not communicate with the esophageal lumen and are demonstrated on barium swallow. They can be seen as an extrinsic mass on endoscopy or ultrasonography. They frequently lie to the right and posterior to the esophagus. As the differential is limited and the risk of infection and hemorrhage is high, these lesions should not be biopsied with EUS.

Surgical management of these lesions is similar to that for other benign esophageal tumors, with thoracic exposure of the esophagus, dissection between the muscular planes, and avoidance of mucosal injury. Postoperative care should include nasogastric drainage and follow-up contrast imaging to demonstrate mucosal integrity.

Esophageal stenosis / webs

Although more commonly found in adulthood, congenital esophageal stenosis and webs have been described usually affecting the distal esophagus. They can be described in three histologic groups: tracheobronchial rests (with cartilage and respiratory glands), membranous diaphragm, and fibromuscular stenosis. Workup should begin with endoscopy, biopsy and pH monitoring to exclude reflux as a cause of the stricture. Pneumatic dilation with fluoroscopy will also provide additional information as well as treatment. With the exception of cartilaginous rings, which will need to undergo resection, good outcomes are found with dilation of the membranous or fibromuscular types.

27. Esophageal reflux disease
Siva Raja, Aundrea L. Oliver

Gastroesophageal reflux disease (GERD) is a common clinical condition in the western world with a prevalence of 14-20%.[1] While its presence can be physiologic, it is considered a pathologic state if symptoms such as heartburn are persistent or lifestyle limiting, or if signs of mucosal damage occur. The definition remains vague due to the broad spectrum of presentation of GERD in patients.

Pathophysiology

The pathophysiology of GERD relates to the patients' inability to limit the exposure of esophageal mucosa to gastric refluxate. This can be due to inability of the esophagus to clear the refluxate due to altered esophageal motility or to the loss of reflux barriers. The latter is usually due to the anatomic changes caused by the presence of a hiatal hernia (or shortened esophagus), intrinsic LES hypotension, or increased intra-gastric pressure from obesity or delayed gastric emptying. While the normal esophageal protective mechanisms such as mucous secretion can guard against the harsh effects of gastric acid and enzymes, pathologic reflux overwhelms these mucosal barriers resulting in esophagitis, ulceration, peptic strictures and Barrett's esophagus (BE) (columnar metaplasia of the squamous epithelium). The presence of GERD increases the risk of BE. The histologic changes in BE represent a pre-malignant lesion that can undergo dysplasia and eventually progress to esophageal adenocarcinoma. The increased risk of cancer is 40 fold in patients with BE.[2]

Clinical presentation

The symptoms of GERD are often non-specific. The most common symptoms are heartburn, regurgitation, and to a lesser degree, dysphagia. Other less common symptoms include odynophagia, hypersalivation (waterbrash), asthma, laryngitis, persistent cough, globus sensation, noncardiac chest pain, and persistent nausea. While symptoms are common, a significant number of patients may also have symptom-free reflux but have evidence of mucosal injury on further incidental testing.

Diagnosis

As the prevalence of GERD is significantly greater than any other esophageal pathology, the initial diagnosis is based primarily on the history of symptoms. For patients who have typical symptoms of heartburn or regurgitation and have relief of symptoms with the use of proton pump inhibitors (PPI), the treatment is both diagnostic and therapeutic. When

PPI therapy fails to completely relieve symptoms, further testing is warranted. The first invasive diagnostic test should be an endoscopy with biopsy of any areas of esophagitis and Barrett's mucosa, or in the absence of visible lesions, random biopsies. This step is crucial in eliminating other conditions in the differential diagnosis such as eosinophilic esophagitis, esophageal cancer and complications of GERD such as peptic strictures. Endoscopy can also identify anatomic causes of GERD such as hiatal hernias. In the case of atypical chest pain, a cardiac source must always be ruled out.

Other tests that can be useful in the diagnosis are a high-resolution esophageal manometry to diagnose esophageal motility disorders and achalasia and a 24-hour pH monitoring study to confirm the presence of gastric acid in the esophagus. These last two tests and endoscopy should always be considered prior to embarking on any surgical anti-reflux procedure.

Patients with BE should have periodic endoscopic surveillance for dysplasia. Biopsies should be obtained in the four quadrants of the esophagus, every 2 cm for no dysplasia or low-grade dysplasia and every cm for high-grade dysplasia. The timeline for surveillance depends on the grade of dysplasia encountered. Patients with no dysplasia in two separate occasions are followed with endoscopy every 3-5 years. If low-grade dysplasia is found, a repeat endoscopy is performed to confirm it and repeat endoscopy is then performed annually. Patients with high-grade dysplasia should be offered surgical resection (esophagectomy) given the high likelihood of occult cancer although intensive surveillance every 3 months and local endoscopic therapy are alternative options.

Treatment

Medical therapy

The mainstay of GERD therapy is medical management. The use of histamine antagonists (H_2 blockers) and PPIs has shown significant improvement in GERD symptoms. However, many recent studies have shown PPIs to have better efficacy in resolving heartburn symptoms (77% vs. 48%)[3] as well as improved rates of healing esophagitis (83% vs. 52%).[4] All attempts to medically control GERD should also include counseling on diet and lifestyle modifications. Patients should be advised to avoid fatty foods and alcohol that can decrease LES tone, as well as acidic/irritating foods such as citrus fruits and carbonated beverages. Lifestyle modifications such as smoking cessation, weight reduction to a BMI of 20-25, and avoidance of meals within 3 hours before bedtime should also be encouraged.

Surgical therapy

Surgical therapy should only be considered when two specific conditions have been satisfied. First, the patients should have failed medical therapy either due to the persistence of symptoms or due to the continued documented presence of mucosal injury. Second, the preoperative studies have to demonstrate a loss of barrier function that may subsequently respond to surgical restoration. The goals of surgery, be it via laparoscopic or open surgery, are to ensure the intra-abdominal location of the gastroesophageal junction (GEJ), reconstruct the extrinsic sphincter (i.e. reduce the esophageal hiatus to a normal physiologic size in the setting of a hiatal hernia), and reinforce the intrinsic LES with fundoplication.[5]

BE itself is not an indication for surgery. Patients with BE tend to have acid reflux or biliary regurgitation that is difficult to control with medical therapy. As with other patients, surgical therapy in patients with BE is aimed at controlling reflux that has failed medical therapy.

In the setting of long-standing reflux disease, the esophagus is often shortened due to scarring. As such, the GEJ is often translocated into the thorax and exposed to negative pressure rather than the physiologic intra-abdominal positive pressure. This can be corrected by mobilizing the esophagus around the hiatus up to the inferior pulmonary veins. If this maneuver does not deliver the GEJ into the abdomen, then a Collis gastroplasty should be performed. In this procedure, a 3-6 cm selectively vagotomized proximal stomach is tubularized to create a neo-esophagus. Upon restoring the GEJ into the abdomen, the crura should be approximated with deep non-absorbable sutures without causing obstruction. Lastly, a fundoplication is added to complete the repair. This is most commonly seen in the form of either a Nissen fundoplication (360 degree posterior wrap) or a Toupet fundoplication (270 degree posterior partial wrap).

It is important that at least 2.5-3.0 cm of esophagus remain in the abdomen without tension, the fundus is completely mobilized with division of the short gastric vessels in order to reduce tension, the vagi nerves are preserved, any diaphragmatic crural defects are closed, and a floppy fundoplication is performed.

The overall success of surgical therapy in resolving GERD symptoms is about 80-90%.[5] This is particularly seen in studies evaluating heartburn and regurgitation. However, when looking at rates of healing for esophagitis, the surgery and medical therapy are likely equivalent. As such, the use of surgery in patients who have incomplete response to medical therapy is likely to have the best yield.

Surgery for GERD can result in persistent bloating, inability to belch, severe dysphagia (from the fundoplication), and need for re-operation. There is no definitive evidence to show that surgical treatment of GERD reduces or reverses BE. Thus, the management of GERD should primarily involve medical management with selective use of surgical therapy.

28. Esophageal motility disorders

Daniela Molena

The esophagus is a muscular tube that actively propels the food bolus from the pharynx to the stomach. Esophageal motility disorders impair the motor function of the esophagus resulting in abnormal esophageal transportation. It is important to differentiate between primary and secondary motility disorders since many systemic diseases can affect the normal esophageal peristalsis. One of the most common causes of esophageal dysmotility is gastroesophageal reflux disease, which should therefore be ruled out before the correct diagnosis of altered motor function, since the treatment would be completely different. Other diseases that might affect the normal esophageal motility are connective tissue disorders, DM, dermatomyositis, amyloidosis, chronic idiopathic intestinal pseudo-obstruction, alcoholism, and Chagas' disease. Some authors think that the only "true" motility disorder is achalasia and there is some controversy regarding the clinical significance of some manometric abnormalities especially after the introduction of high-resolution manometry.

Achalasia

Epidemiology and pathophysiology

Esophageal achalasia is a primary motility disorder characterized by aperistalsis of the distal esophagus and the failure of the LES to completely relax with swallowing. However, early achalasia findings may consist of disordered peristalsis in the presence of normal LES function. It is a rare disorder affecting 1 in 100,000 patients per year with a similar male to female ratio and onset at any age. The motor abnormality is the result of inhibitory activity loss due to the degeneration of the ganglion cells in the myoenteric plexus. The destruction of the inhibitory neurons, which contain nitric oxide and vasoactive intestinal peptide, seems to be the result of an inflammatory process. Indirect evidence suggests that the initiating agent may be viral and the inflammatory process autoimmune in its origin. Elevated antibody titers for neurotropic viruses like the herpes class, predominant T-lymphocyte inflammatory infiltrates, as well as autoantibodies to myoenteric plexus neurons, have been described in patients with achalasia. The loss of propulsion of the esophageal body and the lack of relaxation of the LES cause stasis of the food bolus in the esophagus until enough intraesophageal pressure is generated to allow the transit into the stomach. This process over time will lead to esophageal dilation.

Clinical presentation

The primary symptom of achalasia is dysphagia. Dysphagia is usually progressive to both liquids and solids and can be exacerbated by emotional stress and fast eating. Patients, with time, learn to adapt their dietary habits and maintain reasonable nutritional requirements. Regurgitation of undigested food and saliva and aspiration pneumonia are more common in the advanced phase of achalasia when the esophagus is dilated. Chest pain and indigestion are common symptoms and can mislead to the wrong diagnosis of gastroesophageal reflux disease.

Diagnosis

Barium swallow is helpful for diagnosis by showing the classic "bird's beak" narrowing of the esophagogastric junction and air-fluid level in the distal esophagus, but also for staging the severity based on the degree of esophageal body dilation. Endoscopy can be normal or might show a closed gastroesophageal junction that will open with the passage of the scope. In advanced phases, the esophagus will appear dilated with retained food and saliva. Endoscopy is particularly important when pseudoachalasia is suspected due to esophageal, gastric or pancreatic cancer involving the distal esophagus or the esophageal diaphragmatic hiatus.

Esophageal manometry is the gold standard for diagnosis of achalasia. Aperistalsis and failure of the LES to completely relax to swallow are diagnostic findings of achalasia. The LES is classically defined as hypertensive, but normal or hypotonic sphincters are frequently found in early-stage achalasia. The resting pressure within the esophagus is usually elevated and non-peristaltic, simultaneous contractions are seen in response to swallow. When the esophagus is very dilated, only very low amplitude simultaneous pressure waves are recorded. Rarely, the simultaneous contractions can have high amplitude and duration defining a condition called vigorous achalasia, which is believed to be a characteristic of an early stage disease more than a specific pathological condition. With the recent development of high-resolution manometry and high-resolution esophageal topography plots, a better understanding of esophageal physiology in achalasia will soon be available future. In fact, a subcategorization of achalasia based on esophageal pressurization patterns has already been proposed.

Treatment

Medical therapy with drugs that decrease the LES pressure (anticholinergics, nitrates, calcium channel blockers, β-blockers and phosphodiesterase inhibitors) has been disappointing due to high side effects and low efficacy. Endoscopic balloon dilation was considered the first line of treatment before the laparoscopic era. In experienced hands, dilation has a success rate of 50-70% and up to 90% with multiple sessions. The risk of perforation is about 2-5% per dilation and it is less effective in young patients. In a prospective, randomized trial of balloon dilation versus surgical myotomy, near complete relief of symptoms was obtained in 51% with dilation and 95% with surgery at a follow-up of 5 years. Intrasphincteric injection of botulinum toxin has been reported to have 60-70% success rate but it is usually short lived, repeated injections are required, and treatment can lead to reflux.

Laparoscopic myotomy of the distal esophagus (Heller myotomy) associated with a partial fundoplication (typically a Dor or Toupet) is now considered the standard of care for treatment of achalasia. The myotomy should be extended onto the stomach for at least 1.5 cm and should be attempted even in advanced stages when the esophagus is dilated and tortuous. A recent prospective, randomized study showed that the incidence of postoperative gastroesophageal reflux disease is significantly higher when a myotomy is done without adding a fundoplication. Rarely, esophagectomy and reconstruction with gastric pull-up or colonic interposition is necessary for end-stage achalasia or failure of previous treatments. Although, the most frequent reason for performing an esophagectomy in achalasia remains iatrogenic perforation. Patients with achalasia are at risk of developing esophageal cancer and endoscopic surveillance should be offered even after resolution of symptoms.

Diffuse esophageal spasm

Epidemiology and pathophysiology

Diffuse esophageal spasm (DES) is a very rare motility disorder characterized by non-peristaltic, simultaneous contractions of the distal esophagus, which occur either spontaneously or in response to swallow. Little is known about the pathophysiology of DES, which is thought to be caused by the dysfunction of inhibitory nerves like in achalasia. Many authors believe that DES represents an early stage of a myoenteric plexus denervation disease and it is reported that about 3-5% of cases will evolve into achalasia.

Clinical presentation

The classical symptoms of DES are chest pain and dysphagia. Chest pain can occur at rest or after swallow and is usually associated with high amplitude and long duration contractions. Dysphagia to both solids and liquids is intermittent and non-progressive.

Diagnosis

Radiographic findings in a barium swallow vary from a completely normal appearance to altered progression of the bolus due to uncoordinated simultaneous contractions that give the esophagus the shape of a "corkscrew". An esophageal pulsion diverticulum can be present as well. Upper endoscopy is usually normal. The diagnosis is obtained with manometric evidence of more than 20% simultaneous contractions (with amplitude greater than 30 mmHg) in response to a wet swallow. Typically, the LES is thought to be spared in DES. Recent reports on high-resolution manometry and high-resolution esophageal topography plots suggest that DES diagnosed with conventional manometry is most often a variant of esophageal achalasia.

Treatment

The treatment of DES has been overall disappointing. Pharmacologic treatment with calcium channel blockers, nitrates or phosphodiesterase inhibitors may relieve dysphagia and low dose tricyclic antidepressants seem to be a better option in cases of chest pain. Botulinum toxin injection or balloon dilation have been used to relieve dysphagia with poor results. Surgical treatment has involved long myotomy of the esophagus with contradictory results. Different techniques have been described with access either through the chest or the abdomen and an open or minimally invasive approach. An antireflux procedure is usually added to decrease the postoperative incidence of gastroesophageal reflux. Better results are usually obtained for dysphagia relief rather than chest pain.

Nutcracker esophagus

Epidemiology and pathophysiology

A subgroup of patients evaluated with manometry for non-cardiac chest pain was identified as having high contraction amplitudes and were called "super squeezer" by Pope in 1977. Manometric characteristics of nutcracker esophagus have been described in about 27-48% of patients with non-cardiac chest pain, are more common in females and are associated with psychiatric disorders. However, the concept of nutcracker esophagus has been evolving over the last 20 years and controversy exists today regarding its clinical significance. The pathophysiology of this manometric abnormality remains unclear and it has been suggested that it might be due to an imbalance between excitatory and inhibitory innervation or an impaired inhibitory component. Recently it has been shown that the baseline esophageal muscular thickness, evaluated with EUS, correlates with peak contraction amplitudes and it has been suggested that the increase in muscle thickness might be the reason for high-amplitude peristalsis.

Clinical presentation

Chest pain is the most common symptom, but dysphagia can be reported as well. Depression and anxiety are frequently associated complaints. It has been shown in several studies that the correlation between episodes of chest pain and high amplitude contractions is weak, therefore some authors believe that the hypertensive contractions are a marker for a hypersensitive esophagus rather than the cause of pain.

Diagnosis

The diagnosis of nutcracker esophagus is done with manometry. Radiographic and endoscopic studies are usually normal. The manometric feature that defines this motility disorder is the presence of high amplitude contractions (mean >180 mmHg) in the distal esophagus. Prolonged contractions of more than 6 seconds are common but are not required for diagnosis. The peristaltic waves are normally propagated and are often repetitive and persistent.

Treatment

The management of nutcracker esophagus is very similar to diffuse esophageal spasm. Medical therapy is the mainstay and consists of anticholinergic and smooth muscle relaxing agents. A randomized double-blind study showed significant improvement of dysphagia with diltiazem when compared to placebo. Antidepressants have been shown to be effective as well, likely by modifying visceral sensory perception. Botulinum toxin, esophageal dilation, and surgery have been used in selected cases.

Hypertensive lower esophageal sphincter

Isolated hypertensive LES is an esophageal motility disorder characterized by a resting LES pressure greater than 45 mmHg (or >95th percentile of normal subjects). Some patients also have incomplete relaxation of the LES and elevated intrabolus pressure suggesting outflow obstruction. Up to 50% of patients have peristaltic waves characteristic of nutcracker esophagus. Dysphagia and chest pain are the most common symptoms. Indigestion is also a common complaint. Abnormal esophageal acid exposure and large paraesophageal hernias have been shown to be often associated with a hypertensive LES. Radiographic and endoscopic assessments of these patients are therefore important in order to identify anatomic abnormalities or complications from gastroesophageal reflux disease. A 24-hour pH-monitoring test will identify those patients with pathological esophageal acid exposure. The treatment for isolated hypertensive LES has been controversial and has been focused on reducing the LES pressure by medical and surgical means. Good results with distal esophageal myotomy and partial fundoplication have been reported for relief of dysphagia.

Scleroderma

Scleroderma results in smooth muscle atrophy and subsequent replacement with scar. This leads peristaltic dysfunction and the weakening of the LES. Notably, normal peristalsis is maintained in the upper third of the esophagus, which is lined by striated muscle.

29. Esophageal injury
Daniel C. Wiener

Esophageal injury can be simplified by considering the following key issues:

- Characteristics of the injury

    - Etiology (e.g., caustic, penetrating trauma, foreign body, iatrogenic)

    - Location / relevant anatomy (e.g., cervical, upper-, mid-, lower thoracic, intraabdominal)

    - Severity (e.g., stricture, foreign body, partial thickness tear, perforation, frank contamination with mediastinitis, peritonitis)

    - Timing of injury relative to presentation

- Characteristics of the patient (e.g., age, comorbidities, immune status)

- Characteristics of the pre-existing esophagus (e.g., tumor, achalasia, distal obstruction)

Controversies in management exist and the key to making the right decision comes down to doing what is safest.

Strictures

Strictures can be divided in benign and malignant. Benign strictures can be subdivided into congenital and acquired. Acquired strictures have multiple causes: peptic (Schatzki's rings), pill-induced, autoimmune (eosinophilic esophagitis, Crohn's, scleroderma), iatrogenic (anastomotic, RT induced), and infectious (fungal, bacterial, mycobacterial). Patients present with progressive, persistent dysphagia that is refractory to medical treatment once the esophageal lumen is narrowed by ~ 50%. Evaluation includes esophagogram and EGD. Most can be treated with dilation, which may need to be repeated. Long segment strictures or near total obstruction may require dilation under fluoroscopy with a guide wire. Strictures not responsive to dilation may ultimately require resection and reconstruction.

Corrosive injuries

Ingestion of corrosives can be accidental or intentional. It is a potentially fatal injury that needs immediate attention. *Alkalis* (e.g., lye), often viscous, have a long exposure, deep tissue penetration, and result in liquefactive necrosis. *Acids* are typically less viscous with a rapid transit time and result in a more superficial coagulative necrosis.

Phases of corrosive injury and healing are:

1. Inflammation / necrosis

2. Sloughing / ulceration

3. Fibrosis / scarring

Patients present with dysphagia, odynophagia, chest/abdominal pain, and may be in septic shock depending upon the severity of the injury. IVF resuscitation and empiric broad-spectrum antibiotics are initiated. Plain films of the chest and abdomen can help determine frank perforation. The oropharynx and airway need evaluation with laryngoscopy and intubation is indicated if there are signs of airway involvement. Early endoscopy is important to assess upper GI involvement. Blind NGT placement is contraindicated.

There should be no attempts to "neutralize" the corrosive agent. Injury is graded similar to burns. Third degree injuries with full thickness involvement, perforation, mediastinitis, or peritonitis require emergent resection and delayed reconstruction. More commonly, patients develop late complications with long segment strictures that may not respond to dilations. Resection and reconstruction are indicated. The stomach can be used if not involved in the initial injury.

Perforation

Clinical presentation

There are a number of ways to perforate the esophagus and hence a number of ways that patients can present. Iatrogenic injuries from endoscopy or dilatation are the most common. The most common site of perforation during endoscopy on a patient with a hiatal hernia is the gastroesophageal junction or the gastric cardia. The next most common cause of perforation is "spontaneous" (Boerhaave's syndrome, usually after a bout of vomiting) followed by penetrating trauma (cervical > thoracic). With an esophageal injury, patients may have crepitus though airway injury is higher on the differential. Esophageal perforation from a penetrating injury to the chest is rare and almost always associated with other injuries.

Evaluation

CXR is often the first modality used and may show an effusion, a pneumothorax, or pneumomediastinum though sensitivity is quite low (~10-20%). An esophagogram with water soluble contrast should be obtained. If negative, the study should be repeated using thin barium. Esophagogram has a sensitivity of ~ 80%. CT scan with oral contrast right before scanning is useful in evaluating surrounding structures both in terms of additional injuries in the case of penetrating trauma and to assess for pleural effusions, mediastinal or peritoneal fat stranding. In some institutions, CT is used instead of the initial esophagogram. Endoscopy is particularly useful in cases of foreign-body perforation or penetrating trauma and in equivocal cases.

Management

Management depends upon the cause of injury, timing, the patient's overall condition, comorbidities, and any underlying esophageal pathology. Non-operative management is appropriate if the patient is clinically stable, the injury is recent, there is no evidence of extraluminal contrast, and no distal obstruction. Treatment consists of empiric broad spectrum antibiotics, NPO, and IV hydration. Operative management is warranted in the presence of extraluminal contrast, mediastinal or peritoneal contamination, and sepsis.

Cervical perforation can often be treated with debridement and drainage via an oblique incision anterior to the sternocleidomastoid on the side where contrast was seen on the studies. Intrathoracic injury is more complex. Upper and middle third injuries are approached via right thoracotomy while lower third injuries are approached through the left. Primary repair can be attempted in the setting of early diagnosis, limited contamination, and treatable underlying pathology. Adequate assessment of the perforation requires extension of the myotomy to visualize the extent of mucosal damage and assure adequate closure. Primary closure can be accomplished in one or two layers with absorbable suture. The repair should be buttressed with a pedicled intercostal muscle, pleura, pericardium, or omentum. In some situations, closure over a T-tube may allow for the development of a controlled esophageal fistula that will close over time as the tube is withdrawn in the setting of improved physiology. In cases of perforation resulting from dilatation for achalasia, an esophagomyotomy should be performed 180 degrees opposite to the perforation site, in addition to closure of the perforation defect. Debridement and wide drainage are crucial. In the setting of delayed diagnosis, unrepairable tissue, or poor patient physiology, repair must be delayed. Initial intervention is geared towards debridement, drainage, and controlling further contamination (proximal and distal diversion). Esophageal stents can be used to exclude the perforation and minimize contamination of the mediastinum in poor-risk patients.

Foreign bodies

The ingestion of foreign bodies is a misnomer. Obviously, everything we ingest is foreign. It is the ingestion of non-food items or poorly-chewed food items that can become problematic. More appropriately, this section ought to be labeled esophageal impaction. Most commonly, ingestion of non-food items occurs accidentally in children, elderly, or in the psychiatric patient population. Impaction of food can occur at any age and typically results from inadequate mastication, occasionally in the setting of poor esophageal motility.

Management strategies depend upon the type of object, its location, size, sharpness, and orientation. Evaluation generally starts with a CXR. Occasionally, a swallow study is performed to define the anatomy though often times it is reasonable to proceed with upper endoscopy. Typically, foreign bodies can be removed with flexible endoscopy and an assortment of instruments ranging from grasping forceps to an expandable net, basket, or snare. Some advocate using a Foley catheter much like a Fogarty balloon is used for thrombus removal. Sharp objects obviously cannot be removed in this manner. If the sharp end is pointed distally, flexible endoscopy is a reasonable technique. If the object's orientation is such that removal is likely to cause an esophageal laceration, rigid esophagoscopy can be used. The esophagus is protected by bringing the object into the scope and removing the scope and ingested material as a unit. Depending upon the size and shape, certain objects can be advanced into the stomach and allowed to pass distally.

30. Esophageal diverticula

Jeremiah T. Martin

Nomenclature

An esophageal diverticulum is an abnormal outpouching of the esophageal wall. True diverticula contain all the layers of the esophageal wall whereas false diverticula consist of an outpouching of mucosa and submucosa between splayed muscular fibers. Most esophageal diverticula fall into the latter category.

Classically, esophageal diverticula are also subdivided into "pulsion" and "traction" diverticula. *Pulsion diverticula,* such as Zenker's and epiphrenic, result from an increased pressure gradient across a muscular sphincter and are associated with motility disorders. They occur as the esophageal mucosa is essentially forced through the muscular layers. *Traction diverticula* result from an inflammatory process outside the esophageal wall, which draws all layers of the esophagus into a true diverticulum. This is most commonly seen in the mid-thoracic esophagus due to chronic lymphadenitis. While not usually linked to an esophageal motility disorder, traction diverticula have been associated with fistulas.

Pathophysiology

Zenker's diverticulum is the most common and occurs above the cricopharyngeus muscle. It is typically a lateral projection near the C6 or C7 vertebral body. Hypertonicity of the cricopharyngeus and upper esophageal sphincter can be demonstrated in these patients. Lower esophageal motility and LES dysfunction remains normal.

Epiphrenic diverticula are usually associated with an esophageal motility disorder and are usually within 4 cm of the gastroesophageal junction.

Mid-thoracic diverticula are usually within 4 or 5cm of the carina and are often associated with a chronic inflammatory process in the posterior mediastinum.

Clinical presentation

Patients with esophageal diverticula will present initially with dysphagia, which is initially minor. As the diverticulum enlarges, dysphagia will progress, with the diverticulum itself acting as an extrinsic source of compression on the true lumen of the esophagus. As ingested material accumulates within the diverticulum, patients will also complain of fetor, and regurgitation of food. Zenker's may also present as a neck mass. As with all proximal diverticula, the risk of aspiration is high.

Diagnosis

After yielding a classic history, the diagnosis is best made with barium esophagogram. In addition to demonstrating the diverticulum and mass compression, fluoroscopy may demonstrate an underlying motility disorder, which contributes to the problem. Endoscopy can be helpful in characterizing the extent of the diverticulum, whether or not it has a wide opening, and in particular address any concerns for mucosal abnormalities and rule out concurrent malignancy. Workup should include manometry in the setting of distal/epiphrenic diverticula due to the high association with motility disorders, which might have implications for surgical management.

Treatment

Surgical management depends on the location of the diverticulum:

- *Zenker's diverticulum.* As the underlying problem is the cricopharyngeus, any surgical management of Zenker's must include a cricopharyngomyotomy to decrease the resting pressure of the muscle. The classic approach includes an open exploration of the lateral esophagus at "Killian's triangle", resection of the diverticulum, and performance of a myotomy. As an alternative to resection, suspension of the diverticulum such that it opens dependently into the esophagus has also been described and is effective. More recently, the diverticulum may be approached via a transoral route and passage of a stapler. This serves the dual function of opening the diverticulum widely and dividing the cricopharyngeus.

- *Mid-thoracic diverticulum.* These are best approached through the right chest, which gives excellent exposure of the esophagus at the level of the carina. The diverticulum may be stapled at its base, with performance of a myotomy on the contralateral esophageal wall if a motility disorder is suspected.

- *Epiphrenic diverticulum.* Similarly to a mid-thoracic diverticulum, the esophagus is exposed and the diverticulum is stapled or resected and the mucosa oversewn. The muscular layers should be re-approximated at this level, and a myotomy performed remote from this repair given the high association with motility disorders.

31. Paraesophageal hernias

Shamus R. Carr

Types of hiatal hernia

Hiatal hernias are classified into four distinct types. *Type I*, the most common, account for nearly 95% of all hiatal hernias. These are commonly referred to as sliding hiatal hernias and are characterized by an enlargement of the esophageal hiatus and lengthening of the phreno-esophageal ligament. This combination allows the normal intraabdominal location of the gastroesophageal junction to become intrathoracic.

The other three types of hiatal hernias are broadly classified as paraesophageal (PEH). Compared to a type I hernia, which has no hernia sac, all paraesophageal hernias have a circumferential covering of a layer of peritoneum that forms a true hernia sac. A *type II* PEH is the least common. These hernias are characterized by preservation of the gastroesophageal junction at its normal and expected anatomic position within in the abdomen, but with an enlargement in the esophageal hiatus. The fundus of the stomach tends to be in the thoracic cavity. When there is a combined picture involving both displacement of the gastroesophageal junction with at least 30% of the stomach also being above the diaphragm, this is classified as a *type III* PEH. When there is herniation of other organs into the thoracic cavity along with the stomach, this is termed a *type IV*.

Epidemiology

In the largest series on PEH, 75% of patients are females. About half of all patients are over the age of 70. The proposed reason for this is that there is loss of elasticity and muscle weakening as people age. Additionally, other etiologies that cause increases in intraabdominal pressures are also implicated: obesity, constipation, and abdominal ascites.

History and physical exam

Reflux and dysphagia symptoms occur about 40-70% of the time, but multiple other symptoms are also commonly experienced: regurgitation, dyspnea, or chest/abdominal pain. Additionally, about 40% of patients with a PEH have a chronic anemia that may be the result of either mucosal venous engorgement or a Cameron's ulcer (a peptic ulcer within a hiatal hernia).

If a patient presents with an acute onset of severe abdominal pain with vomiting, one needs to keep in mind the possibility of gastric volvulus, especially in patients with a known PEH. Urgency is of the essence as timely diagnosis and emergent operative intervention can mean the difference between reduction of the hernia and repair versus subtotal gastrectomy.

Evaluation

The first study should be an upper GI series with contrast. This will clearly define the position of the stomach in relationship to the diaphragm and how much stomach is herniated through the hiatus into the chest, and can demonstrate organoaxial rotation of the stomach. Endoscopy is invaluable when there is concern for incarceration or strangulation as it allows direct examination of the gastric mucosa. In the more elective setting, the value lies in confirming that there is not some unexpected pathology such as stricture or malignancy. Some authors advocate using esophageal manometry and pH probe testing as part of the evaluation but their utility for PEH is limited. Pulmonary function testing, if obtained, can be expected to improve by about 15% once the PEH is repaired and the abdominal contents are no longer in the thoracic cavity. For patients that have previously undergone surgical repair of PEH, it is important to know if the vagus nerves have been injured, and gastric emptying studies should be obtained.

Surgical treatment

Surgery for PEH is reconstructive in nature with a two-fold goal: restore normal anatomy by returning the gastroesophageal junction once again into the abdomen and correct the condition that contributed to the development of the anatomic problem, in this case gastroesophageal reflux disease. The sac should be removed, the hiatus closed, and some type of antireflux reconstruction performed. Operative options include transthoracic, transabdominal, and laparoscopic techniques.

Operative outcomes of the various open techniques are all similar. The length of stay (4-5 days) and postoperative complication rate (20-25%) are similar between transthoracic and transabdominal approaches. The reported range of CXR recurrence is 2% to 18% with 86% to 94% of patients reporting good to excellent outcomes. The original papers utilizing the laparoscopic approach had recurrence rates as high as 40% with mortality rates of 5%. However, recent publications demonstrate outcomes that rival open techniques (15% recurrence) and shorter length of stay.

An esophageal lengthening procedure such as a Collis gastroplasty should be used when one is unable to obtain at least 2-2.5 cm of tension-free intra-abdominal esophagus. Some authors advocate the routine use of gastroplasty in all cases. The use of mesh to reinforce the hiatal hernia repair is controversial.

Emergency surgery for paraesophageal hernias

In patients that undergo non-elective surgery, the risk of any complication is at least double compared to elective surgery. In these patients, flexible endoscopy is the first step to evaluate the mucosa of the esophagus, stomach, and duodenum. In some situations, it will allow decompression of the stomach and placement of a NGT, which may allow the patient to be resuscitated and further stabilized, which may increase the likelihood of a primary repair the following day. However, any signs of ischemia mandate proceeding with operative intervention. If the stomach is not grossly ischemic and can be reduced, the option of gastropexy versus primary repair can be considered based on how well the patient is doing clinically during the operation. Any hemodynamic lability, poor urine output, use of inotropes, changes to the EKG, or a persistently elevated lactate mandate reducing the hernia and performing a gastropexy with the addition of a feeding tube, as long as the stomach is viable.

In cases where there are gross ischemic changes, an immediate subtotal gastrectomy needs to be performed expeditiously. In these cases, there is normally a small portion of the antrum that is healthy for placement of a gastric tube. The esophagus is left stapled off with a NGT in the blind pouch. The patient can then be brought to the ICU for resuscitation and a staged procedure with a mandatory "second look" in a day or two, once the patient is stable. This repair can be either an esophagojejunostomy with a Roux-en-Y reconstruction or, if enough stomach remained viable to perform a tension-free anastomosis, an esophagogastrostomy. Either way, durable enteral feeding access should be obtained prior to completion of the operation.

Complications

The two most dreaded complications are almost entirely due to technical errors: recurrence and gastroparesis. If the patient does not have at least 2.5 cm of tension-free intraabdominal esophagus, recurrence is almost assured without an esophageal lengthening procedure. Mobilization of the fat pad also allows evaluation of the vagus nerves. Any injury to them will cause gastric dysfunction, early satiety, and bloating.

When dissecting around the hiatus, attention needs to be paid to the peritoneal lining over the crux. Disruption of this lining will result in poor crural approximation and eventual failure.

If a Collis is performed, there is the possibility of a leak from the staple line. Therefore, leaving a drain may be prudent when a Collis is performed.

Occasionally, the fundoplication is too tight causing dysphagia. Most of the time, this is related to post-operative swelling of the tissue and resolves in a few weeks. If this does not resolve by the first post-operative visit, dilation should be performed.

If a patient complains of recurrent heartburn, dysphagia, or regurgitation the first step should be an upper GI study to assess whether the repair has failed and there is a recurrence. If a patient has a recurrence or a slipped wrap, medical therapy will be futile and the patient should undergo a reoperation. A reoperation should likely require performing an esophageal lengthening procedure.

In cases where the primary symptom is bloating, a radionuclide gastric emptying study will help to provide critical data. If, the upper GI and gastric emptying studies are both normal despite continued complaints of symptoms, endoscopy should be performed. Since nearly all patients with PEH have a previously long-standing history of reflux, they are at risk for esophageal cancer. Thus, endoscopy can visually confirm an intact wrap and a properly appearing recreated esophageal flap valve. It also rules out intraluminal lesions and may identify other causes for the symptoms such as gastric or duodenal ulcers.

32. Tracheal stenosis and postintubation injury
Samuel J. Youssef

The adult trachea measures 11 cm in length from cricoid to carina. There are 18-22 tracheal rings. The only complete ring is the cricoid cartilage of the larynx; the remainder are C-shaped with membranous trachea posteriorly. The blood supply enters the submucosa of the trachea laterally: the upper trachea by branches of the inferior thyroid artery, the lower by branches of the bronchials. Non-neoplastic diseases of the trachea may result in tracheal stenosis and airway obstruction:

- *Congenital tracheal stenosis* most often presents as a web-like diaphragm at the subcricoid level. There also may be a generalized hypoplasia, a funnel-like narrowing, or segmental stenosis due to complete circular cartilaginous rings that are associated with bronchial anomalies such as a RUL bronchus origin from above the stenosed segment.

- *Infectious lesions* such as TB involve the lower trachea and/or main bronchi. There is a lengthy circumferential submucosal fibrosis with narrowing of the distal trachea. Acute ulcerative TB tracheitis should be treated pharmacologically before intervention. Repeated dilatation is the preferred method for treating inflammatory strictures. Histoplasmosis may cause mediastinal fibrosis with enlarged lymph nodes resulting in compression, invasion, or erosion into the right main stem bronchus or carina.

- *Extrinsic compression* may be seen with large goiters, vascular rings, aneurysms of the innominate artery, anomalous subclavian artery, or mediastinal masses. Postpneumonectomy syndrome occurs after a right pneumonectomy where the mediastinum moves to the right and posterior, leading to angulation and compression of the tracheobronchial tree with obstruction at the carina or proximal left main bronchus.

- *COPD* patients may present with "saber-sheath" trachea where the side-to-side diameter of the trachea diminishes progressively and the antero-posterior diameter increases. The posterior part of the cartilages approximate with attempts to cough and the patient cannot clear secretions. Surgical interventions are not indicated. Tracheomalacia may occur also in COPD patients with the tracheal rings taking the shape of an archer's bow where the posterior membranous trachea elongates, becomes redundant, and approaches the anterior flattened cartilage, causing near total obstruction. Surgical intervention with tracheoplasty and Marlex mesh restores rigidity to the tracheal cartilage and plicates the redundant posterior membrane.

- *Postintubation injuries* include granulomas and strictures, cuff stenosis, tracheomalacia, and tracheoinnominate and tracheoesophageal fistulas. Tracheal granulomas and strictures result from proliferative and cicatricial response to tracheal injury. This occurs when the tracheostomy stoma is made too large either by turning a large flap, excising a large window, placing excessive leverage on the tracheostomy tube, or with infection and stoma erosion. The edges of the anterior or lateral tissue defect then approximate during healing, resulting in an A-shaped stricture. Cuff stenosis, most commonly, is attributed to pressure necrosis by the cuff resulting in a circumferential, transmural erosion of all layers of the trachea. The inflated cuff deforms the trachea, destroys the mucosa, compromises the submucosal blood supply, and the cartilage necroses and sloughs off. The endotracheal tube initially stents the airway open. Upon removal of the tube, the transmural weakness in the trachea undergoes cicatricial healing resulting in a tight circumferential stenosis manifesting 3-6 weeks post-tube removal. Tracheomalacia may occur in the tracheal segment between the stoma and the cuff. The mucosa reveals a squamous metaplasia and the cartilage is thinned, but not destroyed. Bacterial infection during the time of ventilatory support contributes to this process.

Presentation

Patients with tracheal stenosis and malacia develop symptoms and signs of airway obstruction consisting of dyspnea on exertion, stridor, cough, and obstructive episodes. A patient with a history of recent intubation or ventilation must be considered to have a postintubation tracheal stenosis rather than adult-onset asthma. Physical exam will demonstrate tachypnea and use of accessory muscles of breathing. An abnormal voice or stridor is suggestive of glottic or subglottic stenosis.

Tracheoinnominate fistula is caused by angulation of a tube tip or erosion of a high pressure cuff directly through the trachea. Rarely, it is seen in young adults with a low placed tracheostomy that is in immediate proximity with the innominate artery. The inner curve erodes through the arterial wall. Presentation is with a premonitory bleed that must be distinguished from granulation bleeding/irritation. When bleeding occurs, bronchoscopy is performed with temporary removal of the tube. Exsanguinating bleeding may be controlled by overinflating the tracheostomy cuff. If unsuccessful, digital pressure is applied through the tracheostomy site to tamponade the innominate artery against the sternum. The patient is reintubated orally. Once bleeding has been controlled, the mainstay for surgical treatment, and that with the least morbidity and mortality, involves proximal debridement of the artery to obtain healthy tissue followed by vessel ligation.

Tracheoesophageal fistula occurs most commonly in patients who have a ventilating cuff in the trachea as well as a feeding tube in the esophagus. The two foreign bodies compress the common wall leading to inflammation and perforation. Often there is circumferential cuff injury. Presentation will be with increased tracheal secretions. Gastric distension may appear if the patient is ventilated. Management includes placing a new, longer tracheostomy tube with the balloon below the fistula and placing a draining gastrostomy tube as well a feeding jejunostomy tube. Once the patient is weaned from ventilation, single stage repair involves deciding whether the fistula can be simply resected or whether tracheal resection and reconstruction will be required. Typical repair involves tracheal resection, closure of the esophagus and insertion of a muscle flap between the two.

Diagnosis

Tracheal lesions are often recognized late. Radiographic studies include lateral films of the neck with chin raised, inspiratory and expiratory CT scans to evaluate for tracheomalacia, MRI for soft tissue evaluation, and virtual bronchoscopy with 3-D reconstructions from CT. Bronchoscopy may precipitate complete obstruction, and should be done with preparations for definitive treatment of the lesions.

Management

Temporizing maneuvers may be necessary for critical situations. Steroids and racemic epinephrine can minimize airway inflammation, edema, and bronchospasm. Heliox can reduce the work of breathing. Accurate assessment of the tracheal lesion is performed in the operating room with rigid bronchoscopy. Anesthesia is by inhalation technique without muscle relaxants. The airway is controlled by direct intubation and serial dilation is performed. This allows for proper assessment of the distal airway and placement of an endotracheal tube. Stents are not used as they may cause severe granulations and stenosis.

Tracheal resection and reconstruction is the preferred treatment for benign obstruction. Reasons to delay definitive surgery include acute airway inflammation, pneumonia, and high dose steroids (>10 mg prednisone/day). Accurate preoperative assessment of location and length of the stenosis allows for planning. Precision and meticulous technique with preservation of lateral blood supply and avoidance of recurrent laryngeal nerve are fundamental. A low-collar incision is used. Intraoperative bronchoscopy can identify the strictured segment. Anterior dissection is performed to identify the strictured segment and to preserve blood supply. Circumferential dissection is limited to 1-1.5 cm in length at the stricture. Traction sutures are placed at the distal trachea, it is transected and then intubated. Cervical flexion will allow for assessment of tension. The proximal trachea is lifted and separated from the esophagus, then resected. An end-to-end tension free anastomosis is performed. Strap muscles are placed over the suture line.

33. Tracheal tumors

Bryan A. Whitson, Shawn S. Groth

Epidemiology

Most tracheal tumors are malignant. Primary tracheal tumors are more common than metastatic tumors. The most common primary tumors are squamous cell carcinomas and adenoid cystic carcinomas. These histologies are more common in men and in smokers. Adenoid cystic carcinomas tend to occur earlier in life (mean age of presentation: 40-50 years old) than squamous cell carcinomas (mean age of presentation: 60-70 years old). Squamous cell tends to invade lymph nodes and the mediastinum whereas adenoid cystic carcinomas are more likely to spread submucosally and less likely to metastasize to lymph nodes. Less common primary tumor histologies include carcinoids, bronchogenic carcinomas, and sarcomas. Laryngeal, lung, thyroid, and esophageal carcinomas are the most common tumors to metastasize to the trachea.

Clinical presentation

These tumors typically manifest with slowly progressive obstructive respiratory symptoms (i.e., wheezing or stridor) and may be misdiagnosed as adult-onset asthma. Less commonly, patients may present with hemoptysis and hoarseness. In patients with a previous thoracic malignancy, the concern for secondary tumor is heightened.

Diagnosis

Diagnosis may be suspected with the clinical history but is more reliably made with imaging (CT and bronchoscopy). Rigid bronchoscopy is useful for accurately identifying tumor location, external compression, and to obtain biopsy for pathologic evaluation. Biopsies should be obtained proximal to and distal to the gross lesion in order to accurately map tumor size and involvement. There may be an emerging role for EBUS to evaluate for radial depth of invasion.

Pertinent anatomy

The trachea is a tubular c-shaped structure 11 to 13 cm in length and approximately 2 to 2.5 cm in diameter. The trachea is comprised of 12 to 16 tracheal rings with an anterior cartilaginous component and a membranous posterior component. The first ring (cricoid cartilage) is the only completely cartilaginous ring. Even though most of the trachea is within the mediastinum, half of the length can be delivered into the neck with cervical hyperextension.

Blood supply is an arcade that typically runs along the lateral borders and is comprised of the fusion of the inferior thyroid arteries (main suppliers of the cervical trachea), the bronchial arteries (main suppliers of the lower trachea), and the internal thoracic artery. The thyroid overlies the cervical trachea. The esophagus typically lies posteriorly and occasionally to the left. Recurrent laryngeal nerves are commonly found in the tracheoesophageal groove. The right recurrent laryngeal nerve lies along the trachea for the upper to mid tracheal while the left runs the majority of the length of the trachea.

Surgical treatment

Primary indications for tracheal resection and reconstruction are a lack of metastatic disease and ability to determine resectability. Resectability depends on the length of trachea needed to be resected, extent of invasion (if any) into adjacent structures, and the patient's functional status. Up to half of the length of the trachea (6cm) may be resected. However, a hallmark of the repair is the ability to have a durable tension-free anastomosis.

A cervical collar incision allows access to the upper trachea adequate for most resections. A T extension including an upper sternotomy may allow further access. A right thoracotomy can be used for tumors of the lower third of the trachea and carina. Excessive lateral longitudinal dissection should be kept at a minimum in order to avoid tracheal devascularization as well as to minimize inadvertent injury to the recurrent laryngeal nerves. If a recurrent nerve is involved with the tumor, it may need to be sacrificed. Intimate collaboration with the anesthesiology team is critical in order to maintain adequate oxygenation, ventilation, and hemodynamic stability. Cross-table ventilation is typical and periods of apnea may need to occur in order for completion of the anastomosis. If periods of apnea are used with the concomitant hypercapnea, a careful eye on progression of acidosis and coagulopathy is required.

Classically, there are 5 release maneuvers described to adequately mobilize the trachea when needed in order to secure a tension free anastomosis. They are (in preferred order):

- Pretracheal dissection

- Neck flexion up to 30° with concomitant chin-to-sternum stitch

- Laryngeal release to "drop" the larynx, cricoid, and trachea

- Release of the inferior pulmonary ligament

- Hilar release of the right lung by incision of the pericardium and if necessary, mobilization of the right PA and superior pulmonary vein

A more advanced maneuver is the transection of the left main bronchus with subsequent re-implantation onto the right bronchus.

The most serious complication after tracheal resection is anastomotic dehiscence. It usually presents days to weeks after resection with signs of wound infection, subcutaneous air, voice changes, stridor, or airway obstruction. Treatment of this complication is centered around maintaining an open airway with a tracheostomy, draining the infection, and controlling the defect (with the same tracheostomy tube or soft tissue / muscle flap). A delayed reoperation can then be performed..

Overall survival is better for adenoid cystic than for squamous cell carcinoma. In addition to histology, the most important prognostic factor is completeness of resection. However, in the event of a positive distal margin, if there is inability to resect more without leaving undue tension, it is often better to leave the anastomosis tension-free and follow resection with adjuvant RT.

Palliation and adjuvant therapy

In those patients who have distant metastatic disease, are non-resectable, or not candidates for complete resection, there are roles for surgical intervention for improving quality of life and controlling local symptoms. The rigid bronchoscope has an invaluable role for dilating stricture and coring out tracheal and main bronchial tumors. Laser ablation can be used for more distal tumors, those that are bleeding, or not amenable to rigid bronchoscopy. Compressive tumors may be palliated by tracheobronchial stents. There are a few caveats for tracheobronchial stents: they are only useful in the proximal airways (trachea and mainstem bronchi), they can be prone to migration, there is little role for silicone removable stents in the palliative setting, an aggressive mucolytic regimen should be employed to minimize the risk of stent occlusion (especially if used too distally).

After the resection has healed, squamous and adenoid cystic carcinomas (as well as other histologies) likely would benefit from adjuvant RT. Patients who are unresectable would also likely derive benefit from external beam RT either alone or in addition to one of the palliative procedures described. The role of chemotherapy is unclear.

34. Anatomy and surgical approaches to the mediastinum

James M. Isbell

Mediastinal anatomy

The mediastinum is bounded anteriorly by the sternum, posteriorly by the spine, superiorly by the thoracic inlet, inferiorly by the diaphragm, and laterally by the pleurae. Several 3- and 4-compartment models of the mediastinum have been proposed. The simplest is the 3-compartment model consisting of anterior, middle and posterior compartments where all 3 compartments are bounded superiorly by the thoracic inlet, inferiorly by the diaphragm and laterally by the pleura:

- *Anterior compartment.* Bounded by the sternum anteriorly and the great vessels and pericardium posteriorly. It houses the thymus gland, the internal mammary arteries and adipose tissue.

- *Middle compartment.* Bounded posteriorly by the anterior surface of the thoracic spine and contains the great vessels, pericardium, heart, trachea, proximal main-stem bronchi, vagus and phrenic nerves, esophagus, thoracic duct and descending aorta.

- *Posterior compartment.* Mostly a potential space that lies laterally along the spine and contains the sympathetic chain, its ganglia, as well as the proximal intercostal neurovascular bundles.

Mediastinal lymph nodes are those contained within the mediastinal pleura, which include stations 1 through 9.

Cervical mediastinoscopy

The most common indication for mediastinal lymph node biopsy is to assess for N2 nodal involvement in stage I-III NSCLC. A 5% mediastinal PET false negative rate serves as rationale for pursuing mediastinal lymph node sampling. Other indications include obtaining a tissue diagnosis in the setting of mediastinal lymphadenopathy (e.g., sarcoidosis, lymphoma) or mediastinal masses.

Preoperative assessment prior to mediastinoscopy should include a history and physical exam with particular attention paid to prior neck or chest surgery and/or radiation. The presence of certain anatomic obstacles such as a severe kyphosis of the cervical spine, tracheostomy, large thyroid goiter, aortic arch or innominate artery aneurysms are relative contraindications to mediastinoscopy. The procedure should not be attempted in patients with superior vena cava (SVC) syndrome due to the high risk of hemorrhage. Caution is also warranted for patients with significant innominate artery calcification as they are at risk for embolic stroke.

Only lymph nodes from stations 2, 4 and 7 are accessible via classic cervical mediastinoscopy. The most common complications of cervical mediastinoscopy are major bleeding (0.1-0.6%), recurrent laryngeal nerve injury (0.5%), pneumothorax, airway injury and esophageal perforation. The most common biopsy site associated with major hemorrhage is 4R with the azygos vein and SVC being the most frequently injured vessels followed by the right main pulmonary artery and bronchial artery at station 7. Major bleeding should initially be addressed with immediate packing through the mediastinoscope, which should be left in position even if visualization is lost. If major bleeding persists after packing, major vessel injury should be suspected. Median sternotomy may be necessary for vascular control. Recurrent laryngeal nerve injuries typically involve the left nerve with biopsies at station 4L. Minimal use of electrocautery at this lymph node station is therefore recommended.

Another technique for assessing mediastinal lymph nodes that is gaining popularity is EBUS-TBNA. With this technique, mediastinal lymph nodes 1, 2, 3, 4 and 7 can be assessed.

Anterior mediastinotomy

Left anterior mediastinotomy (Chamberlain procedure) provides access to level 5 and 6 lymph nodes. Anterior mediastinotomy can also be used to biopsy left or right-sided mediastinal masses. Typically, the mediastinum is entered by making a small transverse incision just lateral to the sternum in the second or third intercostal space. In some instances, resection of the costal cartilage will provide better exposure. Care should be taken to avoid injury to the internal mammary artery and the phrenic nerve.

Median sternotomy

Median sternotomy is quite versatile, providing excellent access to most areas of the mediastinum. Besides its utilization in cardiac procedures, median sternotomy is the traditional approach for thymectomy. The sternal retractor should not be placed too superiorly as this can result in brachial plexus injury.

Transcervical approach

The transcervical approach provides excellent access to the anterior mediastinum. This technique is most commonly used for thymectomies but can also be useful for biopsy or resection of other anterior mediastinal tumors (e.g., parathyroid adenomas). Thymomas that are noninvasive and less than 4 cm may be safely resected with transcervical thymectomy.

Briefly, the transcervical approach is performed by making a 4-5 cm collar incision just above the sternal notch and lifting the sternum with a Cooper thymectomy retractor. Most other small to moderate-sized anterior mediastinal masses can be accessed for biopsy or resection via this approach after removal of the thymus.

Bilateral thoracosternotomy (clamshell)

This approach provides excellent exposure for resection of large anterior mediastinal tumors, especially if there is pleural extension. An incision is made in the inframammary crease bilaterally. Subcutaneous flaps are made on the anterior surface of the pectoralis major fascia up to the level of the third or fourth intercostal spaces. The pectoralis muscle fibers are then split and bilateral anterior thoracotomies are performed. The sternum is then divided with a saw transversely and exposure is achieved with the placement of bilateral rib spreaders. The internal mammary arteries must be ligated and divided.

Unilateral thoracosternotomy (hemi-clamshell)

The hemi-clamshell is useful for anterior Pancoast tumors, large thymomas with lateral extension, and some neurogenic tumors arising from the proximal brachial plexus. The approach requires a partial upper sternal split and an anterior thoracotomy, usually in the fourth intercostal space.

Video-assisted thoracoscopic surgery (VATS)

VATS is being utilized more frequently for biopsy and resection of anterior, middle and posterior mediastinal tumors. Most commonly, VATS is used to resect posterior mediastinal tumors (e.g., neurogenic), but many thoracic surgeons are performing thymectomies with this approach as well. As with transcervical thymectomy, most experts recommend restricting the use of this approach to noninvasive thymomas.

35. Mediastinal masses

Kendra J. Grubb

Table 35-1 is a summary of the mediastinal compartments and associated masses.

Table 35-1. Mediastinal masses.

Compartment (organs)	Masses
Anterior/Superior (thymus)	Thymic neoplasm (thymoma, thymic carcinoma, thymic carcinoid) Lymphoma Germ cell tumor (teratoma, seminoma, non-seminomatous tumor) Thyroid adenoma Parathyroid adenoma Carcinoma Lymphoma
Middle (heart, trachea/bronchi, ascending aorta, esophagus)	Bronchogenic cyst Pericardial cyst Enteric cysts Lymphoma
Posterior (esophagus, descending aorta)	Neurogenic tumors Esophageal/Enteric cyst Lymphoma

Clinical presentation

Most mediastinal masses are asymptomatic and found on routine imaging. Chest pain, cough, dyspnea, and constitutional symptoms can be present. Pain and neurologic deficit tend to accompany neurogenic tumors in the posterior mediastinum.

Diagnosis

A mediastinal mass can often be seen on CXR, but CT is the diagnostic study of choice. CT reveals the location of the mass, morphologic characteristics, and the relationship to other structures, and is essential for surgical planning. Small masses, less than 5cm, with characteristic features, (i.e. thymoma, teratoma, or benign cyst), can be surgically resected for diagnoses. For larger tumors or signs of invasion, a tissue diagnosis is necessary to dictate treatment. CT-guided or percutaneous biopsy offers the least invasive approach. Open biopsy can be performed via mediastinoscopy, VATS, Chamberlain mediastinotomy, or thoracotomy. Serum tumor markers, β-HCG, AFP, and LDH, can be helpful for lesions suspicious for germ cell tumors.

Anterior mediastinal masses

The most common tumors of the mediastinum are in the anterior mediastinum. 95% of all tumors in the anterior mediastinum are one of the "Four T's": thymic neoplasm, teratoma, "terrible" lymphoma, and thyroid goiter.

Thymoma

Thymoma is the most common anterior mediastinal mass in adults. Incidence is equal in males and females and usually in the third to fifth decade of life. Up to half of patients will be asymptomatic and the mass will be found incidentally. The other half may have pain, dyspnea, cough, hoarseness, or other associated syndromes (e.g., myasthenia gravis, red cell hypoplasia, hypogammaglobulinemia, SLE, rheumatoid arthritis, ulcerative colitis, thyroiditis). On CT, benign thymomas are usually < 5 cm, appear well-circumscribed and round. Thymomas are malignant in 50% of patients and are usually > 5 cm, irregular in shape, and may invade neighboring structures.

The treatment of a thymoma is complete excision. This may require *en bloc* resection of structures to which the tumor may be adherent to (e.g., pleura, pericardium, innominate vein, SVC, lung). If both phrenic nerves appear to be involved, one nerve may be excised while the tumor is dissected from the other nerve; pathological frozen examination may help in differentiating tumor from surrounding inflammatory reaction. Median sternotomy is the most common approach, but cervical and VATS approaches are described.

Survival is based on stage. Stage I disease is completely encapsulated, 95% 5-year survival. Stage II has microscopic invasion into mediastinal fat or mediastinal pleura (IIa) or through the capsule (IIb), 85% 5-year survival. Stage III disease invades an adjacent organ, 70% 5-year survival. Stage IV is metastatic to pleura or pericardium (IVa) or distant (IVb), 50% 5-year survival. Increased survival is reported with adjuvant and neoadjuvant therapy for stage III-IV disease with RT and cisplatin-based chemotherapy.

Myasthenia Gravis (MG)

MG is an autoantibody disorder affecting 5-12 per 100,000 in the population. The disease is twice as common in women and usually occurs in the second to third decade of life. For men, MG manifest in the sixth to seventh decade. The antibody targets the acetylcholine receptor (AChR) and binding causes decrease transmission of the action potential at the neuromuscular junction. Clinically, this manifests as decreased contraction of the muscle fibers resulting in weakness.

Symptoms are graded: (I) focal disease - ocular muscle weakness, (II) generalized mild to moderate disease, (III) severe generalized weakness, and (IV) life-threatening weakness - respiratory failure. After a physical exam identifying the level of weakness, an edrophonium (short acting anticholinesterase) test is confirmatory if the patient shows improvement. Assay for AChR antibody is also available.

The treatment of MG includes anticholinesterase therapy (pyridostig-mine) and if needed, corticosteroids for immunosuppression. Plasma-pheresis and IVIG are short-term therapies used for myasthenic crises, preoperatively, or intermittently in patients with poor control of MG de-spite immunosuppression. Thymectomy is indicated in patients with thymic hyperplasia or a thymoma. 30-50% of patients with a thymoma have MG and 10-15% of patients with MG have a thymoma. Further, there is a role for thymectomy in any MG patient with early, generalized, moderate to severe disease, especially if refractory to medical manage-ment. Thymectomy should not be performed emergently for a myasthen-ic crisis / class IV disease.

Primary mediastinal lymphoma

Primary mediastinal lymphoma is rare, only 5-10% of cases of anterior mediastinal masses. T-cell, Non-Hodgkin's lymphoma, is the most common; Hodgkin's and lymphoblastic lymphoma also occur in the me-diastinum. The mediastinum is a common site for more disseminated lymphoma associated with mediastinal lymphadenopathy. A tissue diag-nosis is necessary, and may be accomplished with nodal biopsy. Survival outcomes are based on the grade of the tumor. Treatment is chemothera-py and RT. The only role for surgery is to obtain histological diagnosis.

Germ cell tumors

Germ cell tumors account for 10-15% of mediastinal masses. Males are affected more often. *Teratomas* are the most common germ cell tumor in the mediastinum and affect men and women equally. They are usually asymptomatic but can occasionally become infected or rupture into the pleura or the airway (resulting in coughing of hair or sebum). Serum tumor markers are negative. Biopsy reveals well-differentiated tissue from more than one germ cell line. Surgical resection is the treatment.

Seminoma is the most common malignant germ cell tumor in the medias-tinum and occurs almost exclusively in males, in the third to fourth dec-ade of life. Serum tumor markers can reveal slightly elevated β-HCG levels. CT will reveal a characteristic large, homogeneous mass, with smooth borders. Seminomas tend to grow slowly and are sensitive to RT, traditionally the primary treatment. Cisplatin-based chemotherapy is used for metastatic disease and some authors advocate using it as a first-line treatment. Surgical resection is reserved for any residual disease manifested as local growth of a residual mass.

Non-seminomatous germ cell tumors occur most often in young men 20-30 years old and are associated with elevated β-HCG, AFP, and LDH. There are 3 main subtypes (in order of frequency): yolk sac carcinoma, embryonal carcinoma, and choriocarcinoma. These tumors tend to grow rapidly and compress neighboring tissues, thus most patients are symptomatic at presentation. Metastatic disease is common at the time of presentation and overall prognosis is poor. The first line treatment is cisplatin-based chemotherapy with surgical resection of any residual mass (regardless of response in markers).

Intrathoracic goiter

Intrathoracic goiter can appear as a mediastinal mass, usually associated with cervical goiter. Non-contrast CT shows enhancement of the thyroid gland because of its iodine content and confirms the diagnosis. Most intrathoracic goiters are removed from the neck although an upper sternal split may be required.

Middle mediastinal masses

The majority of middle mediastinal masses are cysts. *Bronchogenic cysts* are the most common cysts (60%) in the mediastinum and are associated with the airway, most often located posterior to the carina. The cysts have the histologic characteristic of the airway and lung. Most patients are symptomatic at time of presentation due to airway or esophageal compression. After tissue diagnosis is obtained, the treatment is complete transthoracic surgical resection.

Pericardial cysts are rare benign cysts that occur at the cardiophrenic angle most often on the right. CT imaging is key to diagnosis as these cysts have a thin wall, are non-enhancing, and have a characteristic density similar to water. If symptoms arise, the treatment is surgical resection. Some argue all pericardial cysts should be resected due to the potential for rupture, erosion, or compression of the heart or great vessels.

Posterior mediastinal masses

Neurogenic tumors account for 15-20% of all mediastinal tumors and often present with pain or neurologic dysfunction. Arising from neural crest cells, the tumors can be divided into three main groups:

- *Nerve sheath tumors.* Most common tumors overall, representing 40-70% of mediastinal neurogenic tumors. They usually present in the costovertebral sulcus. They tend to be benign with the two most common tumors being neurilemmomas (also called schwannomas) and neurofibromas. Neurofibrosarcomas are the malignant counterpart and are differentiated from the benign ones by level of mitotic activity and lack of encapsulation.

- *Ganglion cell tumors.* These tumors arise from the sympathetic chain and adrenal medulla. The benign tumor in this category is the ganglioneuroma, which can secrete vasoactive intestinal peptide (VIP). Ganglioneuroblastomas are malignant tumors that can present with metastases and are more common in children. These tumors are usually resectable. Neuroblastomas are the most common solid extracranial malignancy in children and the most aggressive of the ganglion cell tumors. They can secrete VIP and catecholamines. Treatment of localized disease is surgical with adjuvant chemoradiation for residual tumor. Metastatic disease is treated with chemotherapy. Factors associated with poor prognosis in neuroblastoma are: presence of metastatic disease, age (< 18 months), degree of histologic differentiation, DNA ploidy, presence of residual disease, N-*myc* amplification, and high levels of neuron-specific enolase and LDH.

- *Paraganglionic tumors.* These tumors arise from paraganglionic tissues in the costovertebral area and include pheocromocytomas (which produce catecholamines) and chemodectomas (hormonally inactive). Resection is the treatment of choice. Chemodectomas may also respond to RT.

CT is the best imaging modality for these tumors. A percutaneous FNA biopsy may be obtained for tissue diagnosis (spindle cell neoplasm). Surgical excision, usually through a posterolateral thoracotomy, is the treatment of choice. The tumor capsule should be left intact if possible.

36. Thoracic sympathectomy

Bryan A. Whitson

Clinical syndromes

Thoracic dorsal sympathectomy is performed for hyperhidrosis, complex regional pain syndrome (CRPS), and Raynaud's phenomenon.

Patients with *hyperhidrosis* present with excessive sweating that interferes with their livelihood or quality of life. The incidence of hyperhidrosis is generally felt to be < 3% and can have familial association. The diagnosis of hyperhidrosis is based on H&P. Some accepted criteria include focal sweating for > 6 months, bilateral, symmetric, that impairs quality of life, occurs at least once a week, starts prior to 25 years of age, does not occur during sleep, and may be associated with family history. Thyroid disease should be excluded.

CRPS is a term now used to describe reflex sympathetic dystrophy (RDS, type I) and causalgia (type II). Patients with CRPS have pain, hypersensitivity to minimal stimuli, burning, cutaneous muscular atrophy, fatigue and/or weakness, vasomotor instability with sweating, and patchy bone demineralization. Physical exam reveals edema, stiffness, discoloration, tenderness, atrophy, and decreased motor function from flexion contractures. CRPS type I (RDS) usually occurs after tissue trauma and the symptoms are not confined to a specific nerve or dermatomal distribution. CRPS type II (causalgia) usually occurs after injury to a peripheral nerve and symptoms start within the territory of the nerve but may eventually spread outside the nerve distribution. Diagnosis may be supported with autonomic testing, bone scintigraphy, X-rays, and MRI.

Raynaud's phenomenon presents with numb and cool extremity as a response to stress or cool temperatures. It is believed to be caused by abnormal vasoconstriction of digital arteries and arterioles. History of classic symptoms (sharply demarcated biphasic response – pallor and cyanosis) is sufficient for diagnosis since there is no widely accepted test.

Treatment

Prior to surgical treatment for hyperhidrosis, non-operative approaches should be attempted (e.g., Drysol, iontophoresis, botulinum toxin and/or glycopyrrolate). Drysol solution (aluminum chloride hexahydrate) may be effective but can cause paradoxical hyperhidrosis. Iontophoresis (introducing ionized substances like water or anticholinergic agents through the skin by applying electrical current) needs to be performed relatively frequently (several times a week) and can have adverse cutaneous symptoms (dryness). Botulinum toxin has a longer duration of 6-9 months, when effective, but can cause intrinsic muscle weakness. Glycopyrrolate may have some anticholinergic side effects. Thoracic dorsal sympathectomy is the treatment of choice for patients who are refractory or unable to use the non-operative techniques.

Patients with CRPS should be treated with physical and occupational therapy, smoking cessation (smoking is a risk factor), medications (anticonvulsants, bisphosphonates, steroids, calcitonin, topical capsaicin, sympathicolytics) prior to considering invasive therapies. Invasive treatments include steroid injections for pain control, electrical nerve stimulation, regional sympathetic nerve blocks, and dorsal column spinal cord stimulation. Sympathectomy is considered for patients refractory to other treatments.

Treatment of patients with Raynaud's phenomenon includes general measures to prevent attacks, smoking cessation, and medications (calcium channel blockers, sympathicolytics, vasodilators, and prostaglandins). Surgical intervention is reserved for those patients that are resistant to other treatment modalities.

Patients with CRPS and Raynaud's should undergo a diagnostic sympathetic nerve block to ensure diagnosis and improvement prior to surgical intervention. Some have advocated this nerve block approach prior to sympathectomy for hyperhidrosis as well.

Surgical approach

Thoracoscopic sympathectomy is performed with 1 or 2 trocars. In women, the medial trocar site can be hidden in the inframammary crease at roughly the anterior axillary line. The superior-lateral trocar can be placed at the hairline. On insertion, respirations should be held and the patient unhooked from the ventilator in order to minimize inadvertent injury to the lung. Careful attention to accurately counting rib levels is needed. The pleura overlying the rib lateral to the sympathetic chain should be incised with cautery for 2-3 cm. The chain can be dissected and freed from circumferential attachments. For facial hyperhidrosis, a T2 isolation is performed. Palmar can be controlled with a T2 and T3 or a T3 isolation alone. Axillary hyperhidrosis warrants T3 and T4 isolation. Isolation can be by transection or clipping. Nomenclature is such that the T level is from above that number rib to below the subsequent rib (e.g., a T3 sympathectomy involves isolating above the 3rd and 4th ribs so the T3 ganglia is excluded or removed.

For severe CRPS or Raynaud's, a first rib resection can be performed, either via a transaxillary or posterior approach. The transaxillary approach is preferred and the posterior thoracoplasty type incision is reserved for recurrent or reoperative approaches. A neurectomy (lysis of the axillary to subclavian artery adventitial tissue) should be employed. The stellate ganglia's T1 component should be isolated, clipped, and the ganglia transected at that location. T1-T3 ganglia are then removed in a similar fashion with nerves clipped. A transthoracic approach can be performed as well, similar to that for hyperhidrosis. If the C7-C8 neural fibers are disrupted, a Horner's syndrome may occur.

II. Adult Cardiac Surgery

37. Cardiac anatomy

Ashok Babu, Ramesh Singh

Overview

Two thirds of the cardiac mass lies to the left of midline. The RV is anterior, LA is posterior, LV is to the left, and RA is to the right.

The aortic valve occupies a central position and is wedged between all 3 of the other valves. Its non-coronary leaflet has fibrous continuity with the anterior leaflet of the mitral valve.

The atrioventricular (AV) groove is obliquely oriented closer to vertical than horizontal. This is evidenced when palpating the coronary sinus (traveling in the AV groove) for retrograde cannula placement.

Pericardium

The heart lies within the pericardial sac, which is attached to the great vessels. The heart is enveloped in visceral pericardium, which also is adherent to the first several centimeters of the great vessels. Parietal pericardium lines the inner surface of the fibrous pericardial sac.

There are two pericardial recesses: transverse sinus and oblique sinus. The transverse sinus is bounded anteriorly by the posterior surface of the aorta and PA and posteriorly by the inter-atrial groove. The oblique sinus exists behind the LA, between the IVC and pulmonary veins.

Mediastinal nerves

Phrenic

Descends anterior to the anterior scalene muscle, just posterior to the internal mammary artery. It is at risk for injury during internal mammary artery takedown. It then passes anterior to the pulmonary hilum and travels to the diaphragm.

- *Left.* If there is a persistent left SVC, it will be plastered to its lateral aspect.

- *Right.* Attached to the lateral surface of SVC and can be injured during dissection for SVC cannulation.

Vagus

Enters the thorax posterior to the phrenic nerve and courses along the carotid arteries.

- *Right.* The right recurrent laryngeal nerve (RLN) branches from the right vagus under the right subclavian artery and passes anteriorly to ascend out of thorax. The vagus continues posterior to the pulmonary hilum.

- *Left.* The left vagus descends between the left common carotid and the left subclavian arteries, posterior to the aortic arch. The left RLN comes off and hooks anteriorly around the *ligamentum arteriosum* and ascends to the trachea-esophageal groove.

Coronary arteries

The coronary orifices are in the upper third of the Sinuses of Valsalva. There are 3 main coronary arteries: RCA, LAD, and circumflex. Dominance of left or right is defined by the supplier of the posterior descending artery (PDA), which is from the RCA in 85-90%.

The left main coronary artery (LMCA) courses off the left Sinus of Valsalva, behind the PA and anterior to the LA appendage, and bifurcates into the LAD and circumflex (or trifurcates in the setting of a ramus artery). The LAD is the interventricular artery and courses along the anterior interventricular groove towards the apex. It gives off septal perforators that dive down perpendicularly into the septum, diagonals that course over the LV anterior wall, and RV branches to the anterior surface of the RV.

The circumflex artery travels in the left AV groove and ends near the obtuse margin of the LV. In 10-15% of people it continues in the groove and gives rise to the PDA (left dominance). In this case, it also supplies the AV node. The circumflex gives rise to obtuse marginal (OM) branches, which supply the lateral wall of the LV and the posteromedial papillary muscle. The circumflex supplies the sinoatrial (SA) node in 50% of people.

The RCA courses from the aorta anteriorly and descends in the right AV groove, giving off RV acute marginal branches that supply the RV free wall and may continue in 10-20% of patients across the diaphragmatic surface to supply the distal interventricular septum. The SA nodal artery arises from the RCA in 50% of patients and is usually the first branch. The RCA may give off an early conal branch that courses to the left of the infundibulum. The RCA bifurcates into the PDA and right posterolateral artery. The PDA courses along the interventricular groove towards the apex and gives off septal perforators that typically supply the posterior one third of the septum. The right posterolateral artery gives off branches to the posterior wall of the LV.

Coronary veins

These veins usually have no valves. The coronary sinus largely drains the LV and receives 85% of coronary blood flow. The rest drains via Thebesian veins into the RA. One of the main tributaries is the anterior interventricular vein (analog to the LAD). The great cardiac vein travels in the AV groove and turns into the coronary sinus. The posterior inter-ventricular vein (analog of the PDA) is the last tributary and drains near the coronary sinus orifice. This explains why RV protection from retro-grade cardioplegia can be marginal as the cardioplegia catheter is usually inserted beyond the entry point of this vein. In addition, a persistent left SVC will drain into the coronary sinus, making it ineffective to adminis-ter retrograde cardioplegia in these patients.

Anterior RV veins drain into the right AV groove to form the small cardi-ac vein, which drains directly into the RA or coronary sinus. Thebesian veins are small veins, which drain directly into chambers, mainly the RA and RV.

Right atrium and tricuspid valve

The SA node lies on the right side of the junction of the RA and SVC. It is between the RA appendage and the SVC. 10% of patients have a horseshoe SA node, which is draped along the SVC / RA junction.

The *fossa ovalis* is the true interatrial septum and is the location where the LA should be entered for a trans-septal approach. It is also the loca-tion of a PFO.

The Thebesian valve is the valve of the coronary sinus. The Eustachian valve is the valve of the IVC. The tendon of Todaro is the continuation of the Thebesian valve to the Eustachian valve.

The AV node lies within the triangle of Koch. The triangle of Koch is bounded by the tendon of Todaro, the orifice of the coronary sinus, and the septal leaflet of the tricuspid valve. The bundle of His is located at the apex of the triangle of Koch prior to branching on the interventricular septum.

The trabeculated muscle surrounding the RA appendage makes an abrupt transition to smooth atrial muscle at a well defined band of muscle called the *crista terminalis*. The smooth atrial muscle marks the vestibule of the RA, which funnels blood into the tricuspid valve.

The tricuspid valve has septal, anterior, and inferior leaflets. It does not have a true fibrous annulus. The AV node is at the base of the septal leaflet. The aortic valve is nearby to the junction of the septal and anterior leaflets.

Left atrium and mitral valve

The LA has a large venous component (part of chamber into which pulmonary veins drain), an appendage, and a vestibule funneling blood into the mitral valve. The LA is the most posterior chamber of the heart. Surgical access is gained via an incision anterior to the right pulmonary veins, an incision in the dome, or a trans-septal approach via the RA.

The mitral valve has an anterior and posterior leaflet. The anterior leaflet has fibrous continuity with the aortic valve and is anterior in the surgeon's view as well. It covers only one third of the annular circumference but is the longer leaflet. The posterior leaflet covers two thirds of the annulus but is short with respect to depth of orifice coverage.

Though they may be divided by scallops, the leaflets are somewhat arbitrarily divided into 3 segments (A1, A2, A3 and P1, P2, P3) by the Carpentier classification. A1 and P1 are most medial or to the surgeon's left.

The leaflets are attached via *chordae tendinae* to the posteromedial and anterolateral papillary muscles.

The left side of the posterior leaflet is adjacent to the circumflex artery and the right side is adjacent to the coronary sinus. These can be injured with deep bites through the annulus.

The right and left fibrous trigones are dense collagenous tissue that bound the central fibrous body and are at approximately at 10 o'clock and 2 o'clock on the annulus with respect to the anterior leaflet. They are both anterior to the valve commissures.

Right ventricle and pulmonic valve

The RV outlet is composed of the infundibulum and the tricuspid pulmonic valve. The pulmonic valve does not have a fibrous annulus but is rather suspended in muscle. The apex consists of trabeculated muscle and is quite thin. There is an anterior and medial papillary muscle to suspend the tricuspid valve.

Left ventricle and aortic valve

The LV chamber is composed of fine trabeculated muscle extending all the way to the apex. The mitral valve and subvalvular apparatus compose the inflow portion. The outflow tract is lined by smooth muscle and fibrous tissue. The septal portion of the LVOT includes the membranous ventricular septum. The LVOT also contains a fibrous sheet, which extends from the anterior leaflet of the mitral valve to the mitral-aortic continuity supporting the left and non-coronary leaflets of the aortic valve. The AV bundle and left bundle branch enter the LVOT posterior to the membranous septum and between the right and non-coronary cusps of the aortic valve. This can be injured during aortic valve surgery.

The aortic valve is trileaflet. The leaflets coapt along a semilunar plane. The coaptation surface is thin except centrally where the nodule of Arantius is present on each leaflet. The aortic wall bulges out from each leaflet to form the Sinuses of Valsalva. The "aortic root" is composed of the aortic annulus, valve leaflets, Sinuses of Valsalva, and sinotubular junction. The sinotubular junction is at the top of the commissures and is the point where the sinuses neck down to form a tubular aorta.

38. Cardiopulmonary bypass

Ramesh Singh, Ashok Babu

CPB may be required in patients with CAD, valvular heart disease, aortic dissections, congenital heart defects, aneurysms (aortic, ventricular), transplantation (heart, lung, liver, trachea) undergoing surgery or for hypothermic rescue.

CPB facilitates surgical intervention with a motionless and/or a bloodless field. The bypass machine can isolate the heart and lungs while maintaining organ perfusion. It both serves as a pump and an oxygenator, with pressure and oxygenation easily modulated by increasing flow rates on CPB. Unfortunately, the synthetic interface of the circuit also causes activation of blood components and cytokine release. Specifically, the membrane oxygenator exerts the most damage on blood components. Another, more infrequent complication with blood components occurs in patients with cold agglutinins that precipitate out with cooling on bypass. If recognized, every attempt should be made to do the procedure at normothermia.

The ischemic myocardium of the arrested heart is protected in 3 ways: electrochemical silence, cold temperature, and lack of distension.

Cardioplegia

Cardioplegia is the most common method of accomplishing asystole. It can be given antegrade and/or retrograde. Antegrade cardioplegia is usually quicker at arresting the heart (30-60 sec). This is done using a cardioplegia cannula inserted directly into the ascending aorta or, alternatively, directly down the coronary ostia following aortotomy. Delay usually indicates a problem with delivery of the solution or unrecognized aortic regurgitation.

Retrograde cardioplegia takes longer to induce electrical arrest (2-4 min) and may provide incomplete protection to the RV due to the delivery of cardioplegia into the coronary sinus beyond the site where the first few veins drain the RV. However, it does serve the advantage of flushing out air and emboli from the coronaries.

The heart arrests in diastole and does not use ATP during this period of heart isolation. The cold fluid (usually at 4 °C) cools the heart thus slowing down its metabolism. The cardioprotective effects of hypothermia are often expressed using the Q10 rule, which says that for every 10°C drop in temperature, metabolic rate decreases by 50%.

Venous cannulation and drainage

Drainage amount is determined by CVP, the height differential, resistance in cannulas/tubing, and the absence of air within the system. Inadequate blood volume or excessive siphon pressure may cause venous walls to collapse against the cannula intake producing "chattering". Volume corrects this. Most commonly, bicaval or cavoatrial venous cannulation is used. Elevation of the heart may kink the cavo-atrial junction and partially obstruct the venous drainage.

Femoral and iliac vein cannulation can also be used and is especially useful in the following scenarios: emergency closed cardiopulmonary assist, prevention or management of bleeding during sternotomy, re-operative heart surgery, certain types of aortic and thoracic surgery, and applications of CPB that do not require a sternotomy or thoracotomy.

Complications of venous cannulation

Venous cannulation can lead to several complications including atrial arrhythmias, atrial or caval tears and bleeding, air embolization, injury or obstruction due to catheter malposition, reversing of arterial and venous lines, unexpected decannulation, and obstruction of the cavae with tying of improperly placed purse-string sutures. In addition, there may be complications when placing tapes around the cavae such as lacerating venous branches, nearby vessels (e.g. right PA) or the cava itself.

Arterial cannulation

Arterial cannulation is used to support the circulation. The cannulation site is influenced by the planned operation and the distribution of atherosclerotic disease. Cannulas are usually placed in the proximal aorta but can also be placed in any major artery (innominate artery, distal aortic arch, axillary/subclavian artery, femoral/external iliac artery).

Complications of arterial cannulation

High velocity jets out of the cannula tip can cause a sand-blasting effect. This can damage the aortic wall, dislodge atheroemboli, produce dissections, disturb flow to nearby vessels, and cause cavitation and hemolysis. The debris is preferentially directed into the left common carotid artery, which explains the predominance of left sided strokes following cardiac surgery. Other complications include difficult insertion, bleeding, intramural or other type of malpositioning of the cannula tip, failure to remove all air from the arterial line after connection, injury to the aortic back wall, obstruction to flow, inadequate or excessive cerebral perfusion, and delayed complications (late bleeding and infected or non-infected false aneurysms).

Epiaortic US is the best method for assessing atherosclerosis of the ascending aorta. Calcified aorta ("porcelain aorta") occurs in 1.2% to 4.3% of cases and is an indication for changing location of the aortic cannula.

Aortic dissection occurs in 0.01 to 0.09% of all aortic cannulations and it's more common in patients with aortic root disease. First clues are discoloration beneath the adventitia near the cannulation site, an increase in arterial line pressure, and a sharp reduction in return to the venous reservoir. Prompt action is necessary to limit dissection and maintain perfusion. The cannula must be promptly transferred to a peripheral artery or uninvolved distal aorta. Blood pressure should be controlled medically. Perfusion cooling to a temperature < 20°C is initiated. During deep hypothermic circulatory arrest (DHCA), the aorta is opened at the original site of cannulation and repaired by direct suture, patch, or circumferential graft. Early recognition brings survival rates up to 66% - 85%. If recognized after surgery, the survival is approximately 50%.

Lower body cannulation is associated with many complications such as tears, dissection, late stenosis or thrombosis, bleeding, lymph fistula, infection in the groin, cerebral and coronary atheroembolism. Malperfusion can also be a problem in those with prior aortic dissections. Ischemic complications of the lower extremity can occur with prolonged retrograde perfusion unless a side-arm is used to perfuse the distal leg.

Retrograde arterial dissection is the most serious complication and may extend to the aortic root. The incidence is 0.2% to 1.3% and is associated with a mortality of about 50%. It is more likely to occur in diseased arteries and in patients over 40 years of age. It is confirmed by echocardiography of the descending thoracic aorta and antegrade perfusion in the true lumen needs to be resumed either by the heart itself or by cannulation in the distal aorta or axillary-subclavian artery.

Venting the heart

If the heart is unable to contract, distention of either ventricle is detrimental to subsequent contractility. LV distention can be insidious unless a vent catheter is used. Blood can enter this cavity from multiple sources: blood escaping atrial or venous cannulas, coronary sinus and Thebesian veins (via pulmonary circulation), bronchial arterial and venous blood, regurgitation through the aortic valve, or undiagnosed abnormal sources (PFO or PDA). There are 4 main vents that can be used for this purpose: aortic root vent, an LV vent via the right superior pulmonary vein, direct venting of the LV via the apex, and venting of the main PA (no valves in the pulmonary circulation).

Persistent left superior vena cava (PLSVC)

PLSVC is present in 0.3 to 0.5% of the population. It usually drains into the coronary sinus. However, in 10% of cases it drains into the left atria. It should be suspected when the (left) innominate vein is small or absent and a large coronary sinus or PLSVC is seen on baseline echocardiography. If these signs are missed, it should be considered with inadequate venous cannula flow with bicaval cannulation. It may complicate retrograde cardioplegia or surgical entry into the right heart. If an adequate sized innominate vein is present (30% of patients), the PLSVC can be occluded during CPB, if the ostium of the coronary sinus is present. If the innominate vein is absent (40%) or small (33%), occlusion of the PLSVC may cause venous hypertension and possible cerebral injury. In these patients, a cannula is passed retrogradely into the PLSVC through the coronary sinus ostium and secured. If the right SVC is not present (approximately 20% of patients with PLSVC), the left SVC cannot be occluded.

39. Coronary artery disease
Kendra J. Grubb

CAD is the single largest killer of Americans, accounting for nearly 500,000 deaths per year and affecting 1.5 million in the population. Classic symptoms of angina need not be present as CAD can present with dyspnea, dizziness, syncope, and pulmonary edema. Reduced coronary blood flow, under conditions of increased demand, results in ischemia and symptoms. Coronary angiography is the gold standard for diagnosis with the goal to identify hemodynamically significant atherosclerotic lesions. A 75% reduction in cross-sectional area (stenosis) results in a 50% loss of arterial diameter and is sufficient to impair coronary blood flow and cause symptoms of angina with activity. A 90% stenosis results in a 75-80% loss in diameter and will cause reduced blood flow at rest.

Patients with CAD may present with chronic CAD (stable angina) or with an acute coronary syndrome (ACS). ACS can itself present in different ways: ST elevation MI (STEMI), non-ST elevation MI (NSTEMI), or unstable angina. A STEMI (evidence of myocardial necrosis based on cardiac biomarkers and ST changes in the EKG) usually occurs when an atherosclerotic plaque ruptures and a mural thrombus forms acutely at the site of the plaque, occluding the vessel. Unstable angina or a NSTEMI (evidence of myocardial necrosis based on cardiac biomarkers in the absence of ST changes in the EKG) can occur as a consequence of different scenarios: plaque rupture and thrombosis (most common), coronary spasm (Prinzmetal's angina), progressive coronary obstruction, or increased oxygen demand (e.g. tachycardia) and/or decreased oxygen supply (e.g., anemia) on a patient with an existing coronary obstruction.

CAD can result in LV dysfunction due to 3 different mechanisms: loss of muscle due to an MI (irreversible), "hibernating" myocardium, or "stunned" myocardium. *Hibernating myocardium* is a state of myocardial dysfunction at rest due to CAD that will partially or completely resolve after revascularization. *Stunned myocardium* is defined as transient myocardial dysfunction after reperfusion.

Medical management

AHA/ACC 2006 guidelines[1] focus on the controllable risk factors: smoking cessation, hypertension (goal <140/90, or <130/80 in diabetics or chronic kidney disease), hypercholesterolemia (goal LDL <100 mg/dL, if triglycerides >200 non-HDL should be <130), obesity (goal BMI 18.5 to 24.9), physical inactivity (goal 30 min of exercise, 7 days a week), DM management (goal HbA1c <7%), and anticoagulation (aspirin 75 to 162 mg/day in all patients, clopidogrel 70 mg/day plus aspirin if the patient has had an ACS or PCI). ACE inhibitors are indicated for EF < 40%; ARB should be used for patients with heart failure or MI and intolerant to ACE inhibitors. Beta-blockers are indicated in all patients who have had MI, ACS, or LV dysfunction, with or without heart failure. Aldosterone blockade is indicated after large MI in patients with low EF and without renal dysfunction.

Percutaneous coronary intervention (PCI)

PCI was first introduced in 1977 as angioplasty for stenotic coronary lesions. In March of 2009, the New England Journal of Medicine published data comparing PCI versus CABG for severe CAD (SYNTAX trial).[2] The study was a non-inferiority comparison for patients with left main disease or three-vessel CAD. It showed that adverse cardiac or cerebrovascular events were higher in the PCI group at 12 months, mainly due to an increased rate of repeat revascularization. The rates of MI and death were similar between both groups and the rate of stroke was higher in the CABG group.

Several other randomized trials have been designed over the years to compare PCI and CABG (BARI, EAST, CABRI, GABI, RITA). Overall, these trials have found similar survival between both groups but the incidence of repeat revascularization is much higher among PCI patients (30% at 1 year, 55% at 5 years) than CABG patients (3-15%).

Indications for CABG

AHA/ACC 2004 Guidelines for CABG[3] are based on trials comparing surgical revascularization with medical therapy. In summary, the trials demonstrated the greatest survival benefits for revascularization for patients at highest risk as defined by angina and/or ischemia:

- Left main disease (≥50% stenosis)

- Left main equivalent (≥70% stenosis of proximal LAD and proximal circumflex)

- Triple-vessel disease, especially if EF < 50%

- Two-vessel disease with proximal LAD stenosis and EF < 50%

- Proximal LAD and one- or two- vessel disease

- Disabling angina refractory to medical management

- Failed PCI

Additional indications include pathology not suitable to PCI such as total occlusion, circumferential calcification, bifurcation involvement and diffuse or distal lesions, and obstructive coronary disease associated with other cardiac conditions requiring operation. The guidelines also recommend CABG for diabetics as the disease is usually diffuse, distal, progressive, and associated with sudden death. Patients with STEMI usually undergo non-surgical treatment unless there is ongoing ischemia or cardiogenic shock despite maximal non-surgical therapy.

On- and off-pump CABG

Off-pump CABG (OPCAB) has gained some popularity recently to try to decrease the morbidity of CPB. The procedure uses self-retaining coronary stabilizers and coronary snares to allow for creation of the anastomoses. Hemodynamic instability during the procedure can be due to RV compression (resulting in decreased RV filling and cardiac output) during exposure of the lateral wall of the LV, diastolic dysfunction from excessive downward pressure from a coronary stabilizer, or intraoperative ischemia from the native CAD or coronary snaring. Hemodynamic instability can be improved by using short-acting alpha-adrenergic agents, volume loading the patient, using a Trendelenburg position, creating the internal mammary artery (IMA)-LAD anastomosis prior to manipulating the heart, using coronary shunts as appropriate, and using certain exposure techniques such as deep pericardial sutures, right pleurotomy and pericardiotomy to decrease RV compression, right hemisternal elevation, and use of apical suction devices.

The AHA published a statement comparing on-pump and OPCAB coronary revascularization in 2005.[4] Surgical outcomes are similar. However the following trends were noted: less blood loss and need for transfusion after OPCAB, less myocardial enzyme release after OPCAB up to 24 hrs, less early neurocognitive dysfunction after OPCAB, and less renal insufficiency after OPCAB. CABG is associated with higher number of total bypass grafts constructed, easier grafts to posterior (circumflex) targets, and possibly better long-term graft patency.

Conduit choices

Internal mammary artery (IMA)

The IMA is the first choice of conduit and has been associated with excellent long-term patency. The use of the IMA has showed early and late survival benefit and better event-free survival after CABG. IMA grafts are resistant to development of atherosclerosis as the artery has greater resistance to endothelium harvest injury. Furthermore, the non-fenestrated internal elastic lamina may inhibit cellular migration and prevent intimal hyperplasia. The unique endothelium has higher basal production of vasodilators with favorable response to milrinone. The graft also shows no vasoconstriction in response to norepinephrine, and nitroglycerin causes vasodilatation. 10-year patency is 82-95%.

Radial artery

The radial artery is a secondary choice of conduit. The vessel has fenestrated internal elastic lamina and a thicker wall. It is more likely to have atherosclerotic changes and more likely to spasm. 5-year patency is 83-95%.

Gastroepiploic artery

The right gastroepiploic artery is not typically used in an initial CABG, but can be utilized in reoperation. If no alternative suitable conduits are available, the right gastroepiploic artery can be harvested as a pedicle or free graft. Further, it is a secondary arterial conduit in all-arterial revascularization. The use of the gastroepiploic artery does increase operative time needed to harvest the vessel and has potential for perioperative and long term abdominal complications. There is a lack of consensus on long-term benefit. 5-year patency is 80% and 10-year is 62%.

Other artery

For patients in whom no other conduit is available, the following vessels can be utilized for CABG: inferior epigastric artery, ulnar artery, left gastric artery, splenic artery, thoracodorsal artery, and the lateral femoral circumflex artery.

Greater saphenous vein (GSV)

One of the most common conduits used for CABG. The GSV is easy to harvest, available in most patients, versatile, and resistant to spasm. Unfortunately, there is increased graft failure with GSV conduits as a result of thrombosis, intimal hyperplasia, and graft atherosclerosis. 10 year patency is 61-71%.

Complications

The most common complications after CABG are:

- *Postoperative bleeding.* Approximately 20% of patients receive transfusions and 2% of patients undergo re-explorations for bleeding. Re-exploration is indicated for bleeding > 400 cc/hr, 300 cc/hr for 2 hours, 200 cc/hr for > 4 hours or if tamponade is suspected.[5] Preoperative use of anticoagulant and antiplatelet medications increases the risk of postoperative bleeding. Medications such as aspirin are usually continued up to the day of surgery. Warfarin is discontinued 1 week before surgery and if needed, short-term anticoagulation with low-molecular weight heparin can be started at that time. Ideally, clopidogrel should be stopped 5-7 days prior to surgery although it may be continued in some high-risk patients up to the time of surgery.

- *Perioperative MI / low cardiac output syndrome.* Perioperative MI occurs in approximately 2% of cases. The prevalence of low cardiac output syndrome, defined as need for inotropic or mechanical support for > 30 minutes after surgery, is approximately 5-10%. It is associated with a mortality risk of 17%.

- *Renal failure.* Incidence of postoperative renal failure is approximately 8% with 1-2% of patients requiring dialysis. Risk factors include age > 70 years, DM, CHF, preoperative renal dysfunction, prior CABG, and long pump run.

- *Neurological complications.* Type 1 deficits (major focal neurological deficits) occur in 1-3% of patients while type 2 deficits (global deterioration of memory or function) occur in approximately 3%. Risk of stroke is higher in older patients (>70 years), with prior strokes, hypertension, renal failure, DM, smoking, and a carotid bruit.

- *Arrythmias.* Atrial fibrillation presents in 20-40% of patients after CABG. Risk factors include advanced age, prolonged cross-clamp time, COPD, and beta-blocker withdrawal. Prophylactic regimens with beta-blockers, amiodarone, or biatrial pacing may reduce the risk of atrial arrhythmias.

- *Sternal wound infection.* Mediastinitis and deep sternal wound infection occur in 1-3% of cases and carry a mortality of 15%. Risk factors include use of bilateral pedicled IMAs in diabetic patients, obesity, DM, advanced age, male gender, and perioperative hyperglycemia.

Overall mortality after CABG is 1-3% and it may be lower on low-risk patients. Risk factors include urgent status, advanced age, female sex, DM, poor EF, CHF, preoperative renal dysfunction, PVD, pulmonary disease, and left main disease.

Redo CABG

Redo CABG operations are becoming more common but convey an increased risk than primary operations. Some accepted indications for redo CABG are:

- Significant stenoses on vein grafts to the LAD or multiple vein grafts, especially among patients with abnormal LV function, a positive stress test, and myocardium in jeopardy

- Highly symptomatic patients with severe stenoses on grafts supplying viable myocardium

The use of PCI vs. CABG for patients with a prior CABG is unclear and should be individualized depending on anatomy, symptoms, and comorbidities.

Preoperative workup on these patients should include: coronary angiography, angiography of IMA vessels (if intended to be used), copy of the prior operative report, myocardial viability studies, venous and/or arterial conduit vascular studies to assess possible grafts, and a CT scan of the chest to assess anatomy.

Intraoperatively, manipulation of the grafts should be avoided during dissection of the heart ("no touch" technique) to avoid embolization of debris. A patent IMA graft should be clamped, if possible, for optimal myocardial protection. Retrograde cardioplegia should be used in most cases.

Diseased vein grafts should be replaced with other vein grafts. If an arterial graft will be used to replace a vein graft, the arterial graft should be added but the previous vein graft left intact, as long as the stenosis on the previous vein graft is > 50% (to avoid competitive flow). The distal anastomoses of the new grafts should be performed directly to the native coronary vessel. Proximal anastomoses may be performed to the hood of new or old vein grafts.

Mortality after redo CABG is approximately 3-8%, with the most common cause of mortality being perioperative MI.

40. Mechanical complications of coronary artery disease

Leo M. Gazoni

While the incidence of mechanical complications after MI is uncommon, these complications account for 15-20% of deaths after acute MI. Such complications are less common with improving medical management and catheter based interventions.

Free wall ventricular rupture

Incidence, pathogenesis, and presentation

Free wall ventricular rupture occurs in 2 to 4% of patients presenting with an acute MI and accounts for up to 10% of associated MI related death. Rupture tends to occur at the junction of viable and necrotic myocardium. Patients with rupture commonly have persistent (> 4-6 hours) chest pain, ST elevation (transmural process), and uncontrolled hypertension. Acute rupture uniformly results in severe hypotension from cardiac tamponade and subsequent electromechanical dissociation and death. The term "subacute" rupture is occasionally used and essentially represents cases that do not result in immediate death and offer the opportunity for surgical rescue.

Diagnosis and treatment

When patient status allows for it, echocardiography is used for diagnosis. In subacute forms of free wall rupture, pericardiocentesis can help temporize the patient's hemodynamic status while preparing an operating room. Repair is performed under CPB. Successful repair requires the suturing of healthy myocardium, most commonly with a horizontal mattress buttressed with pledgets. A pericardial, Dacron, or PTFE patch can also be used in an epicardial repair. An IABP is commonly necessary for preoperative stabilization and/or for weaning off CPB.

Post-infarction VSD

Without surgery, 50% of patients with post-infarction VSD will die within 24 hours, and 80% will die within 4 weeks. Approximately 7% of patients live longer than one year. Post-infarct VSDs have the following distribution: apical 20%, anterior 50%, and posteroinferior 30%. LAD occlusions causing anterior/septal MI result in anterior and apical defects. In about 1/3 of patients, the rupture occurs in the posterior septum after an inferior septal infarction. The posterior papillary muscle is often involved in a posterior post-infarction septal defect.

Diagnosis and treatment

Patients with a post-infarct VSD classically have a harsh holosystolic murmur radiating to the axilla. On right heart catheterization there is a step-up in the oxygen saturation between the RA and PA. Currently, Doppler echocardiography can most definitively demonstrate the size and location of the VSD. Echocardiography can also delineate associated mitral valve pathology. The presence of a post-infarct VSD is enough of an indication for an operation. Determining who would benefit from surgery proves to be difficult. Cardiogenic shock in the setting of a post-infarct VSD is a surgical emergency. Often, IABP placement will be required prior to operative intervention. If the patient is already in multi-system organ failure and survival from emergent surgery is highly unlikely, a mechanical bridge or catheter closure can salvage the occasional patient for surgery in a more stable state in the future. Less than 5% of patients can be totally stable and undergo surgery on a semi-elective basis. Operative mortality ranges from 30% to 50%. Mortality after surgical intervention is caused by a low cardiac output state half of the time and by recurrent or residual VSD a quarter of the time. While a residual defect in an unstable patient should be imminently addressed, delayed repair is favored in a hemodynamically stable patient with a residual VSD. Long-term survival is most commonly quoted between 40 to 60%.

Medical management

Medical management revolves around the reduction of the left-to-right shunt by reducing systemic vascular resistance and LV pressure. Placement of an IABP is usually helpful. Percutaneous closure rarely works as the adjacent muscle is fragile and the mitral valve and papillary muscles are in close proximity.

Surgical management

Pre-operative coronary imaging does not convey a survival benefit, as revascularization of full-thickness infarcted tissues is not helpful. When possible, necrotic tissue should be debrided and sutures placed through non-infarcted tissue to maximize suture-line integrity. Perhaps the key principle in surgical intervention is minimizing tension. Prosthetic material is crucial in achieving this end. Small anterior and apical defects can be closed by suturing the free wall of the RV and LV with the septum. The defect is approached by incising the ventricle through the area of the scar. Usually the defect is too large and a prosthetic patch should be used to close the VSD. The LV is then closed in 2 layers with pledgets. Posteroinferior VSDs are the most difficult to fix. The incision is made through the infarcted area on the LV side of the posterior descending coronary artery. In order two minimize tension, 2 patches have to commonly be used, one for the VSD and the other to close the LV.

Perioperative management

If an IABP has not yet been placed, it will almost be universally necessary to wean off CPB. After separating from CPB, right heart failure is more common with posterior defects. PGE_1 and/or inhaled nitric oxide can be helpful in this setting.

Papillary muscle rupture

As with free wall rupture and post-infarct VSDs, the incidence of acute papillary muscle rupture is decreasing with early reperfusion therapy. The posterior papillary muscle is more susceptible to rupture. Unlike the anterior papillary muscle, which is supplied by both the LAD and diagonals, the posterior papillary muscle is supplied by the RCA or circumflex. A new systolic murmur in conjunction with cardiovascular collapse several days after MI should raise the suspicion of papillary muscle rupture. An echocardiogram confirms the diagnosis. IABP commonly helps stabilize the patient. Emergent mitral valve replacement is most commonly undertaken with appropriate coronary revascularization. There are rare circumstances where the papillary muscle can be re-implanted or where neo-chords can be used.

41. Left ventricular aneurysms
Leo M. Gazoni

LV aneurysms are the result of remodeling after MI. Regional contraction is affected by the remodeling. Systolic and diastolic dysfunction results in heart failure. An LV aneurysm in the setting of CHF, embolism, or arrhythmia is an indication for surgery. Surgical ventricular reconstruction (SVR) refers to operations that decrease LV volume and attempt to reestablish the normal geometrical configuration of the ventricle.

Diagnostics

Preoperatively, CAD and MR should be quantified via cardiac catheterization and echocardiography, respectively. Revascularization strategies should be determined preoperatively. 2+ or greater MR is usually surgically addressed with a mitral valve ring as MR usually results from annular dilatation and/or posterior papillary muscle displacement. It is also important to determine the location of the akinetic area and the size of the LV. MRI is becoming more common in delineating the aforementioned anatomy as well as providing information regarding viable myocardium. The aneurysm is classically delineated by thinning of the anterior wall and apex. Ventriculograms are still common and already part of the necessary cardiac catheterization. To benefit from surgery, the patient should not have severe RV dysfunction or too small a LV cavity such that volume reduction would compromise stroke volume.

Surgical intervention

As a ventriculotomy will be performed, the anatomy of the coronary arteries should be well visualized. Once the cross-clamp is applied and LV vent is on, the akinetic segment along the anterior wall will dimple. It is important to minimize LV manipulation prior to the application of the cross clamp as one can dislodge an LV thrombus.

If needed, coronary revascularization is performed first. The LV is then opened, parallel and lateral to the LAD (1-3cm from the LAD). Thrombus, if present, is cleared from the LV and the scar is identified. The major difficulty in the procedure is determining the location of the Fontan stitch, which effectively reduces the volume of the LV. Some advocate the placement of a balloon, 50 mL/m² BSA, in the LV while others use intraoperatively TEE to guide the placement of the Fontan stitch. The Fontan stitch is a 2-0 Prolene suture placed in a running circular fashion in the endocardium at the junction of viable myocardium and scar. The

Fontan stitch is then cinched down such that the volume is reduced but the opening is not closed. The opening itself is closed with a circular piece of Dacron, and the ventriculotomy is then closed over the defect in two layers.

Outcomes

Several studies have supported the benefits of SVR. Long term survival and symptoms are improved as is EF and the incidence of ventricular arrhythmias. The RESTORE (Reconstructive Endoventricular Surgery returning Torsion Original Radius Elliptical shape the LV) group published the most well known study related to SVR. In this study, EF, NYHA class, and LV end systolic volume improved postoperatively. Of note, 95% and 22% of patients underwent concomitant CABG and mitral valve repair, respectively. Preoperative risk factors that increase long-term mortality include older age, degree of CHF, EF < 35%, cardiomegaly, LV end-diastolic pressure > 20 mmHg, and presence of MR. The degree of residual myocardial function is important to determine overall improvement after surgery.

The recent STICH (Surgical Treatment for Ischemic Heart Failure) trial has called into question the utility of SVR. This study compared CABG to CABG + SVR in a randomized controlled trial. After 48 months, the study demonstrated no difference in the primary outcomes of death and cardiac related hospitalizations between SVR + CABG versus CABG alone. This study has been largely criticized.

42. Combined carotid and coronary artery surgery
Stephen H. McKellar

Atherosclerosis occurs throughout the body and has different clinical manifestations. In coronary arteries, it can present as chronic, stable angina or MI. In carotid arteries, it can present as a transient ischemic attack (TIA) or stroke. In the peripheral arteries, it can present as claudication or chronic limb ischemia. Given the disease process is the same, up to 15% of patients with clinical manifestations in one location are harboring subclinical, or concomitantly clinical manifestations of the disease. This chapter will focus on the clinical decision making involved in treating patients with atherosclerosis in both carotid and coronary arteries.

Pathophysiology

The vascular risk factors of hypertension, hyperlipidemia, tobacco use, and increasing age play important roles in disease of both the coronary and cerebral arterial beds. In addition, the presence of atherosclerosis in one location is associated disease in other locations. Risk factor modification is beneficial in treating carotid and CAD.

The presence of both diseases dramatically increases perioperative risk for patients undergoing either CABG or carotid endarterectomy (CEA). The presence of carotid artery disease increases the risk of perioperative stroke in patients undergoing CABG. Similarly, the presence of CAD increases the risk of perioperative MI in patients undergoing CEA.

It is important to note that carotid artery disease is only one of the causes of perioperative stroke during CABG. Carotid stenosis is implicated in cerebral hypoperfusion (cerebral perfusion pressure < 60 mmHg during CPB). Additional causes include atherosclerotic embolism from aortic manipulation (clamping, cannulating). MI during CEA is attributed to the hemodynamic strain and instability associated with general anesthesia, which can theoretically be minimized by performing CEA without general anesthesia.

Diagnosis

A detailed history and physical examination are important for diagnosis of both carotid and CAD. Symptoms suggestive of TIAs, or strokes, or angina pectoris should direct further investigation. Of note, studies have found that increasing age, female gender, PVD, history of stroke or TIA, smoking history, DM, and left main coronary disease are independent predictors of concomitant, severe, carotid artery disease in patients preparing for CABG. EKG and pharmacologic stress echocardiography are useful initial screening tests for CAD. If positive, coronary angiography is needed to diagnose flow-limiting stenoses. Similarly, carotid duplex ultrasonography is useful in detecting asymptomatic carotid artery disease, particular in patients with carotid bruit on physical exam. Duplex ultrasonography is sufficient to make the diagnosis of carotid artery disease in most patients. In general, CEA is indicated for patients with asymptomatic carotid stenosis > 70% and for symptomatic patients > 50% with the greatest benefit among patients with higher-grade stenoses and/or ulcerated plaques. In patients with equivocal duplex studies or high (distal) lesions CT or MRA can be useful.

Treatment

There are several options for treating combined severe carotid and coronary occlusive disease but no clinical guidelines to direct clinical decisions. Options include staged carotid and coronary operations (CEA followed by CABG), reversed staged (CABG followed by CEA), and combined (simultaneous) CEA and CABG. It is important to note that carotid artery stenting and PCI are also beginning to be used in this setting but little data exists about their efficacy.

The decision about staged versus reversed staged intervention is usually based on which lesion is most symptomatic. For example, patients presenting with acute coronary syndrome should undergo coronary revascularization prior to carotid artery intervention. Similarly, patients presenting with TIA or crescendo TIA should be offered carotid surgery prior to coronary revascularization. The combined risk of stroke or MI with staged or reversed staged procedures is reported to be around 3%. The decision becomes more complicated in patients with chronic stable angina and concomitant high grade lesion(s) or unilateral or bilateral internal carotid artery occlusion. Unfortunately, there are no well-established guidelines.

Combined CEA and CABG is often reserved for patients who are at high risk for either staged or reversed staged intervention due to increased risk of stroke and MI (often reported around 6%). This increased risk is likely a marker of higher-risk patients with more severe disease rather than the two operations *per se*. Better studies are needed to clarify this issue. Carotid artery stenting may be most applicable for this high-risk cohort. During combined intervention, CEA is usually performed with minimal systemic heparinization while the conduits for CABG are being harvested. The neck incision is usually left open during CPB and then closed over a drain after protamine administration.

43. Aortic valve disease

Ravi K. Ghanta, Bryan M. Burt

Anatomy and pathophysiology

The aortic valve is a tricuspid semilunar valve that allows unidirectional flow from the LV to the aorta when LV pressure exceeds aortic pressure. Aortic stenosis (AS) or insufficiency (AI) affects an estimated 700,000 people in the United States requiring 70,000 aortic valve replacements (AVR) per year.

Key surgical anatomy includes an understanding of the relationship of the aortic valve to the coronary arteries, atrioventricular (AV) conduction system, membranous septum, and mitral valve. The three semilunar valve cusps are termed the left, right, and non-coronary cusps based on their position relative to the coronary ostia. The cusps have a parabolic attachment to the aorta creating the Sinuses of Valsalva between the cusps and the aortic wall. The junction points between the cusps are termed commisures. Although there is no true aortic annulus, the valve cusps are supported by a fibrous skeleton that is in continuity with the anterior leaflet of the mitral valve between the left and non-coronary valve cusps. The AV conduction system lies between the right and non-coronary cusps. The membranous septum can be found below the right coronary cusp.

Pathology of the aortic valve results in stenosis and/or insufficiency. AS increases LV afterload during systole resulting in increased LV pressure and wall stress. Over time, AS leads to LV remodeling and hypertrophy. The etiologies for AS are calcific degeneration (most common), congenital valve abnormality (i.e. bicuspid valve), or rheumatic heart disease. The main symptoms of AS are: angina, syncope, and CHF. If untreated, death may ensue from LV failure. The interval from onset of symptoms to death tends to be 2 years for CHF, 3 years for syncope, and 5 years for angina.

AI results in regurgitant flow from the aorta into the LV during diastole. Acute AI leads to decreased cardiac output and heart failure. Progressive, chronic AI results in progressive LV dilation, elevated wall stress, and heart failure. Prognosis of patients with chronic AI is determined by symptom status and LV size and function. Insufficiency is secondary to poor valve cusp coaptation due to valve cusp pathology or a dilated aortic root.

Grading

AS is graded by echocardiography (most common) or cardiac catheterization to estimate the aortic valve area (AVA) using mean aortic flow (AF), the transvalvular gradient (AVG), and the Gorlin Formula (that uses cardiac output, systolic ejection period, heart rate, and mean gradient to calculate AVA). Valve gradient can easily be calculated from the peak blood velocity measured by Doppler using the simplified Bernoulli equation (pressure gradient (mmHg) = 4 x peak velocity (m/s) squared). In addition, the continuity equation can be used to calculate AVA based on cross-sectional area (cm^2) and velocity (cm/s) of the blood at the LVOT, and velocity of blood at the aortic valve.

AS is graded as mild (AVA > 1.5 cm^2), moderate (1-1.5 cm^2), or severe (< 1 cm^2). An important caveat to this grading system is that patients may have severe anatomic AS but have low flow and low gradient due to poor ventricular function. In these patients, the calculated AVA by the Gorlin formula will underestimate their disease. Use of the continuity equation or dobutamine stress echocardiography (allowing estimation of valve area and gradient at a higher cardiac output) may be useful for these patients.

AI is graded by echocardiography based on the severity of the regurgitant jet. Severe AI is defined by a regurgitant fraction $\geq$ 50%, vena contracta width (narrowest diameter of the flow stream) > 6 mm, regurgitant volume $\geq$ 60 mL, jet width / LVOT $\geq$ 65%, and an effective regurgitant orifice (ERO) area $\geq$ 0.3 cm^2.

Surgical indications

All symptomatic patients with AS should undergo AVR. Symptoms include syncope, angina, or dyspnea. AVR is also indicated in asymptomatic patients with severe AS with LV systolic dysfunction or those undergoing cardiac surgery for coronary or other valvular heart disease. For other asymptomatic patients, recommendations regarding AVR are controversial. According to the 2006 ACC/AHA guidelines,[1] AVR may be considered in asymptomatic patients with AVA < 0.6 cm^2, mean gradient > 60 mmHg, rapidly progressing disease resulting in severe AS, and mild AS with moderate to severe calcification at time of CABG.

For patients with AI, AVR is indicated for symptomatic patients with severe AI, asymptomatic patients with severe AI and LV dysfunction or severe LV dilatation, and patients with severe AI undergoing other cardiac surgical procedures. Patients with acute-onset AI should also be operated on to avoid decompensation.

The bicuspid aortic valve

Bicuspid aortic valve (BAV) disease is a disease of the aortic valve and the aorta. It is present in 2% of the population and does not shorten life expectancy. Bicuspid aortic valves usually have three Sinuses of Valsalva and two cusps due to the fusion of two of the leaflets (most commonly the right and the left coronary cusps). Symptoms usually present with valve pathology in the 5th to 6th decades of life. According to 2006 ACC/AHA guidelines,[1] surgical indications for BAV are similar to tricuspid aortic valve disease. During AVR for BAV, aortic replacement should be performed if aortic diameter is greater than 4.5 cm.

Choice of prosthesis

Valve replacement devices are characterized by their effective orifice area (EOA), device profile (or size), durability, and thromboembolism risk. The calculus of prosthesis choice is a function of anatomy (annular size, location of coronaries), hemodynamic requirements (EOA, supra-annular position), valve availability, and patient preferences. Undersizing the valve results in patient prosthesis mismatch (PPM), which may increase morbidity and mortality and fail to alleviate symptoms. Maintaining an EOA to BSA ratio of 0.85 cm^2/m^2 minimizes the risk of PPM-related morbidity. Profile height may limit replacement options depending on coronary orifice position.

Enlargement of the aortic root may be necessary in order to avoid PPM. In adults, the aortic root is usually enlarged up to 4 mm using the Manougian technique (extending the aortotomy incision through the commissure between left and non-coronary cusps and enlarging the root with a patch) or the Nicks technique (similar to the Manougian technique but extending the incision through the non-coronary cusp). The Konno procedure is used more commonly in children and involves making a vertical aortotomy (instead of a horizontal one) and extending it downwards through the right Sinus of Valsalva, just to the left of the RCA orifice, and into the RVOT with incision of the ventricular septum.

Table 43-1 indicates prosthesis options, advantages, and disadvantages. In general, bioprosthetic valves have less durability, higher profiles, and lower EOA than mechanical valves. Mechanical valves, however, have a higher thromboembolism risk than bioprosthetic valves and require permanent anticoagulation. Bioprosthetic valves are composed of fixed biologic tissue (pericardium or porcine valve) on stent. The presence of the stent increases valve profile, decreases EOA, and increases transvalvular gradient. This has spurred development of stentless bioprosthetic valves, which are usually fixed tissue derived from porcine aortic roots. Placement involves replacement of the entire valve apparatus and sometimes the entire aortic root. Technical complexity with this operation has limited its use.

Table 43-1. Overview of AVR options.

Prosthesis	Description	Advantages	Disadvantages	Lifespan
Mechanical	Caged Ball, Tilting Disk, Bileaflet*	Higher EOA Lower Gradient Best Durability Easiest Insertion	Anticoagulation Increased Noise	Lifetime
Stented Bio-prosthetic	Porcine Pericardial*	High EOA Low Gradient Low thromboembolism	Durability Higher profile	~15 years
Stentless Bioprosthetic	Porcine Aortic Root Homograft	Highest EOA Lowest Gradient Low thromboembolism Lowest infection risk	Technical complexity Durability Availability	~15 years
Autograft	Pulmonic Valve	Highest EOA Lowest Gradient Low thromboembolism Lowest infection risk Growth	Technical complexity Two valve replacements	~20 years

* Most common option. EOA: Effective orifice area.

The Ross procedure

First performed in 1967, the Ross Procedure involves replacement of the aortic valve with an autograft of the patient's own pulmonary valve followed by homograft replacement of the pulmonary valve. The primary advantages of the Ross procedure are favorable hemodynamics and the capacity for growth, making this a promising option for younger patients. The procedure may be performed with or without aortic root replacement. The primary disadvantages are technical complexity and requirement for pulmonic valve replacement. Care should be placed not to injure the LAD and the first septal perforator branch during the removal of the pulmonary root. Up to 30% of patients may develop hemodynamically significant pulmonic valve homograft stenosis. At present, use of the Ross procedure is declining with an estimated 200 procedures performed in 2000 according to the International Ross Registry.

Outcomes of AVR

Mortality after AVR is approximately 2-5%. Risk factors include advanced age, low EF, CHF, CAD, renal failure, endocarditis, female gender, emergent operation, concomitant surgery, and previous heart surgery. Causes of early mortality include MI or cardiac failure, hemorrhage, infection, arrhythmias, and stroke.

Late complications include:

- *Thromboembolic events* (1% per patient-year with bioprostheses and 2% for mechanical valves)

- *Significant bleeding* (0.3% per patient-year for bioprostheses and 2-3% for mechanical valves)

- *Structural valve deterioration.* Rate of deterioration is inversely proportional to patient's age. Current generation bioprosthetic valves have a 90% freedom of deterioration at 12 years with a high increase in deterioration rates after 15 years.

- *Paravalvular leak* (0.2-0.5%)

- *Hemolysis* (rare)

44. Tricuspid valve repair and replacement

Lucas M. Duvall

Anatomy

The tricuspid valve is a tri-leaflet valve located near the entrance to right side of the heart. Because of this, many of the symptoms related to tricuspid disease are extracardiac. The three leaflets are 1) septal, 2) anterior, and 3) posterior. They are separated by three clefts, or commissures, that do not extend to the annulus and thus have small "commissural leaflets". The leaflets are typically attached to three papillary muscles: anterior, posterior, and septal (absent in 20%). Ancillary anatomic considerations include the close proximity to the coronary sinus, the conducting system near the base of the septal leaflet, the relationship to the membranous septum, central fibrous body and the RCA.

Pathophysiology

For the purposes of this review, pathologies will be classified as either tricuspid regurgitation or tricuspid stenosis. The disease processes can be organic or functional. Organic tricuspid disease includes: infective endocarditis (*S. aureus*), rheumatic fever, degenerative (myxomatous), traumatic injury, postinfarction damage, carcinoid (characteristic retracted leaflets), SLE (inflammatory disorders), and tumors. The tricuspid valve is the valve most commonly affected by carcinoid disease. Functional tricuspid regurgitation usually involves annular dilation, primarily along the attachments of the anterior and posterior leaflets, and dysfunction. Most commonly, this results from an underlying left sided valvular heart disease. Carpentier devised a classification of three types of disease based on leaflet mobility:

- *Type I.* Normal motion with annular dilation

- *Type II.* Increased leaflet motion due to prolapsed from chordal rupture or elongation

- *Type III.* Reduced leaflet motion due to thickening, fused commissures or tethering.

Diagnosis

Tricuspid regurgitation manifests with weakness and fatigue related to reduction in cardiac output. Right-sided failure will lead to ascites, jugular venous distention (JVD), hepatosplenomegaly, peripheral edema and atrial fibrillation. Later sequelae include cardiac cachexia, cyanosis and jaundice. On exam, an S_3 may be auscultated as well as a parasternal pansystolic murmur. CXR may demonstrate RA and RV enlargement, pleural effusion and a prominent azygos vein. Cardiac catheterization will demonstrate elevated right-sided pressures and "ventricularization" of the RA tracing.

Echocardiography remains the gold-standard. Severity of regurgitation can be based on the height of the regurgitant jet into the RA. A jet of 2 cm is mild, 3-5 cm is moderate, and > 5 cm or reversal of hepatic vein flow is severe. The proximal iso-velocity surface area (PISA) radius can also be useful. A radius of 1-4mm, 5-8mm, or >9mm relates to mild, moderate, and severe regurgitation. Echocardiography is also very useful in evaluating transvalvular gradients, structural abnormalities, and other etiologies of right heart failure.

Tricuspid stenosis is usually related to rheumatic disease, and remains an absolute indication for replacement over repair. More often than not there is a component of regurgitation. Clinical features are consistent with reduced cardiac output. Fatigue, malaise, JVD, hepatomegaly, peripheral edema and atrial fibrillation can all occur. The underfilling of the left heart may mask additional mitral disease. CXR reveals an enlarged RA. EKG will show prominent P-waves, assuming sinus rhythm. Echocardiography will reveal an elevated transvalvular gradient, reduced leaflet mobility, reduced orifice of flow, chordal shortening, thickening of the leaflets, fusion along the leaflet edges and calcific deposits on the valve.

Surgical treatment

The indication for surgery for tricuspid valve disease should be determined by the severity of the lesions and its reparability. Severe lesions warrant surgery, whether repair or replacement. Moderate lesions should be treated if repair is expected. This, of course, is subject to debate and relies heavily on a precise preoperative diagnosis.

The tricuspid valve is visualized via a midline sternotomy or a right thoracotomy. Bicaval cannulation strategy is endorsed, with an atrial incision beginning at the appendage and directed toward the posterior aspect of the atrium between the IVC and the right inferior pulmonary vein. The procedure can be done in the beating heart, under fibrillation or full arrest.

Advanced techniques such as chordal resuspension, neo-cords, triangular resections and patching of leaflet perforations can be done as in mitral disease, but the bulk of operative interventions are done secondary to functional disease, essentially annular dilation. Bicuspidization involves suture plication of mild annular dilation by obliterating the posterior leaflet. A double pledgeted nonabsorbable suture is placed from the anteroposterior commissure to the posteroseptal commissure and tied. An annuloplasty ring is then often placed for further support. The DeVega suture annuloplasty involves a single running suture along the annulus from the anteroseptal commissure to the posteroseptal commissure and back with a pledget at either end. The suture is then cinched down and tied, providing the appropriate reduction.

Significant degrees of reduction are often best accomplished with rigid rings, flexible rings or partial bands. The length and size of the septal leaflet and its base determine the ring size. These devices involve placing sutures through the annulus and the fabric of the prosthetic. The plication is mostly along the length of the posterior leaflet. Suture placement is avoided at the AV node region (apex of the triangle of Koch) to prevent conduction injury. Clinical experience has shown that risk factors for worsening regurgitation include poor LV function, permanent pacemaker, higher degree of preoperative regurgitation, and repair type other than ring annuloplasty.

Tricuspid valve replacement is reserved for situations in which the valve cannot be repaired with satisfactory results. Replacement of the valve is not unlike the technique for mitral valve replacement. Choices for replacement include homografts, stented porcine or pericardial valves, or a mechanical valve. Porcine and pericardial valves are the most common used. The valve leaflets are left in place to preserve the subvalvar apparatus. The durability of bioprosthetic valves is an issue. Mechanical valves are extremely durable, but the risks of anticoagulation must be addressed.

Heart block is a known complication and a reason that mechanical valves can be less desirable. If a permanent pacemaker is required, the ventricular lead across a mechanical valve is not generally well tolerated. Furthermore, pannus formation on the ventricular side of the valve can limit the long term effectiveness of the valve.

45. Mitral regurgitation

Tom C. Nguyen

Background

MR is defined as retrograde flow from the LV into the LA due to impaired systolic coaptation between the anterior and posterior mitral leaflets.

Causes of MR are broadly grouped as ischemic or non-ischemic. Mechanisms of MR are grossly classified as "functional" (i.e. structurally normal mitral valve) or "organic" (i.e. intrinsic valve abnormality). The mechanisms of functional MR can be further broken down according to Carpentier's classification based on leaflet coaptation and leaflet or chordal motion:

- *Type I:* mitral annular dilatation with normal mitral leaflets

- *Type II:* leaflet prolapse or excess motion

- *Type IIIa:* leaflet restriction on systole and diastole from leaflet or chordal retraction or thickening

- *Type IIIb:* leaflet restriction or tethering on diastole from papillary muscle displacement

The major cause of MR in western countries is degenerative (primary myxomatous disease, primary flail leaflets, annular calcifications) representing 60-70% of cases, followed by ischemic MR (20%), endocarditis (2-5%), and rheumatic (2-5%). In developing areas of the world, the leading cause of MR is rheumatic heart disease.

Ischemic MR (IMR) represents a subset of functional MR whereas the mitral leaflets are structurally normal and disease is due to ischemic injury to the myocardium. Leaflet closing forces are reduced due to LV systolic dysfunction. After acute MI, 17% to 55% of patients develop a mitral systolic murmur or echocardiographic evidence of IMR. Many of these murmurs, however, are transient and disappear at time of discharge. It is important to distinguish between acute IMR from chronic IMR. Patients with acute IMR often present with hemodynamic distress in which prompt surgery affords the best chance for survival. Chronic IMR represents the majority of patients with IMR in which presentation is more progressive and insidious, often associated with decremental decline in LV function.

Pathophysiology

Patients with MR may be asymptomatic or present with signs of acute severe MR, chronic compensated MR, or chronic decompensated MR. Patients with chronic MR can remain asymptomatic for years. Acute severe MR usually manifests as symptomatic heart failure because the LV is unable to tolerate the sudden increase in volume overload. In patients that survive the insult, LV remodeling ensues, resulting in compensatory changes. The adaptive compensatory changes of the LV to the volume overload include LV dilatation, with new sarcomeres added in series, and resultant eccentric LV hypertrophy. MR can also beget MR. With this phenomenon, progression of MR dilates the LV, which dilates the atrium and mitral annulus, thus worsening the preexisting MR.

In patients with MR, EF may be a misleading measure of LV function. The measured LV EF in chronic MR may be greater than normal because of the increase in preload and afterload-reducing effect of ejection into a low-resistance LA. Significant myocardial dysfunction may exist despite a relatively normal LV EF. Outcomes after mitral valve surgery are, thus, poorer in patients with a preoperative EF < 60%.

Diagnosis

On physical exam, the murmur of MR is usually heard best at the apex with the patient in the left lateral decubitus position. With severe degenerative MR, the murmur is holosystolic radiating to the axilla.

CXR may demonstrate cardiomegaly and/or LA enlargement. On EKG, LA enlargement and/or atrial fibrillation may be seen.

Echocardiography is the most useful study in evaluating MR, yielding insight into the mechanisms and severity, LV function and size, LA size, degree of pulmonary hypertension, presence of associated valvular disease, effective regurgitant orifice (ERO), and regurgitant volume. Severe MR is characterized by a vena contracta width (narrowest diameter of the jet flow) $\geq$ 0.7 cm, ERO $\geq$ 0.4 cm2, regurgitant volume $\geq$ 60 mL, regurgitant fraction $\geq$ 50%, and a jet area > 40% of LA area.

Surgical indications

In general, mitral surgery for MR is reserved for patients with symptoms or asymptomatic patients with evidence of LV dysfunction, new onset atrial fibrillation, or pulmonary hypertension. Isolated mitral surgery is not indicated for patients with mild or moderate MR.

Based on the 2008 ACC/AHA Guidelines,[1] mitral valve operation is indicated (Class I) in:

- Symptomatic patients with acute severe MR

- Patients with chronic severe MR and NYHA class II, III, or IV, in the absence of severe LV dysfunction (i.e., EF < 30% and/or end-systolic dimension (ESD) > 55mm)

- Asymptomatic patients with chronic severe MR and mild-moderate LV dysfunction (EF 30-60% and/or ESD ≥ 40mm)

Mitral surgery is reasonable (Class IIa) in:

- Asymptomatic patients with chronic severe MR and preserved LV function (EF > 60% and ESD < 40 mm) in experienced surgical centers, in whom the likelihood of success is > 90%

- Asymptomatic patients with chronic severe MR, preserved LV function, and new onset atrial fibrillation or pulmonary hypertension (PA systolic pressure > 50mmHg at rest or > 60mmHg with exercise)

- Patients with chronic severe MR due to a primary abnormality of the mitral apparatus and NYHA class III-IV symptoms and severe LV dysfunction in whom MV repair is highly likely

Mitral repair may also be considered (Class IIb) for patients with chronic severe secondary MR due to severe LV dysfunction who have persistent NYHA class III-IV symptoms despite optimal therapy for CHF, including biventricular pacing.

Treatment

Mitral repair is preferred over mitral replacement if technically feasible, likelihood of a successful result, and if performed in experienced hands at a high volume center. Patients undergoing repair have an improved survival when compared to those having replacement (10-year survival of 68% vs. 52%, respectively). To consider whether a patient is a candidate for mitral repair, a Wilkins Score may be used, with components that include leaflet mobility, leaflet thickening, and leaflet calcification. Scores less than 8 and no more than mild MR have the best prognosis.

Basic techniques for mitral valve reconstruction include annuloplasty rings, quadrangular or triangular resection of the posterior leaflet, chordal transposition, chordal shortening, artificial chordae, and triangular resection of the anterior leaflet. The use of each particular technique depends on the anatomy of the valve. An annuloplasty ring should be used as part of every repair.

Posterior leaflet prolapse is traditionally treated with a quadrangular resection. However, triangular resections and artificial chords have been used successfully. When the posterior leaflet prolapse occurs from excessive tissue in Barlow's disease, the best strategy is a quadrangular resection of P2 and a sliding plasty of P1 and P3 to avoid postoperative systolic anterior motion (SAM) of the mitral valve leading to LVOT obstruction. *Commissural prolapse* can be treated with either a commissuroplasty or a resection of the prolapsed area with sliding plasty. The most common strategies to treat *anterior leaflet prolapse* include: triangular resection, placement of artificial chords, chordal transfer from the posterior to the anterior leaflet, and less frequently chordal or papillary muscle shortening.

In some situations, mitral valve repair is not possible and replacement is necessary (e.g., heavy calcification of the leaflets and subvalvar apparatus from rheumatic disease, extensive leaflet destruction). In these cases, it is important to try to preserve the posterior leaflet and its chordal attachments in order to preserve LV shape and function.

Left atriotomy is the most common technique to expose the mitral valve, but a trans-septal approach can also be employed via a right atriotomy followed by a trans-septal incision in patients with a reoperation, aortic prosthesis, a small LA, or if access is difficult. The latter approach may divide the artery to the sinus node and thus affect sinus node function.

Minimally invasive surgery (MIS) for mitral disease may also be employed with absolute mortality and morbidity similar to open techniques. Postoperative atrial fibrillation, renal failure, and respiratory complications are the same with MIS, however some studies indicate increased aortic, neurologic, and embolic complications. Transfusion requirements and wound infections are lower for MIS, while postoperative incidence of pleural effusion is higher. Contraindications to MIS include severe aortoiliac disease, previous right thoracotomy, and severe COPD.

There are several potential injuries/complications from mitral valve surgery including injury to the circumflex artery and coronary sinus injury. However, the most dreaded complication is atrioventricular groove disruption, which involves separation between the LA and ventricle. This can occur with elevation of the LV following mitral replacement and is more common if the mitral annulus is calcified, in women, and in the elderly. If this occurs, most advocate reinstitution of CPB, cardioplegic arrest, and internal repair using a pericardial patch followed by implantation of a low profile mechanical prosthesis.

SAM is another adverse sequelae following mitral valve repair where the anterior mitral leaflet obstructs the LVOT due to a coaptation point that is displaced towards the LVOT. There is an increased risk of SAM with redundant leaflet tissue, a small annuloplasty ring, and long posterior leaflet that can push the anterior leaflet into the LVOT. SAM can also occur in patients with Hypertrophic Obstructive Cardiomyopathy (HOCM) and in patients after MI. Diagnosis is established by echocardiography by visualizing the anterior mitral leaflet extend into the LVOT during systole. The LV often appears small and septal bulging may be present. The initial management of SAM involves volume loading to fully expand the LV (minimizing LVOT obstruction) and treatment of tachyarrhythmias with beta-blockers. Inotropes should be used with caution since they can narrow the LVOT. Afterload reduction by IABP or drugs can also exacerbate SAM and, thus, should be avoided. If medical therapy is not adequate, surgical intervention involves removal of the annuloplasty ring and subsequent mitral replacement or shortening of the posterior leaflet size, depending on the original surgery. The use of a larger annuloplasty ring may decrease the likelihood of SAM.

46. Mitral stenosis

Tom C. Nguyen

Pathophysiology

Rheumatic fever is the most common cause of mitral stenosis (MS) worldwide with 60% of patients with pure MS reporting a history of exposure. After an episode of rheumatic carditis, the progression of MS is usually slow. Although rare, other causes of MS include congenital anomalies, chest RT, mucopolysaccharidosis, severe mitral annular calcification, and LA myxoma.

Diagnosis

MS can be classified as mild (valve area > 1.5 cm^2, gradient <5 mmHg), moderate (valve area 1.0-1.5 cm^2, gradient 5-10 mmHg), or severe (valve area < 1.0 cm^2, gradient > 10mmHg). Narrowing of the mitral valve orifice decreases LV filling and increases LA and pulmonary venous pressures, which ultimately results in CHF. Patients with MS can present with exertional dyspnea, fatigue, pulmonary edema, atrial fibrillation, and/or an embolic event. Symptoms usually develop when the valve area decreases below 2.5 cm^2 during exercise and below 1.5 cm^2 when at rest.

LA enlargement is the most common finding on CXR in patients with severe MS. A normal EKG is common in early MS, but in advanced MS, the P waves become wide, notched, and shaped like an "M". This finding of "P mitrale" is most common in patients with MS and often prominent in lead II and biphasic V1. Echocardiography remains the primary imaging tool for patients with MS, providing structural insight into the mitral leaflet, mitral annular size, LA size, LV function, degree of pulmonary hypertension, and mitral annular gradient. The anterior mitral leaflet may demonstrate a "hockey stick" deformity due to restricted leaflet motion.

Treatment

Therapeutic options for MS include percutaneous mitral balloon valvotomy (MBV) or mitral valve surgery. MBV has become the first-line treatment for most patients with MS.

Based on the 2008 ACC/AHA Guidelines,[1] MBV is indicated (Class I) in:

- Symptomatic patients with moderate or severe MS and favorable valve morphology, as long as there is no LA thrombus.

- Asymptomatic patients with moderate or severe MS and favorable valve morphology if there is evidence of pulmonary hypertension

(PA systolic pressure > 50 mmHg at rest or > 60 mmHg with exercise), in the absence of LA thrombus.

MBV is reasonable (Class IIa) in symptomatic patients (NYHA class III-IV) with moderate to severe MS who are either not candidates for surgery or are at high risk for surgery.

MBV is contraindicated in patients with moderate-severe MR or LA thrombus.

Mitral valve surgery is indicated (Class I) for symptomatic patients (NYHA class III-IV) with moderate or severe MS when MBV is unavailable, MBV is contraindicated because of LA thrombus despite anticoagulation or concomitant moderate to severe MR, or when there is unfavorable valve morphology for MBV.

47. Combined valve / coronary artery bypass grafting
Ahmet Kilic

A consequence of the advancements in diagnostic and therapeutic interventions on CAD and valvular pathology of the heart has been the referral of older and sicker patients to the cardiac surgeon. The result has been an increase in combined valvular and coronary arterial revascularization procedures. Estimates of concomitant CABG and valvular surgery have ranged between 4-50% of all operative revascularizations in a given institution. The trend of operating on more complex pathology with increased co-morbidities has necessitated better pre-, intra- and post-operative optimization of patients to achieve acceptable outcomes. Currently CABG is most commonly performed with aortic valve repair / replacement (AVR) surgery, followed by CABG and mitral valve repair / replacement (MVR) and finally CABG + AVR/MVR.

Pathophysiology

Aortic valve and CAD
Aortic stenosis leads to LV hypertrophy from pressure overload whereas aortic regurgitation leads to LV failure from volume overload. Common reasons for aortic stenosis are degenerative valve calcification, congenital abnormality of cusp anatomy (bicuspid, unicuspid or quadricuspid) and rheumatic disease. Aortic regurgitation can be a consequence of degenerative valve calcification, bicuspid valve, dilatation of the aortic root, aortic dissection, iatrogenic injury, trauma and endocarditis. Aortic stenosis is the most common physiologic abnormality associated with need for coronary revascularization.

Mitral valve and CAD
The mitral valve is intimately involved with the LV via its chordal attachments to the papillary muscle and hence the LV wall. As a result of this relationship, MR can be secondary to annular dilatation from either ischemic or nonischemic cardiomyopathy. The other most common pathophysiologic pathway for MR is an abnormality in any of the components of the valvular / subvalvular apparatus. Degenerative valve disease (Barlow's disease, Marfan's disease or fibroelastic deficiency), rheumatic heart disease, trauma / iatrogenesis, annular calcification and endocarditis are the leading etiologies. Regardless of the underlying cause of MR, volume overload of the LV ensues with a drop in preload as well as a decrease in afterload.

Mitral stenosis is often cause by rheumatic heart disease and can be classified into mild (valve area ≥ 1.5 cm^2), moderate (1-1.5 cm^2) or severe (<

1.0 cm^2 or transvalvular gradient $\geq$ 10 mm Hg). Pressure overload of the LA ensues with pulmonary arterial hypertension leading to RV dysfunction as well as tricuspid valve regurgitation.

Mitral / aortic valve and CAD

These usually present a little earlier than isolated mitral / CAD or aortic / CAD cases. In the setting of aortic stenosis and CAD, mitral valve repair / replacement is indicated for moderate to severe insufficiency. Insufficiency of both valves with CAD can be sequelae of rheumatic heart disease and it is imperative to determine underlying cardiac function as the presenting symptoms may be irreversible heart failure.

Preoperative evaluation

An assessment of LV function in cases of combined valvular and CABG cases should always be carried out. Along with a thorough history and physical focusing on heart failure, edema and pulmonary hypertension, echocardiographic and angiographic work-up needs to be exhaustive as the intra- and postoperative care will be dictated by the complex interactions between effects of preload, afterload and intrinsic heart function. In select cases, preoperative evaluation should include a myocardial viability study. Patients that have irreversible damage to their ventricular function will be high risk and may not tolerate repair/replacement of their valves and hence not good operative candidates.

Combined coronary arterial bypass grafting and aortic valve surgery

Indications

- Moderate to severe aortic stenosis and CAD

- Rapid progression of transvalvular gradients (>10 mm) in stenosis and CAD

- For regurgitation – err of fixing valve earlier when combined CAD is present as LV failure can lead to a vicious circle with the end point of irreversible heart failure

Operative sequence

1. TEE

2. Aortic and single venous cannula with systemic hypothermia

3. Antegrade / retrograde cardioplegia, LV/root vent. In AI, antegrade cardioplegia should be given directly into the coronary ostia with hand-held catheters after an aortotomy

4. Distal anastomoses except for internal mammary artery (IMA) anastomoses

5. Aortotomy w/AVR and closure of aortotomy

6. IMA anastomoses

7. Proximal anastomoses

Combined coronary arterial bypass grafting and mitral valve surgery

Indications

If patients have irreversible cardiomyopathy with a profound global LV dysfunction with mitral valve regurgitation they should not be operated on as the ventricle will not be able to function with the increase in after-load and inability to use the lower pressure LA as a pop-off. Recently a push towards mitral valve repair whenever feasible has been made with mitral valve replacement reserved for irreparable valves or valves with severe organic dysfunction. All effort should be made regardless of re-pair/replacement to not disturb the annular – papillary muscle relationship to preserve LV geometry / function.

Any mild mitral stenosis (i.e. patient with mitral valve area of $\geq 1.5 \text{cm}^2$) and ischemic MR may be treated with CABG alone whereas moderate functional MR is somewhat controversial and is actively being investigated in clinical trials. Patients with any non-ischemic pathology of the mitral valve leading to MR that is moderate – severe should be treated with MVR at the setting of CABG. Patients with mitral stenosis have increased pulmonary hypertension and a propensity for tricuspid insufficiency with resultant RV dysfunction.

Operative sequence

1. TEE

2. Aortic and bicaval (although some use single) venous cannula with systemic hypothermia

3. Antegrade (optional retrograde) cardioplegia, root vent, then aortotomy. Retrograde cardioplegia if AI

4. Distal anastomoses

5. Left atriotomy vs. biatrial (transseptal) approach with MVR

6. Ablation +/- LA appendage ligation in concomitant atrial fibrillation

7. Dor / remodeling procedure in large akinetic low EF patients

8. IMA anastomoses

9. Proximal anastomoses

Combined coronary arterial bypass grafting and both aortic and mitral valvular surgeries

Indications
As per previous sections.

Operative sequence
1. TEE

2. Aortic and bicaval (although may use single venous) venous cannulation with systemic hypothermia

3. Antegrade (and retrograde with AI) cardioplegia, root vent

4. Distal anastomoses

5. Aortotomy with excision of aortic valve to allow exposure of mitral valve easier and to prevent accidental disruption of mitral valve sutures during aortic valve debridement / excision

6. Left atriotomy / transseptal approach with mitral valve repair/replacement. Leave a vent in place via the left atriotomy to serve as a LV vent for the aortic portion of the procedure

7. Aortic valve replacement

8. IMA anastomoses

9. Proximal anastomoses

48. Endocarditis

Zain Khalpey

Endocarditis is an inflammation of either the heart muscle, the endothelial lining of the heart, the heart valves, or their connective tissue bed. This condition is commonly caused by infectious agents such as bacteria or fungus (infective endocarditis (IE)).

Epidemiology

IE is a relatively uncommon condition in the U.S. with approximately 15,000 cases annually. The incidence of IE worldwide is estimated at 2-10 cases per 100,000 patient years and accounts for 1 in 1,000 hospital admissions. Untreated IE is fatal despite recent advances in diagnosis and therapy.

Over the past several decades the incidence of IE has been stable but the nature of this disease has changed dramatically. IE was previously related to rheumatic heart disease and poor dental hygiene. It is now more commonly found associated with structural heart disease and prosthetic cardiac valves, nosocomial infections due to invasive medical procedures, IV drug abuse and previous episodes of IE, among others. IE is more common among men (2-3:1 male/female ratio) and is associated with increasing age.

Pathophysiology

IE is often associated with pre-existing valvular abnormalities. Congenital or acquired structural damage of heart valves cause turbulent blood flow and ulceration of the valvular endothelium. These endothelial ulcers accumulate thrombus to which the infectious agent adheres. Local inflammation induces downstream inflammatory protein cascades leading to the progressive growth of infected valvular vegetations. In mature vegetations, bacteria often locate below the surface thus becoming protected from antibiotics and phagocytes. The mitral valve is most commonly infected (40%), with the aortic valve next (36%), and multivalvular involvement third. The pulmonary valve is rarely involved.

Causative agents

Many bacteria are causative agents of IE. *Staphylococci* and *Streptococci* are the most commonly identified. For patients with native valves that are not IV drug users, *Streptococcus viridans* is the most common agent, followed by *Staphylococcus* and *Enterococcus*. For IV drug users, *Staphylococcus* is most common, followed by *Streptococcus*, and *Entero-*

coccus. Other less common microorganisms include HACEK organisms (*Hemophilus, Actinobacillus, Cardiobacterium, Eikenella, Kingella*) and fungus. HACEK organisms tend to cause a subacute form of the disease and can be difficult to isolate.

Diagnosis

The diagnosis of IE depends on complete medical history with emphasis on past medical procedures, previous IE, presence of structural heart disease, incidence of IV drug use, and other known risk factors followed by a physical examination of the heart, skin, eyes, dentition, neurologic areas, and sites of any recent medical procedures. New regurgitant heart murmurs occur in 85% of cases. Evidence of new CHF is a poor prognostic finding. Physical signs of small and large emboli in the eye, conjunctivae, skin, and digits are common. Some classic manifestations of IE include splinter hemorrhages (longitudinal dark red streaks under the nails), Janeway lesions (irregular painless small nodes in palms and soles), Osler nodes (tender larger nodes with central pallor in hands and feet) and Roth spots (oval retinal hemorrhages with central pallor).

Laboratory studies include blood cultures (3 done within 1 hour but from 3 separate sites), other blood chemistry studies (polymerase chain reaction analyses), EKG, CXR (CT and/or MRI), and echocardiography (transthoracic vs. transesophageal).

Comprehensive IE diagnosis is based on both microbiologic and endocardial involvement as well as other minor criteria, as shown in Table 48-1 (commonly known as Modified Duke Criteria).

Management

Successful management of IE to facilitate the best possible outcome for the patient involves the use of a multidisciplinary approach including therapy with antimicrobial agents and surgery. The use of such an approach is necessary since only 50% of all IE cases are successfully managed with antibiotic therapy. Surgery is most clearly indicated in patients with life threatening CHF and/or cardiogenic shock.

Antimicrobial treatment is the first-line treatment for IE. Antibiotics should be selected based on the isolated organisms. For patients with suspicion of IE in which no organism has been isolated yet, empiric antibiotics are used. For stable patients with native endocarditis and no history of IV drug use, penicillin and gentamicin are a good combination. If *Staphylococcus* is suspected, such as on IV drug users, nafcillin can be used instead of penicillin. Patients with penicillin allergy, hemodynamically unstable, or that reside in communities with high prevalence of MRSA, vancomycin is used instead of penicillin or nafcillin. Antifungals and/or ampicillin (for HACEK organisms) may be used for patients that show no improvement despite adequate antibiotic treatment.

Table 48-1. Modified Duke Criteria for diagnosis of infective endocarditis *(Adapted with permission from McDonald JR. Acute infective endocarditis. Infect Dis Clin North Am. 2009; 23: 643–664. Copyright W.B. Saunders Co.).*

Definite endocarditis requires 2 major, or 1 major and 3 minor, or 5 minor criteria.	
Possible endocarditis requires 1 major and 1 minor, or 3 minor criteria.	
Major Criteria	
1. Microbiologic evidence of IE	Typical organisms cultured from 2 separate blood cultures: • Viridans streptococci, Staphylococcus aureus, HACEK organism, or Streptococcus bovis, OR • Community-acquired enterococcus in the absence of an alternative primary site of infection
	Persistently positive blood cultures with other organism: • At least 2 positives drawn >12 hours apart, OR • All of 3 or majority of 4, with first and last drawn >1 hour apart • One culture (or phase 1 IgG >1:800) for Coxiella burnetii
2. Evidence of endocardial involvement	Echocardiogram showing: • Oscillating intracardiac mass without alternative explanation, OR • Abscess, OR • New partial dehiscence of a prosthetic valve, OR • New valvular regurgitation
Minor Criteria	
1. Predisposition to infective endocarditis	Previous IE, injection drug use, prosthetic heart valve, or cardiac lesion causing turbulent blood flow
2. Fever >38° C	
3. Vascular phenomenon	Arterial embolism, pulmonary infarct, mycotic aneurysm, intracranial or conjunctival hemorrhage, or Janeway's lesions
4. Immunologic phenomenon	Glomerulonephritis, Osler's nodes, Roth's spots, or rheumatoid factor
5. Microbiologic finding not meeting major criteria	

Indications for surgery

Strict indications for surgery on IE are not standardized. Widely accepted indications include:[1]

- Indications for emergent surgery

    - Acute AI with early closure of the mitral valve

    - Rupture into the pericardium or a heart chamber

- Indications for urgent surgery

    - Heart failure with acute AI or MR

    - Aortic or perivalvular abscess, aneurysm (as defined by echo-cardiography, usually TEE)

    - Valve obstruction

    - Conduction disturbances

    - Ineffective antimicrobial therapy

    - Unstable prosthetic valve

    - Septal perforation

- Indications for elective surgery

    - Progressive paravalvular prosthetic leak

    - Persistent valve dysfunction and infection after 7-10 days of appropriate treatment

    - Fungal endocarditis

Using embolism as an indication for surgery is somewhat controversial, since embolism often exists concurrently with other conditions, such as perivalvular extension or multidrug-resistant microorganisms. Patients have a greater risk of embolizing before the endocarditis is diagnosed and during the first week of antimicrobial treatment. The risk of embolism generally decreases after the second week of antimicrobial treatment. Therefore, the presence of embolism should not be the sole criteria for surgery.

There are several factors associated with increased mortality in patients with *prosthetic* valve endocarditis: CHF, early prosthetic valve endocarditis (commonly defined as < 60 days after valve implantation), *S aureus* infection, and complicated endocarditis (persistent bacteremia, renal failure). Early surgical therapy should be considered on these patients.

Surgical treatment

Surgery for IE involves excision of all infected tissue, reconstruction including repair (preferable) or replacement, and postoperative antibiotic treatment. Surgical techniques vary with the etiology and type of IE as well as its severity. For example, mitral valve repair is indicated for patients with less severe damage, whereas mitral valve replacement is reserved for patients with more severe damage for whom mitral valve repair is not feasible. In patients with IE associated with implantation of pacemakers or cardioverter-defibrillators, the surgical procedure consists of removing the device. Similarly, in patients who have endocarditis associated with placement of prosthetic mitral valves, the infected tissue is removed and valves replaced again. For aortic valve endocarditis, any annular defects are closed with a patch. Most aortic valve endocarditis cases are treated with either a prosthetic valve, aortic homograft, or Ross procedure. Mechanical and bioprosthetic valves have essentially the same risk of reinfection.

Operative mortality for endocarditis ranges from 3-15% depending on the preoperative condition of the patient. Risk factors include CHF, renal failure, age, and Staphylococcus involvement. Recurrence rates are approximately 5-12%.

49. Aortic dissection

J. Chad Johnson, Jason A. Williams

Pathophysiology

Aortic dissection is defined as a physical disruption in the intima of the aorta along with degeneration of the media, which in turn leads to a passage or "false lumen" through which blood abnormally flows. This can result in involvement or compression of distal arterial branches, which can in turn lead to malperfusion or life threatening hemorrhage.

The initiating factor involved in intimal disruption is varied. Direct mechanical causes include trauma or iatrogenic injuries (e.g. cannulation). Other causes of "spontaneous" dissection are less well understood, but theories include repetitive hydrodynamic insult/intimal breakdown due to hypertension, intimal disruption due to atherosclerotic plaque ulceration, and possibly adventitial hemorrhage into the media leading to medial breakdown and erosion into the intima. The greatest area of stress on the aorta is the outer curvature and the majority of intimal disruptions occur on the outer aspect of the ascending aorta and proximal arch. The actual incidence of aortic dissection is difficult to estimate, but it is the most common acute disease process of the aorta.

Intramural hematomas are distinguished from acute dissections by an absence of a definable flap or communication between the true and thrombosed false lumen of the aorta. The etiology of this entity is presumed to be secondary to a rupture of the vasa vasorum with associated intramural hemorrhage.

The causes are variable and a high index of suspicion must be maintained in a patient presenting with symptoms suggestive of aortic dissection. The disorder occurs most commonly in the 6th-7th decades of life and afflicts men approximately twice as often as women. Connective tissue disorders that affect the components of the aortic media (such as Marfan's syndrome, Loeys-Dietz syndrome, and Ehlers-Danlos syndrome) have been shown to have a higher association with aortic dissection. Likewise, hypertension and a bicuspid aortic valve are associated with a higher incidence of aortic dissection than the general population.

Classification

Throughout the last 50 years, multiple classification schemes have been proposed to categorize aortic dissections based on anatomic location and/or involvement. The most commonly referenced are the Stanford and DeBakey systems. The principle component that dictates how a dissection is treated is whether or not it involves the ascending aorta/aortic arch or if involvement is limited to the descending aorta (distal to the left subclavian artery). It is important to note that, from the point of intimal disruption, dissections can propagate in an antegrade or retrograde fashion. Dissections are also further subclassified based on acuity with "acute" referring to symptoms less than 2 weeks and "chronic" referring to symptoms lasting more than 2 weeks.

The two common classification schemes for aortic dissection are:

- *Stanford classification*
    - A: involves the ascending arch
    - B: involves only the descending aorta
- *DeBakey classification*
    - I: involves the ascending aorta and arch
    - II: involves the ascending aorta only
    - III: involves the descending aorta (a: descending only, b: descending and abdominal)

Presentation and clinical features

The symptoms and associated clinical signs associated with aortic dissection depend largely on the presence of extra-aortic hemorrhage or whether aortic branches have been compressed or sheared off. Classically, severe tearing pain in the chest and back are present. If hemorrhage has occurred, hypotension and shock may be seen. If branch vessels have been involved, additional signs may be apparent depending on the specific branches involved (i.e. stroke, acute renal insufficiency, visceral ischemia, etc.). Finally, sudden death may be seen in the case of dissection rupture into the pericardium leading to tamponade.

Diagnosis

It is imperative that an evaluating clinician have a high index of suspicion to make an accurate diagnosis and implement timely intervention in acute aortic dissection. This can be very difficult because this disease process shares similar presenting symptoms with clinical problems that are far more common. Other entities that are often considered first include acute MI or PE.

Once the possibility of aortic dissection has been raised in the differential, evaluation of the aorta should be initiated as soon as possible. While a widened mediastinum may be present on CXR, angiography (CTA or MRA) is typically the preferred diagnostic imaging test; both CT and MRI images can be re-formatted into 3-D reconstructions to better appreciate the anatomy and plan therapeutic intervention. CTA or intraoperative TEE are the preferred diagnostic modalities in the emergent setting.

Treatment

Treatment of aortic dissection depends on whether the ascending aorta/arch is involved as well as the acuity of the process. Typically, presentation of a dissection involving the ascending aorta (i.e., Stanford Type A) is an indication for immediate operative intervention, whereas uncomplicated dissections limited to the descending aorta (i.e., Stanford Type B) are treated medically. Intramural hematomas are treated like the corresponding acute dissections (i.e., Type A managed surgically and Type B medically).

Acutely, Type A dissections are approached with blood pressure control followed by expeditious surgical repair. Exceptions may include patients with irreversible stroke, advanced and debilitating diseases limiting life expectancy, advanced age (> 80 years), and patients with significant complications from the dissection that are not expected to survive the operation.

Surgical therapy is generally via an open approach. The choice of approach is influenced by the expertise available at a given medical center, associated valvular or coronary artery abnormalities caused by the dissection, and the proximity of branch vessels to the intimal tear. The principle goals of operative repair include excision/exclusion of the intimal tear to arrest further propagation of the dissection, replacement of the ascending aorta to prevent rupture, resuspension of the aortic valve to address associated aortic valve insufficiency, possible replacement of the aortic arch in cases of malperfusion of the great vessels, and repair or bypass of involved coronary arteries (usually the right as left main coronary involvement is usually fatal).

It should be noted that Type A dissections that involve the descending aorta and more distal branches can result in malperfusion syndromes even after operative repair of the ascending aorta and arch. For situations where a single lower extremity is affected, a femoral-femoral bypass can be performed to restore perfusion to the affected limb. When both lower extremities are involved by the dissection and compromise of perfusion is present bilaterally, axillary-femoral bypass with femoral-femoral bypass or axillary-bifemoral bypass are acceptable options for correction. Malperfusion of visceral vessels can likewise be addressed by percutaneous fenestration techniques. Subjection of the patient to an intra-abdominal revascularization procedure immediately after repair of a Type A dissection is not recommended.

Operative mortality for Type A dissection repair is 10-20%; survival is 55% at 5 years and 37-46% at 10 years after repair. The presence of a persistent false lumen following the repair of a Type A aortic dissection is associated with significant morbidity.

Type B dissections are managed medically. The goal of medical therapy is to control hypertension and prevent propagation of the dissection. This is ideally accomplished in the acute setting using IV agents such as β-blocker agents and the addition of vasodilators such as sodium nitroprusside if the hypertension is not controlled with β-blockers alone. Failure of medical therapy or complicated dissections of the descending aorta (e.g., malperfusion) are indications for surgical repair. Type B dissections treated medically lead to an 80% survival at 1 year, but only 50% at 5 years.

50. Ascending aortic aneurysms
Stephen H. McKellar

The natural history of ascending aortic aneurysms (AscAA) helps determine the timing of intervention as complications of the disease can be life threatening. The goal of treating AscAA is to intervene on patients prior to aneurysm rupture or dissection, the most common sequelae of AscAA. However, all AscAAs are not the same, and are caused by a variety of etiologies, with more "aggressive" forms of the disease. In general, the risk of complications increases proportionally to the size of the aneurysm due to increased wall tension as described by Laplace's law.

Pathophysiology

The final common pathway of all etiologies of AscAA is pathologic dilatation and thinning of the aortic wall. There are three main categories of AscAA. When listed in decreasing order of "virulence" they are: aneurysms associated with connective tissue disorders such as Marfan syndrome, associated with bicuspid aortic valve (BAV), and sporadic aneurysms with tricuspid aortic valves.

Connective tissue disorders

The most common connective tissue disorders associated with AscAA, and in particular aneurysms of the aortic root, are Marfan, Ehlers-Danlos, and Loeys-Dietz syndromes. Aortas of these patients often display younger age of onset and more rapid growth compared to sporadic AscAA. The majority of patients with Marfan syndrome have a mutation of the fibrillin-1 (FBN1) gene leading to a weakened aortic wall known as cystic medial degeneration on histologic examination. Patients with Ehlers-Danlos type IV have a defect in procollagen III synthesis, which predisposes them to AscAA. Patients with Loeys-Dietz syndrome have mutations in the genes encoding TGF-ß receptors 1 and 2 and are associated with a complex phenotype (hypertelorism, bifid uvula or cleft palate, and arterial tortuosity).

Sporadic

Patients with sporadic (non-syndromal, non BAV) AscAA have a much more predictable course. They tend to enlarge at a predicted rate of 0.1cm/year. This frequently predictable rate of growth allows serial follow-up of these aneurysm and elective treatment when size criteria are met.

Bicuspid aortic valve

AscAA among patients with BAV are less predictable and fall some-where in between syndromal and sporadic AscAA in terms of aggressive-ness. This has lead several investigators to recommend intervention on AscAA at smaller diameters than patients with the sporadic form.

Clinical presentation

Patients with AscAA can present in 3 ways: an asymptomatic aneurysm incidentally detected on imaging for another problem, a symptomatic aneurysm, or sudden death from acute rupture. When symptoms are pre-sent, they can be anterior or posterior chest pain, voice changes due to stretching of the recurrent laryngeal nerve, or rarely, stridor. Most pa-tients with AscAA, however, are asymptomatic.

Diagnosis

The diagnosis of AscAA is largely based on imaging. The most com-monly used diagnostic modalities are echocardiogram and CTA. Echo-cardiography is limited by the variable skill of the sonographer and its inability to visualize the distal extent of aneurysm. CT allows more pre-cise measurements and with less variability in technique, allows compari-son of aneurysm growth over time. It does, however, come at the ex-pense of ionizing radiation and IV contrast loads.

Treatment

Symptomatic AscAA is considered an acute aortic syndrome and requires urgent surgical repair to prevent aortic catastrophe. Treatment of asymp-tomatic AscAA is surgical and the indication for surgery depends on the size and etiology of the aneurysm. Additionally, the AscAA is often re-placed during concomitant cardiac surgery such as AVR even though strict size thresholds are not met. Commonly accepted size criteria for surgical intervention of an isolated AscAA are:

- *Connective tissue disorders:* 4.5-5.0 cm

- *Bicuspid aortic valves:* 5.0-5.5 cm

- *Sporadic:* 5.5-6.0 cm

The recommendations for repair are based mostly on natural history stud-ies of sporadic AscAA in which the risk of rupture increased dramatically at 6.0 cm. Therefore, good-risk patients with sporadic AscAA of $\geq$ 5.5 cm should be offered repair. The most appropriate time for intervention on an AscAA in patients with BAV remains controversial with some authors recommending replacement of even normal-appearing ascending aortas while others pursue a more individualized approach. Growth of the aneurysm at a rate > 1 cm/year is also an accepted indication for intervention.

Surgical repair of AscAA is based on the anatomic location of the aneurysm and if there is concomitant aortic valve pathology. Common options are:

- Aneurysm replacement with tube graft. For patients with isolated AscAA and normal aortic root.

- Aortic valve and ascending aortic replacement with separate valve and graft; the aortic root is preserved. For patients with AscAA and abnormal aortic valve but with normal aortic root.

- Combined (composite) aortic valve, root and ascending aortic replacement (modified Bentall) with reimplantation of coronary arteries. This can be done with either biologic or mechanical valve prostheses. For patients with abnormal ascending aorta and aortic root, with a valve that cannot be spared.

- Valve-sparing root procedure with tube graft. For patients with abnormal ascending aorta and aortic root with normal or near-normal aortic valve.

- Aortic homograft. Useful for cases of endocarditis or prior prosthetic infection.

- Ross procedure (controversial in adults). Used on young patients who would benefit from growth of the autograft.

An AscAA with a normal root requires only replacement of the ascending aorta with a tube graft. If the valve is diseased, it can be replaced while leaving the root alone. Marfan patients are exceptions to this rule; the root should be replaced in these patients (with or without valve replacement), regardless of the appearance of the root.

Surgical repair can be done using standard CPB if the distal extent of the AscAA allows sufficient room for placement of an aortic cross clamp. If, however, the distal extent of the AscAA does not allow an aortic cross clamp, then an arch or hemiarch replacement is indicated using deep hypothermic circulatory arrest with or without cervical debranching.

51. Thoracoabdominal aortic aneurysms

Mani A. Daneshmand, Jason A. Williams

Aortic pathology

Aortic pathology can be classified as dissection (disruption of intima from media), aneurysm (dilation to greater than 1.5 times normal size of all 3 layers), or pseudoaneurysm (a defect in the wall resulting in an extravascular hematoma). Aneurysms are further classified morphologically as fusiform (diffuse, circumferential dilatation) or saccular (spherical outpouchings involving only a portion of the vessel wall). Finally, aneurysms are classified according to the segment of the aorta involved as thoracic aneurysms (which include the ascending or descending aorta in the thoracic cavity), and thoracoabdominal (TAAA) or abdominal (involving the infrarenal abdominal aorta).

Pathogenesis of aortic aneurysms

The aorta is a constantly remodeling tissue. Its structural integrity is maintained by constantly synthesizing, degrading, and repairing the extracellular matrix (ECM). Failure of this dynamic system at any point results in aneurysm:

- *Collagen vascular disease*

  - Marfan syndrome (autosomal dominant) - the defective synthesis of fibrillin-1 causes altered TGF-β activity and weakening of elastic tissue. There are more than 125 identified mutations on the human fibrillin-1 gene (FBN1).

  - Loeys-Dietz syndrome (autosomal dominant) - mutations in TGF-β (1 or 2) receptors cause abnormalities in elastin and collagen II and I. Aneurysms in these patients tend to rupture at smaller sizes. It is subdivided into Type 1A, 1B, 2A and 2B. Type 1A is also known as Furlong disease, and Type 2B was previously known as Marfan syndrome Type 2. These patients have widely spaced eyes, cleft palate or bifid uvula, and tortuous aneurysmal aortas that are prone to dissection. Many patients with Loeys-Dietz also have bicuspid aortic valves.

  - Ehlers-Danlos syndrome - defective type III collagen synthesis.

  - Severe vitamin C deficiency - altered cross-linking of type III collagen.

- *Imbalance of collagen synthesis and degradation*

- Atherosclerosis results in inflammatory mediators, which stimulate macrophage production of matrix metalloproteinases (MMP) resulting in ECM degradation.

- Ischemia of the aortic wall causes cystic medial degeneration, characterized by scarring and loss of smooth muscle cells and elastic fibers.

Classification

TAAAs are defined by the Crawford classification system, which takes into account the extent of aortic involvement. There are four Crawford categories described as follows:

- *Type I.* Originates below the left subclavian artery and extends into the abdominal aorta including the celiac axis and mesenteric arteries.

- *Type II.* Involves the same areas as type I, but extends caudally to include the infrarenal abdominal aorta.

- *Type III.* Begins in the lower descending thoracic aorta (T6) and involves the remainder of the aorta.

- *Type IV.* Begins at the diaphragm and involves the abdominal aorta only.

Natural history and clinical presentation

Thoracic aortic aneurysms grow at an average rate of 0.12 cm/year. The rate of growth is 0.3 cm/year for descending and 0.1 cm/year for ascending aorta aneurysms. Aortic aneurysms grow faster in the setting of a chronic dissection or collagen vascular disease. TAAAs grow asymptomatically in approximately 43% of patients. Usually the diagnosis is made incidentally on imaging. Five to 10% of patients present with symptoms. Typical symptoms include pain from aortic wall stretching or extrinsic compression of contiguous structures, depending upon their location. Hemoptysis occurs from erosion of TAAAs into bronchi or lung parenchyma. Hoarseness or dysphagia are caused by compression of the recurrent laryngeal nerve or the esophagus, respectively. Due to its proximity, nerve injury also remains a particular concern in the reoperative setting. In many instances the presenting feature is rupture or dissection.

Indications and timing of surgical intervention

Aneurysm size is the best predictor of rupture risk and thus guides the timing of surgical intervention. The annual rate of rupture or dissection is

2% for aneurysms less than 5 cm, 3% for aneurysms 5 to 5.9 cm, and 7% for aneurysms 6 cm or more in diameter. Advanced age increases the relative risk of rupture by a factor of 2.6 for every decade of life. The presence of COPD is another significant predictor of rupture. Patients with TAAAs and chest or back pain are also at increased risk of aneurysm rupture. Approximately 79% of ruptures occur in women. Due to the increased operative risk in descending thoracic aneurysms, surgery is recommended at an aortic diameter 6 cm or more, or in the setting of an annual growth rate of 1 cm or more.

Procedural morbidity and mortality

The mortality of TAAA repair ranges from 3% to 23%. Paraplegia remains of utmost concern, with the tenuous nature of the spinal cord highlighted by the fact that a single anterior spinal artery supplies 75% of the blood supply to the cord (two posterior spinal arteries supply the other 25%). Paraplegia rates range from 1.5-5%. Frequent neurologic assessment in the postoperative patient is vital to prevent permanent paraplegia, as most episodes of paresis are reversible with blood pressure augmentation and/or drainage of CSF. Postoperative respiratory failure occurs in 25-45% of patients, MI in 7-13%, stroke 1.3-7.5%, acute kidney injury in 3-14%, and reoperation or bleeding in 3-5%. Five-year survival rates are about 65% with mid- and long-term mortality usually unrelated to the surgical intervention.

Open surgical repair

The patient is placed in a partial right lateral decubitus position with the hips almost supine to allow femoral cannulation. The incision, in the left chest, is tailored to complement the extent of the aneurysm. Partial left-heart bypass can serve as a viable perfusion strategy in the setting of a limited proximal descending resection. Cannulation for partial left-heart bypass (LA to femoral artery) is performed with an outflow cannula in the LA and an inflow cannula in the right femoral artery. This technique also enables management of upper extremity hypertension while on bypass by simply increasing flow rates to bring pressures down. For deep hypothermic circulatory arrest (DHCA), cannulation is typically a right femoral venous cannula (placed either through an open approach, or percutaneously); an arterial cannula at the distal arch, proximal descending aorta, axillary artery, or femoral artery (depending on the anatomy of the aneurysm and the planned repair); as well as a LV vent placed at the LV apex or the left inferior pulmonary vein.

Endovascular repair

Endovascular TAAA repair is a less invasive alternative to open repair where the aorta is only briefly occluded and there is minimal hemodynamic and metabolic stress. Candidate aneurysms have 20 mm proximal neck/landing zone and the maximum aneurysm diameter should be no larger than the largest available endograft.

Endovascular stent grafting should follow many of the principles established originally in abdominal aorta. Specifically, stents should be oversized by 15% of the diameter of the landing zone to optimize radial apposition. Additionally, stents should be "built-up", i.e. larger stents placed within smaller stents to account for differences in proximal and distal landing zones. Frequently, the left subclavian artery can be covered to increase proximal neck length. Significant type 2 endoleaks resulting from this practice can be addressed by coiling through left brachial access. Alternately, reversal of flow in the ipsilateral vertebral artery suggests subclavian steal as a consequence of subclavian coverage. Here, a carotid-subclavian bypass is the treatment of choice. "Hybrid" procedures have been developed to increase the applicability of endovascular techniques to patients who previously were not candidates due to aneurysm anatomy.

52. End-stage heart failure
Stephen H. McKellar

End-stage heart failure is a growing epidemic in industrialized nations. Both medical and surgical treatments play important roles in treating this deadly disease.

Pathophysiology

The pathophysiology of CHF is broken into two broad categories: ischemic and non-ischemic. The latter category, however, is comprised of various etiologies of heart failure including congenital heart disease, idiopathic dilated cardiomyopathy, known genetic cardiomyopathies, and restrictive or infiltrative processes such as hypertrophic obstructive cardiomyopathy or amyloidosis and sarcoidosis. Systolic dysfunction is predominantly the etiology of heart failure in ischemic heart failure as well as most non-ischemic etiologies. However, diastolic dysfunction also plays a role in the restrictive and infiltrative cardiomyopathies.

Clinical presentation

The clinical presentation of biventricular heart failure is similar regardless of etiology. Initially, symptoms are often fatigue, dyspnea, and exercise intolerance but progress to symptoms at rest, cachexia, and if untreated, multisystem organ failure and death. The acuity of presentation, however, often varies depending on etiology of heart failure. The most striking example of this is acute cardiogenic shock following MI of a large territory of myocardium. Whereas, the other etiologies of chronic heart failure have a more insidious onset. These patients are frequently hospitalized for CHF exacerbations. They are diuresed, undergo medication changes and then dismissed, but frequently readmitted within a few months.

Diagnosis

The diagnosis of heart failure is predominantly a clinical one with adjunctive use of echocardiography. History and physical examination are suggestive of CHF with the frequent findings of pulmonary and pedal edema, elevated jugular venous pressure, displaced apical impulse, S3 gallop, and evidence of renal and hepatic dysfunction. CXR is helpful in assessing the presence and degree of pulmonary edema and pleural effusions. Echocardiography is the best study for evaluating systolic and diastolic function and should be used liberally. Once obtained, comparison to old echocardiograms is important to measure disease progression or documenting new problems such as valvular insufficiency. Echocardiography, however, does have its limitations as most of its data are estimates. Hemodynamic right-heart catheterization, therefore, remains the standard for assessing the severity of end-stage heart failure, particularly when being evaluated for heart transplantation and/or VADs.

It is important to identify the etiology of heart failure as treatment strategies vary. For this, additional tests are often needed. Coronary angiography is needed to determine the presence and/or severity of ischemic heart disease and to decide if coronary revascularization is indicated. For non-ischemic processes, endomyocardial biopsies and often genetic studies are needed.

Treatment

Medical therapy

All patients with heart failure need optimal medical therapy. For acute cardiogenic shock, inotropes and vasopressors are needed, often in conjunction with an IABP. For patients with chronic systolic heart failure, beta agonists, nitrates and ACE inhibitors / ARBs are the mainstay of medical therapy. If systolic function has deteriorated to a point where these agents fail, chronic IV agents such as milrinone may be needed.

Surgical therapy

The indications for surgical treatment of heart failure include acute cardiogenic shock refractory to less conservative measures or progressive decline of cardiac function with optimal medical therapies. Causes for acute cardiogenic shock include acute MI, postcardiotomy shock, myocarditis, and refractory ventricular arrhythmias.

For patients in acute cardiogenic shock, non-implantable VADs are frequently used to stabilize the patient, await for myocardial recovery in case of transitory causes (e.g., acute MI, postcardiotomy shock, or myocarditis), and determine eligibility for transplant and/or suitability for implantable assist devices. This is often called bridge-to-decision. In contrast, patients with chronic heart failure are considered eligible for implantable left ventricular assist device (LVAD) therapy if they: have an EF of < 25%, peak oxygen consumption of < 14 ml/kg/min, NYHA class IIIB or IV, or IABP or inotrope dependence. Most patients simultaneously undergo transplant evaluation and either undergo transplantation or LVAD implantation as either a bridge-to-transplantation (BTT) or destination-therapy (DT).

Continuous flow LVADs

Preoperative considerations are mostly related to patient selection. Earlier utilization of LVADs have demonstrated improved survival due to prevention of end-organ dysfunction and malnutrition found in the late stages of CHF. Additionally, RV function is important as the RV must be able to pump blood to the preload-dependent LVAD. There is no perfectly predictable measure of adequate RV function but CVP, RV stroke work index (RVSWI), and the degree of tricuspid valve dysfunction are frequently used.

At the time of LVAD implantation certain things need to be addressed to improve outcomes. Moderate-severe aortic regurgitation must be corrected (by either aortic valve replacement or by suturing the aortic valve close) to prevent circular flow from LVAD to ascending aorta and back into the LVAD, thus creating a low cardiac index to the body. Additionally, the LVAD inflow cannula must be positioned properly towards the mitral valve orifice for unobstructed flow dynamics. Finally, any interatrial or interventricular septal defects must be corrected or a pronounced right-to-left shunt with hypoxemia will result due to the presence of vacuum pressures in the left side.

Postoperative considerations include aggressive ICU management, including adequate nutritional support and anticoagulation. In general, an antiplatelet agent and warfarin are used. The decision as to when to start anticoagulation postoperatively is individualized for each patient.

Right heart failure occurs in 20% of patients after LVAD. Early signs include elevated CVP, marginal LVAD flows, and decreased urine output. Right heart failure is managed with milrinone, dobutamine, diuresis, and nitric oxide. Nitric oxide is particularly important with patients with preoperative pulmonary hypertension. In some cases of persistent right heart failure, a right VAD may be required.

The most common complication after implantation of current devices is bleeding. Coagulopathy is usually caused by a combination of causes including alterations in the hemostatic system (e.g., acquired von Willebrand syndrome from loss of von Willebrand multimers from high shear stress), dilutional thrombocytopenia, hypothermia, and the use of other antiplatelet or anticoagulant agents. Sepsis occurs in 10-25% of LVAD patients and accounts for almost a quarter of all LVAD deaths. Thromboembolic events with the current devices occur in approximately 8% of cases.

53. Cardiac transplantation

George M. Comas

Orthotopic heart transplantation (OHT) is the therapy of choice for end-stage heart failure. Technical advances, better immunosuppression and infection control have dramatically improved outcomes in recent decades. Limited donor supply is the primary factor restricting availability to the growing number of patients who would benefit from this therapy. 20-40% of patients on the waiting list die before OHT. Overall, operative mortality for OHT is 5%. One-year survival is 80-90%, with primary graft failure the most common cause of death in the first month, and infection the predominant causative factor from one month to one year post-transplant. Three-year survival is 75%.

Indications for OHT

The indication for OHT is irreversible cardiac disease not amenable to other treatment (optimized medical therapy, revascularization, ventricular remodeling, valve surgery, biventricular pacing). Candidates are patients with NYHA class III-IV heart failure with a predicted 2-year survival < 60%. Most have ischemic or idiopathic dilated cardiomyopathy. Contraindications include: active infection, irreversible renal or hepatic dysfunction, fixed pulmonary hypertension (PAP > 60mmHg, transpulmonary gradient > 15mmHg, PVR > 6 Wood units), advanced age (> 70 years), severe obstructive or restrictive pulmonary disease (FEV_1 < 1.5 L, DLCO < 50% predicted), unresolved, recent malignancy, significant systemic disease (severe PVD or DM with significant end organ dysfunction), psychiatric illness, or medical non-compliance.

Organ allocation

The allocation system is regulated by UNOS and provides the most critically ill patients with hearts, while limiting allograft ischemic time. Patients are classified on the transplant list by status:

- *Status 1A.* Patients that are hospitalized with either IV inotropes, heart assist devices, mechanical ventilation, or have a life expectancy of less than 1 week.

- *Status 1B.* Patients that are not hospitalized but have IV inotropes or a heart assist device.

- *Status 2.* All other active patients, usually seen by a cardiologist every month, with a right heart catheterization performed every 3 months.

Recipient and donors must be ABO compatible to avoid hyperacute rejection. Incompatibility may be tolerated in some pediatric patients less than a year of age (A donor for B recipient). Donor weight should be within 20% of recipient weight (closer size matching required in children).

Echocardiography assesses potential donors. However, there is poor correlation among interpretations of echocardiograms of brain dead donors, so caution should be used. In one study, there was only 77% agreement between local cardiologists at the donor hospital and cardiologists at the transplant hospital regarding major abnormalities. Mild ventricular dysfunction of the donor heart is often reversible after transplant. Catheterization is unnecessary if the donor is young (< 45 years). . Older donors must have catheterization to screen for CAD.

Four to six hours is the recommended cold ischemic time for OHT. Longer ischemic times are tolerated in pediatric donors. Older donor hearts tolerate prolonged cold ischemia less well, and it generally felt that they should be kept under 4 hours to maximize success of the organ. Gender mismatched hearts may not do as well as gender matched organs.

Recipients must appear on the UNOS match-run for a particular donor. If a recipient is a re-transplant, a panel of reactive antibodies (PRA) panel should be done (percentage reactive antibody). If the PRA is greater than 10-15%, then a prospective T-cell crossmatch is recommended before transplant. Recipients with high antibody titers are optimally managed with plasmapheresis and immunoglobulin preoperatively.

Organ procurement

During donor heart procurement, the heart is assessed in the operating room to identify ventricular or valvar dysfunction. If accepted, the heart is mobilized for cardiectomy. The SVC and IVC are encircled. Extra length is useful for bicaval anastomosis. After mobilization, the donor is heparinized. The SVC is ligated, IVC is vented, inferior pulmonary vein or LA appendage is transected for LA venting, and arrest is initiated by cross-clamping the aorta and administering antegrade cardioplegia (single flush cold crystalloid cardioplegia). Topical cooling is used. After donor cardiectomy, the heart is inspected and transported in a sterile saline filled container. To avoid procurement pitfalls, one must monitor the heart during visceral organ dissection, heparinize fully, avoid ventricular distension, ensure myocardial preservation, and maintain hypothermia during harvest and transport.

Organ implantation

During implantation, the recipient heart is bicavally cannulated. Cross-clamp and cardiectomy are completed by the time the donor heart arrives. An adequate recipient LA cuff is necessary. The donor heart is prepared: the LA cuff is trimmed to the size of the recipient's LA. A donor PFO is closed if found. Most centers perform bicaval anastomosis in adults. The typical order of anastomoses is:

1. LA

2. IVC

3. SVC

4. PA

5. Aorta

The heart is de-aired with a root vent. Pulmonary hypertension and right heart failure must be monitored when coming off bypass. Bicaval versus biatrial implantation is controversial. The bicaval technique retains the normal shaped atria, which may preserve atrial contractility, sinus node function and may maintain AV valve competence. Conversely, biatrial anastomosis is faster and decreases the risk of anastomotic caval stenosis (especially in children). In the most recent analysis of the UNOS database, the bicaval technique required less frequent pacemaker implantations and attained a small, yet significant survival advantage over the biatrial approach.

Postoperative management

Donor myocardial function may be tenuous in the postoperative period. In addition, there may be allograft injury from donor hemodynamic instability. Prolonged hypothermia and ischemia from poor preservation can lead to reduced ventricular compliance and contractility. Temporary inotropic support (dobutamine) may be needed. As an alternative, isoproterenol has inotropic with chronotropic effects that mitigate brady-arrhythmias. An IABP can be placed if further support is needed.

Sinus node dysfunction from prolonged ischemia leads to permanent pacing in 2-25% of patients. AAIR pacing is the preferred pacing modality, with DDD reserved for rare cases of AV conduction abnormalities. If the patient had pulmonary hypertension preoperatively (> 3 Wood units), right heart failure is a postoperative concern. The donor heart is not conditioned to pump against high PVR. Rising CVP with worsening ventricular function and falling PAP are indicators of a failing right heart. The RV is particularly susceptible to dysfunction if there is elevated donor PAP, multiple transfusions, or suboptimal preservation. Patient survival is dependent on treating right heart failure. To optimize function of the donor heart, pulmonary vasodilators may be started. These include: inhaled nitric oxide, inhaled prostacyclin, IV milrinone/nitroglycerine/isoproterenol. Particularly effective is milrinone, a phosphodiesterase inhibitor. Milrinone enhances contractility, decreases stroke volume, decreases LV end-diastolic pressure, decreases heart rate, and reverses vasospasm, all without a proportional increase in oxygen consumption. This leads to an increase in cardiac output and a decrease in PAP. For OHT patients, milrinone bridges them preoperatively and manages biventricular dysfunction postoperatively. In addition to pharmacologic measures, right heart failure can be treated with atrial pacing at 110 bpm (tachycardia leads to smaller RV volumes and helps avoid RV dilation and subsequent tricuspid regurgitation). Keeping the oxygen saturation above 95% and avoiding hypercarbia also helps ameliorate pulmonary hypertension.

Acute rejection

Acute rejection is the most common cause of depressed ventricular function associated with fever after OHT. Usually there are subtle clinical manifestations and the patient is without symptoms until rejection is advanced. Frequently, the patient is several weeks to months into the postoperative period with a low-grade fever and an echocardiogram that shows a depressed EF from the initial postoperative period. Due to the effectiveness of calcineurin inhibitors, most episodes of rejection are mild or moderate; it is rare to have rejection that leads to hemodynamic instability. Routine surveillance biopsies over the first year can diagnose early rejection in an asymptomatic patient. An endomyocardial biopsy from the RV septum allows for histologic diagnosis of rejection severity:

- *Grade 0* – no rejection

- *Grade I (mild)* – minimal infiltrate, no or minimal myocyte necrosis, asymptomatic

- *Grade 2 (moderate)* – 2 or more foci of perivascular infiltrates with associated myocyte damage

- *Grade 3 (severe)* – Diffuse infiltrate with multifocal myocyte damage

Occasionally seen are "quilty" lesions, nests of CD4 and CD8 T lymphocytes with histiocytes that are sites of antigen processing and low-grade immune stimulation. Additionally, biopsies may reveal infections transmitted with the transplanted organ, namely toxoplasmosis.

Forty percent of patients have a rejection episode within the first month, 60% within 6 months and 66% by one year. After one year, the risk decreases to a low level. Risk factors for rejection include: female gender, young, black race, +CMV, HLA-DR mismatch, previous serious infection and prolonged ischemic time. Rejection must be treated early to improve long-term survival. Treatment includes increased immunosuppression and pulse steroids.

Chronic rejection

Chronic rejection is manifested as allograft vasculopathy. The incidence is 10% per year after OHT or 50% at 5 years. It represents the most common cause of long-term death following OHT. Allograft vasculopathy develops *de novo* and is not a progression of existing donor disease. Angina is rare because the heart remains denervated. Hence, diagnosis is usually with catheterization, routine surveillance or prompted by EKG changes, echocardiogram changes or clinical deterioration. Sixty percent of patients with severe allograft vasculopathy develop graft loss at 2 years. Risk factors for allograft vasculopathy include: +CMV disease, elevated homocysteine, smoking, obesity, hyperlipidemia, DM.

Statins started within two weeks after OHT can lower cholesterol and lead to less graft CAD and better graft survival. Steroids or blood pressure control do not alter the course of allograft vasculopathy. Treatment options include all forms of revascularization, however, there is rarely a discrete proximal lesion with a well-preserved distal vessel. There exists 50% mortality for re-operative CABG for allograft vasculopathy. If ventricular hypertrophy is present, mortality from post-OHT vasculopathy is especially high. As a result of this dismal prognosis, allograft vasculopathy remains the main indication for retransplantation. Early retransplantation (within 9 months) has prohibitive mortality, but retransplantation after this time has the same survival curve as primary OHT.

Immunosuppression

Immunosuppression medications for OHT have many sequelae: hyperlipidemia, hypertension and coronary vasculopathy. Renal dysfunction is 24% at 4 years and is the most common toxicity associated with calcineurin/IL-2 inhibitors (cyclosporine and tacrolimus). Osteoporosis is also caused by calcineurin inhibitors. The trabecular bone of the spine is at highest risk (20% incidence of vertebral compression fractures). Steroid-induced DM, post-transplant lymphoproliferative disorder and skin cancer also occur in immunosuppressed post-transplant patients.

Post-transplant lymphoproliferative disorder

Post-transplant lymphoproliferative disorder, a proliferation of B-cells (usually monoclonal in origin) after immunosuppression, occurs in 2-10% of OHT patients. It is associated with +EBV, +CMV and certain immunosuppression (tacrolimus, anti-CD3 antibody). There is a higher incidence in children. It appears months to years after OHT (usually 2-3 years) and can present with malaise, fever, or weight loss (symptoms depend on the location of the lymphoid tissue mass). Biopsy is diagnostic. Treatment includes reducing or temporarily stopping immunosuppression. The polymorphic form responds better than the monomorphic form. Advanced disease can be treated with chemotherapy.

54. Arrhythmia surgery

Chad N. Stasik

Non-pharmacologic treatments for arrhythmia include catheter ablation, pacemaker and defibrillator placement, and surgery. This chapter focuses on the surgical treatment of arrhythmias, mainly atrial fibrillation (AF).

Over 2 million Americans have AF and the lifetime risk of developing AF after age 40 is approximately 25%. Current guidelines[1] classify AF as either *paroxysmal* or *persistent*. Paroxysmal AF terminates spontaneously while persistent AF is sustained beyond 7 days. Either can be *recurrent*, meaning that there have been 2 or more episodes of AF. AF is considered *permanent* if it is present for greater than 1 year and cardioversion has failed or has not been attempted.

Patients with AF may experience palpitations, anxiety, dizziness, fatigue, presyncope, and syncope. The loss of atrioventricular synchrony (and the "atrial kick") decreases cardiac output by as much as 15-20%. Stasis of blood in the LA also predisposes to stroke. Antiarrhythmic drugs have limited efficacy in conversion to sinus rhythm and are not without side effects, while rate control alone does not decrease the risk of thromboembolism. In addition, anticoagulation carries a major complication rate of about 2% per year.

Electrophysiology

For AF to occur there must be initiation of an abnormal impulse and perpetuation of the abnormal rhythm. Impulse generation can come from an ectopic focus or a reentrant wave. Paroxysmal AF originates in the pulmonary veins greater than 50% of the time. Reentry is caused by the propagation of an action potential through the heart in a continuous loop. For reentry to occur, there must be a unidirectional block to action potential propagation and the refractory period must be shorter than the time it takes the action potential to propagate around the loop.

Indications for surgery

The Heart Rhythm Society published a consensus statement[2] on catheter and surgical ablation of AF in 2007. Current indications for surgical ablation of AF include the following:

- Symptomatic AF patients undergoing other cardiac surgical procedures.

- Selected asymptomatic AF patients undergoing cardiac surgery in whom the ablation can be performed with minimal risk.

- Stand-alone AF surgery should be considered for symptomatic AF patients who prefer a surgical approach, have failed one or more attempts at catheter ablation, or are not candidates for catheter ablation.

In addition, patients with a contraindication to anticoagulation should be considered for surgical ablation.

Cox-Maze procedure

The Maze procedure, introduced by Dr. James Cox in 1987, was devised to interrupt reentrant circuits in the atria and direct the propagation of currents from the sinoatrial node through both atria. This was done with strategically placed incisions across the atria. By restoring sinus rhythm, it precludes the need for anticoagulation and provides symptomatic relief.

The cut-and-sew Cox-Maze III procedure is the gold standard for the surgical treatment of AF, but it has largely been replaced by procedures that use various energy sources to create linear lines of ablation. These include cryoablation, radiofrequency, microwave, laser, and high-frequency US. The complete Maze lesion set includes the following ablation lines:

- Right and left pulmonary vein isolation

- Right atriotomy

- Intercaval lesion from the SVC to the IVC

- Free wall lesion from RA appendage to intercaval lesion

- Lesions to tricuspid annulus at 10 o'clock and 2 o'clock

- Left atriotomy

- Lesion from LA appendage to left superior pulmonary vein

- Two lesions connecting left and right pulmonary veins

- Line from left pulmonary vein lesion to mitral valve

- Coronary sinus lesion

The LA appendage is also amputated or oversewn. A spectrum of less invasive modifications exists, ranging from partial lesion sets performed off bypass to alternative approaches such as minithoracotomy or endoscopic and robotic techniques.

Long-term freedom from AF following the traditional cut-and-sew Maze procedure has consistently been reported above 90%. There is also a decreased incidence of late strokes. Excellent results have been obtained using alternative energy sources as well, but when an incomplete lesion set is performed, such as in pulmonary vein isolation only, efficacy is significantly decreased.

Other arrhythmias

Atrioventricular nodal reentrant tachycardia (AVNRT) is the most common type of supraventricular tachycardia. It is usually managed initially with drug therapy and responds well to catheter ablation therapies. Atrial tachycardias are supraventricular tachycardias that originate in the left or right atria and tend to be resistant to drug therapy. They are usually treated with catheter electrophysiology mapping and ablation. Patients with inappropriate sinus tachycardia who fail medical therapy may be candidates for surgical isolation or ablation of the sinoatrial node.

With the advent of implantable cardioverter-defibrillators (ICDs), the role of surgery for ventricular tachycardia (VT) has decreased markedly. Surgical ablation or resection of the arrhythmogenic focus is an option for patients with recurrent VT refractory to medical and catheter-based therapies. Surgery should also be considered for patients with ischemic VT and prior MI with LV aneurysms who have significant coronary disease requiring revascularization. Available surgical options include coronary revascularization, ventricular remodeling, and resection of the endomyocardial scar.

55. Pacemakers and defibrillators

Keshava Rajagopal

A pacemaker is a device that electrically paces the heart and is placed due to inadequacy of the endogenous rate and/or rhythm. An implantable cardioverter-defibrillator (ICD) is a device that electrically shocks the heart out of unstable cardiac rhythms.

The basic components of all devices are similar and include:

- *Pulse generator.* Consists of a power source (battery), circuitry, a metal shell, and outlets for the pacing leads.

- *Leads.* Insulated wires that connect the generator to the heart. They can be unipolar (cathode only at lead tip; anode is part of the generator) or bipolar (both cathode and anode at lead tip). The fixation of the lead to the heart can be passive (tines or talons) or active (screw). Defibrillation leads are high-voltage conductor coils.

The *pacing threshold* is the minimum amount of energy required for successful pacing of the heart (*capture*). This threshold is determined by the voltage of each impulse and its duration (usually expressed in milliseconds). Ventricular thresholds should ideally be < 0.7 V with R-wave amplitudes being > 5 mV.

Most pacemakers are placed transvenously. The ventricular lead is placed in the RV, usually at the septum or inferior apical area, avoiding the free wall and the RVOT. The atrial lead is placed in the RA, ideally at the level of the appendage. For cardiac resynchronization (biventricular pacing) in CHF patients, an additional LV lead is placed transvenously through the coronary sinus or epicardially.

Pacing modes

Pacing modes are described according to a four-letter international nomenclature although the first three letters are the most important. The letters refer to the type of pacing, sensing, response, and programmability, respectively.

- *Pacing.* Which chamber(s) are being paced by direct stimulation in the absence of intrinsic cardiac electrical activity: Atrial (A), Ventricular (V), Dual (D), or none (O).

- *Sensing.* Which chamber(s)' intrinsic electrical activity is detected by the pacemaker: Atrial (A), Ventricular (V), Dual (D), or none (O).

- *Response.* What the response of the chamber(s) is in response to sensing intrinsic electrical activity (i.e., pacing algorithm): Triggered (T), Inhibited (I), Dual (D), or none (O). In T mode, sensed intrinsic activity leads to a pacemaker stimulus (used to avoid inhibition of the pacemaker). In I mode, sensed intrinsic activity leads to inhibition of the pacemaker. In D mode, the detection of intrinsic ventricular activity inhibits the pacemaker while the detection of intrinsic atrial activity leads to inhibition of the atrial pacemaker stimulus and triggering of a ventricular stimulus after a predetermined delay.

- *Programmability of rate modulation:* simple programmable (P), multiprogrammable (M), communicating (C), rate modulation (R), or none (O). Permanent pacemakers generally are R as the rate is adjusted depending on different sensors (motion, temperature, etc.) to try to compensate for the activity and metabolic demands of the patient.

For example, temporary epicardial pacing wires used in cardiac surgery are typically fixed-rate and either "A-pace" (AOO(O)), "V-pace" (VOO(O)), or "AV-sequentially pace" (DOO(O)). However, some newer external pacemakers allow AAI(O), VVI(O), DVI(O), and DDD(O) pacing. Permanent pacemakers placed postoperatively for persistent complete heart block are typically DDD(R) ("full service" pacemakers). Permanent pacemakers placed postoperatively for complete heart block in the setting of atrial fibrillation are VVI(R).

ICDs are programmed to detect tachyarrhythmias, deliver the therapy, and detect if the therapy was successful or not. Multiple different zones of detection can be set (e.g., ventricular tachycardia (VT), fast VT, ventricular fibrillation (VF)) and the therapies can be individualized for each particular zone. Delivered therapy can be in the form of high-energy defibrillation shocks, low-energy synchronized cardioversions, or antitachycardia pacing.

Overdrive pacing can be used in a non-ICD pacemaker to treat AV nodal reentrant tachycardia, atrial flutter, ventricular tachyarrhythmias, or Wolff-Parkinson-White syndrome.

When a magnet is applied to a pacemaker, the sensing function is temporarily inactivated, essentially changing the pacing mode to AOO, VOO, or DOO until the magnet is removed. This is used during surgery to prevent inadequate sensing of the pacemaker due to artifacts from the electrocautery. Application of a magnet to an ICD inactivates the delivery of tachyarrhythmia therapy but does not inactive sensing of the pacemaker component.

Indications for placement

Placement of temporary pacemakers is indicated for:

- Bradyarrhythmia with hemodynamic compromise or symptoms

- High risk of important bradyarrhythmia

- Symptomatic sinus bradycardia, sinus pauses > 3 sec, sinus bradycardia with heart rate (HR) < 40 bpm

- Ventricular asystole

- Alternating left and right bundle branch block (BBB)

According to ACC/AHA Guidelines,[1] permanent pacemakers are indicated (Class I recommendations) for particular patients in the following categories:

- *Sinus node dysfunction.* Symptomatic bradycardia for any reason, severe sinus pauses, and "chronotropic incompetence"

- *Atrioventricular (AV) block*

  - After catheter ablation of the AV node

  - Persistent advanced 2nd or 3rd degree AV block after cardiac surgery

  - Asymptomatic 3rd degree heart block if coexistent LV dilatation or dysfunction

  - Advanced 2nd (Mobitz II) or 3rd degree AV block with infranodal escape rhythm, ventricular arrhythmias, periods of asystole > 3 sec, or need for medications that induce bradycardia

  - 2nd (Mobitz I or II) or 3rd degree block with significant bradycardia (HR < 40 bpm or symptomatic)

- *Chronic bifascicular block.* Advanced 2nd or 3rd degree block and alternating left and right BBB

- *Tachyarrhythmias (ventricular).* Prophylactically for sustained pause-dependent VT

- *Post-acute MI:* persistent 2nd or 3rd degree AV block or alternating left and right BBB after ST-elevation MI, and transient 2nd or 3rd degree infranodal AV block with BBB

According to ACC/AHA Guidelines,[1] ICDs are indicated (Class I recommendations) for the following patients:

- Survivors of VF or hemodynamically unstable sustained VT in the *absence* of identified and treated causes that resolved the dysrhythmia (e.g., coronary artery disease, structural cardiac disease)

- Structural heart disease with sustained VT (stable or unstable)

- Sustained or inducible (during study) VT with associated syncope of otherwise indeterminate origin

- EF < 35% (non-ischemic or at least 40 days post-MI), with NYHA Class II or III CHF; EF < 30% if Class I CHF

- Non-sustained VT after an MI if EF < 40%

Cardiac resynchronization therapy (biventricular pacing), with or without an ICD, is indicated for patients with NYHA class III or IV CHF with EF < 35%, QRS duration ≥ 0.12 sec, and sinus rhythm.

Contraindications

The presence of active infection is a contraindication for placement of a permanent pacemaker or ICD. If a pacemaker is needed in the setting of infection, a temporary transvenous pacemaker or an externalized pulse generator is recommended. Placement of cardiac devices is also contraindicated with inadequately treated coagulopathy.

ICDs are not recommended for patients with reversible causes of arrhythmia, those with a life expectancy < 12 months, or psychiatric patients that may be adversely affected by ICD shocks.

Complications

Significant complications occur in < 2% of transvenous devices. Early complications include injury to systemic veins and right-sided cardiac structures (including RA perforation with tamponade or traumatic tricuspid regurgitation), pneumothorax, hemothorax, air embolus, venous thrombosis, arrhythmias.

The most important long-term complication is infection of the pocket or leads, which occur in 3% of patients. Other possible late complications include lead fracture, lead malfunction, pocket erosion, and venous thrombosis. Lead fracture or malfunction is usually detected by an increase in pacing thresholds.

56. Cardiac tumors

Joseph W. Turek, Nicholas D. Andersen

Classification

The vast majority of cardiac tumors are metastatic lesions from another source. In order of decreasing frequency, tumors metastatic to the heart include: lung cancer, breast cancer, leukemia, lymphoma, esophageal cancer, and melanoma. Conversely, primary cardiac tumors are relatively uncommon. Benign lesions account for 75% of primary cardiac tumors, with 25% derived from malignant origin.

Presentation

Obstruction, followed by embolization, represent the two most common acute manifestations of cardiac tumors. Bulky tumors can cause valvular obstruction thereby mimicking symptoms of stenosis associated with a particular valve. With larger pedunculated lesions (classically myxomas) these symptoms are more positional and acute than with calcific valvular stenosis as the neoplasm intermittently occludes the valve orifice.

Embolization occurs frequently with friable intracardiac lesions (i.e. papillary fibroelastomas and myxomas) and is the primary adverse event with papillary fibroelastomas.

Finally, non-specific symptoms such as fever, fatigue, and myalgias can be associated with cardiac tumors. The cause of these symptoms is not always clear. However, tumor excision typically leads to regression of symptoms, suggesting an association with tumor presence.

Echocardiography remains the test of choice for diagnosing cardiac masses. CT and MRI have utility in evaluating the degree of tumor invasion into the myocardium and adjacent structures for malignant cardiac tumors.

Tumors metastatic to the heart

Treatment for tumors metastatic to the heart is largely limited to the drainage of symptomatic pericardial and pleural effusions. Surgical excision does play a role in certain subdiaphragmatic masses that have invaded the RA via the inferior vena cava. In particular, transthoracic / transabdominal operations have shown survival advantages in the treatment of aggressive renal cell carcinomas and neuroblastomas.

Benign cardiac tumors

Myxomas comprise nearly 50% of all benign primary cardiac neoplasms. 75% of these lesions are found in the LA, usually originating from the atrial septum. The remainder originate in the RA, with only a small fraction arising from within a ventricular cavity. Most myxomas are sporadic, more frequently found in women, and occur in adulthood. However, 5% of myxomas follow a familial pattern of autosomal dominant inheritance. In these cases, the tumors tend to be more aggressive, occur earlier in life and are more prevalent in men. Carney's triad is a notable familial syndrome consisting of atrial myxomas, endocrine overactivity, and cutaneous lentiginosis. Symptoms include intracardiac obstruction with CHF including positional dyspnea (60-70%), emboli (30-50%), and constitutional symptoms (20%). However, many patients are asymptomatic. Surgical excision is indicated soon after discovery to prevent obstructive or embolic consequences in these potentially large and friable masses. Sporadic myxomas recur in 1-3% of patients while familial myxomas recur in 12-20%.

Cardiac lipomas are slow-growing, encapsulated fatty tumors. A non-encapsulated variant, known as lipomatous hypertrophy, has an affinity for the interatrial septum. Surgical excision is indicated only if symptoms are present, or if removal can be performed conveniently during a concomitant cardiac procedure. Lipomas most commonly generate obstructive symptoms, whereas lipomatous hypertrophic lesions more commonly produce arrhythmias.

Papillary fibroelastomas account for 15% of benign cardiac tumors, although echocardiography has led to an increased rate of identification. The tumors consist of multiple delicate fronds resembling sea anemones and commonly arise from left-sided cardiac structures, with the aortic valve being the most frequent site. Half of papillary fibroelastomas are asymptomatic and identified incidentally, whereas half are detected following embolization. Surgical resection is indicated upon diagnosis given the high rate of embolization. Valve-sparing shave excision carries a low mortality and recurrence rate.

Rhabdomyomas are the most common primary cardiac tumor in children and occur with tuberous sclerosis in 50% of patients. Lesions are commonly multicentric and found within the ventricles. They are frequently identified in the neonatal period, and place the infant at high risk of cardiac failure due to obstruction and arrhythmia. Resection is indicated following diagnosis if tuberous sclerosis is absent. Given the poor prognosis in tuberous sclerosis patients, resection is contraindicated aside from palliative debulking for symptomatic relief.

Fibromas are the second most common primary cardiac tumor in children and are characteristically large, solitary tumors arising in the ventricles. Fibromas are occasionally identified on CXR given a tendency for calcification. Obstruction and arrhythmia are the most common presenting symptoms. Treatment involves complete surgical removal, although promising outcomes have been achieved from debulking of giant fibromas.

Mesotheliomas of the atrioventricular node are small tumors that have been linked to sudden death due to heart block and ventricular fibrillation. Experience with excision is limited.

Malignant cardiac tumors

Malignant cardiac tumors originating in the heart portend a poor prognosis. They are often rapidly metastatic, thus precluding surgical resection in most cases. Invariably, these lesions are sarcomas, with angiosarcomas representing the most common pathology. Patients present primarily with arrhythmias or symptoms of CHF. Surgical resection has a role in rare cases of a small neoplasm without evidence for metastasis. However, drainage procedures are by far the most common surgical interventions for this disease entity.

Surgical treatment

Lesions should be completely resected with negative margins and direct tumor manipulation should be minimized. For atrial lesions, bicaval cannulation is recommended and vents placed through the pulmonary veins should be avoided. For LA lesions, biatrial incisions may be useful to optimize exposure. Defects can generally be closed primarily, with rare cases requiring pericardial patch closure. Outcomes following myxoma resection are excellent, with mortality rates less than 5%.

Surgical excision is generally indicated as the primary treatment for benign cardiac tumors and is typically curative, with recurrence being uncommon. Conversely, malignant cardiac neoplasms carry a poor prognosis. Prior to resection of a malignant tumor, a full metastatic search should be performed. Evidence of metastases precludes resection. For the few patients with malignancy that undergo surgery, resection is rarely curative, but rather serves a palliative role. Adjuvant chemotherapy can be recommended and provides a modest survival benefit.

57. Acute and chronic pulmonary embolism

Serguei I. Melnitchouk

Pathophysiology

Approximately 90% of pulmonary embolism (PE) cases are associated with lower extremity deep vein thrombosis. The emboli lodge in the PAs, cause mechanical obstruction, and get further coated with platelets and thrombin. Platelets release vasoactive agents, such as serotonin, thromboxane, and adenosine diphosphate, which significantly contribute to the elevation of PVR. Depending on the clot burden, this leads to RV dilation, ischemia, and dysfunction. RV dysfunction leads to reduced LV filling, reduction in coronary blood flow, and systemic hypotension. However, a vast majority of patients with PE are managed medically with aggressive anticoagulation and only a small fraction of PE cases exhibit hemodynamic instability and/or require surgical intervention.

With time, the clot dissolves and becomes clinically insignificant in most of PE cases, but in approximately 4% of patients a chronic thromboembolic pulmonary hypertension develops. Failure to resolve the initial embolus and its development into the dense fibrous tissue, incorporated in the vessel wall, leads to the large- and small-vessel vasculopathy and the development of pulmonary arterial hypertension with subsequent right heart failure. These patients eventually require pulmonary thromboendarterectomy, provided they have surgically accessible disease.

Diagnosis

Few clinical and diagnostic findings are used in the diagnosis of pulmonary embolism:

- *Clinical presentation.* Dyspnea, pleuritic chest pain, low grade fever, tachycardia, tachypnea, cyanosis, neck vein distention, and hypotension.

- *EKG.* Tachycardia, nonspecific T-wave and ST changes; a minority of patients with massive PE may show cor pulmonale, right-axis deviation, or right bundle-branch block.

- *Room air ABG.* Hypoxia, hypocarbia, occasionally acidosis.

- *CXR.* May be normal or with parenchymal infiltrate, atelectasis, pleural effusion.

- *D-dimer.* Specificity reduced in patients with cancer, pregnant women, after trauma or surgery, and in hospitalized/elderly patients.

- *Cardiac enzymes / brain natriuretic peptide.* Elevation of cardiac troponins indicates RV microinfarction.

- *CT pulmonary angiography.* Mainstay of diagnosis, shows intraluminal filling defects in the pulmonary arterial tree.

- *V/Q scanning.* Lesser sensitivity than CT, alternative test in patients with renal failure or allergy to contrast dye.

- *Echocardiography.* RV pressure overload/dysfunction (see below), may demonstrate central thromboemboli.

Pulmonary embolectomy

Indications

Primary indications for acute pulmonary embolectomy include massive pulmonary embolism with systemic arterial hypotension as well as submassive pulmonary embolism, defined as RV dysfunction and troponin elevation despite normal systemic arterial pressure. Other indications include need for a surgical removal of a RA or ventricular thrombus, need for closure of a PFO, and pulmonary embolectomy in failed thrombolysis cases. RV enlargement on echocardiography is characterized by a RV diameter that is 90% or greater the size of the LV diameter. Other echocardiographic findings associated with PE include RV wall hypokinesis, paradoxical septal motion, increased PA pressure, tricuspid regurgitation, and inferior vena cava congestion.

Surgical technique

For acute pulmonary thromboembolectomy, CPB with high ascending aortic and bicaval cannulation is established. Because only a short period of bypass is needed, there is no need for significant hypothermia. To arrest the heart, either cold cardioplegic solution or electrical fibrillation may be used. Alternatively, the procedure can be performed on a warm, beating heart, without aortic cross-clamping or cardioplegic or fibrillatory arrest. The RA is opened if an embolus is in transit and aortic cross-clamping is performed if a PFO is present and requires closure. The main PA is opened longitudinally approximately 2 cm distal to the pulmonary valve and the incision is extended onto the proximal left PA. Care is taken to avoid blind instrumentation of the fragile PAs. The clot should gently be freed from the PA with hand-over-hand type motion (e.g. with open gallstone forceps) to support the extraction from segmental branches and to avoid fragmentation of the embolus. Lifting the apex of the heart upward and to the right will provide a view into the distal branches of the LLL PA. The right PA can be opened longitudinally between the SVC and the aorta for an additional separate exposure. Placing a cerebellar retractor between the SVC and aorta will improve the visualization of the branches of the right PA. Pediatric size bronchoscope may be used to confirm the completeness of the embolectomy. Postoperative long-term ventilation after embolectomy is usually secondary to lung reperfusion injury.

Pulmonary thromboendarterectomy

Indications

Pulmonary thromboendarterectomy (PTE) is considered in patients with chronic thromboembolic pulmonary hypertension who are symptomatic and have evidence of hemodynamic or ventilatory impairment at rest or during exercise. Recent clinical guidelines recommend that the following four basic criteria should be met: 1) NYHA class III or IV symptoms, 2) preoperative PVR of more than 300 dynes×sec×cm^{-5}, 3) surgically accessible thrombus in the main, lobar, segmental, or subsegmental arteries, and 4) no significant comorbidities. The only absolute contraindication to PTE is the presence of severe underlying lung disease, either obstructive or restrictive. Patients with suprasystemic PA pressures can safely undergo PTE.

There are four types of pulmonary occlusive disease:

- *Type I.* Visible clot in the main PA upon opening the arteries

- *Type II.* Thickened intima with webs; proximal disease; most frequent (40-70%)

- *Type III.* Distal disease in the segmental and subsegmental branches; challenging dissection

- *Type IV.* Intrinsic small-vessel disease causing idiopathic pulmonary hypertension; inoperable

Surgical technique

Full CPB is instituted with bicaval and high ascending aortic cannulation. A vent is placed through the main PA 2 cm distal to the pulmonary valve and a LA vent is placed through the right superior pulmonary vein. The patient is cooled down to 18 °C and circulatory arrest is used to have a bloodless field for dissection in the segmental and subsegmental branches. The right PA is approached between the aorta and the SVC by using a cerebellar retractor. A longitudinal incision is extended onto the lower lobe branch. After the loose thrombi and debris are removed, the endarterectomy plane is raised to clear the intima and the endarterectomy specimen is carefully dissected out in each segmental branch and then extracted. Attention is paid to dissect not too deep in the media, as this may lead to an inadvertent perforation. The pulmonary vent is removed and an arteriotomy is extended laterally from the vent cannulation site onto the left PA until the pericardial reflection is reached. Similar endarterectomy technique is performed on the left side as well.

58. Diseases of the pericardium
Gabriel Loor

Anatomy

The pericardium is a serosal sac that covers the heart and origins of the great vessels. The sac is lined by a single layer of mesothelial cells. The normal volume of pericardial fluid is 15-50 ml and normal pressure ranges from -5 to +5 mmHg. The visceral pericardium is in direct contact with the epicardium. The parietal pericardium is covered by a fibroelastic tissue (fibrosa), which determines the compliance.

Pericardial effusion

A pericardial effusion is defined as an abnormal increase in the volume of pericardial fluid. Acute increases in fluid are poorly tolerated by the relatively noncompliant parietal pericardium and result in rapidly elevated filling pressures (see below "Cardiac Tamponade"). Gradual increases in fluid allow elastin fibers to adjust their compliance and result in a lower pressure rise and a greater volume capacity.

Pericardial effusions may be transudative, exudative, chylous, hemorrhagic or purulent. They are easily identified by either transthoracic echocardiography or TEE. It takes 250 ml of fluid to appreciate an enlarged cardiac silhouette on CXR. CT scans and MRIs may also reveal the presence of effusions.

In general, effusions are drained by pericardiocentesis for refractory symptoms or diagnostic uncertainty. Symptoms may range from dyspnea, chest pressure, or tamponade. While history alone may suffice to distinguish transudative from exudative effusions, diagnostic pericardiocentesis may be necessary.

Exudative fluid is characterized by an LDH > 200 U/L, protein > 0.5x the serum protein, LDH > 0.6x the serum LDH, and/or cholesterol level > 45 mg/dl. Exudative effusions result from inflammation of the pericardium due to pericarditis. Transudative effusions are rarely significant and are usually due to volume overload from heart or renal failure. Chylous effusions are rare. They are due to abnormal connections between the thoracic duct and the pericardium most likely from trauma or iatrogenic injuries. These effusions are milky and contain > 110 mg/dL of triglycerides. They are generally treated conservatively with initial percutaneous drainage, NPO and TPN but may require thoracic duct ligation or mediastinal exploration in refractory cases.

Acute pericarditis

Acute pericarditis produces a typical serofibrinous exudate on the pericardium, which may or may not produce an effusion. The typical presentation for acute pericarditis is pleuritic chest pain relieved by leaning forward. A pericardial friction rub is common on exam. EKG findings include diffuse ST elevations in all leads except V1 and aVF along with diffuse PR depressions. Acute pericarditis must be differentiated from an acute MI, which produces more regionalized EKG abnormalities.

Types of acute pericarditis include:

- *Viral pericarditis.* Caused by Coxsackievirus B (most common), Echovirus, Adenovirus, Influenza virus, mumps, varicella, EBV, or HBV. Viral pericarditis may be responsible for "idiopathic pericarditis" and both, viral and idiopathic pericarditis, resolve within 1-3 weeks. Treatment is supportive with NSAIDs +/- colchicine. Large effusions are rare with idiopathic/viral pericarditis and would be drained only for symptoms or diagnostic uncertainty.

- *Bacterial pericarditis.* Most commonly due to Streptococcal, Pneumococcal or Staphylococcal organisms. They are treated with antibiotics and supportive care but purulent effusions may contribute to refractory sepsis and even tamponade. These effusions often require surgical drainage through a pericardial window.

- *Tuberculous pericarditis.* Results in an exudative pericardial inflammation in the setting of an active TB infection. Management is mainly medical with triple drug therapy but they may develop bloody effusions that require drainage for symptoms and prevention of constrictive pericarditis in the future.

- *Fungal pericarditis.* Treated medically with antifungals and NSAIDs.

- *Neoplastic pericarditis.* Rarely due to primary tumors but rather secondary tumors from metastatic disease or contiguous spread. The most common tumors include breast, lung and lymphoma. Neoplastic effusions are drained for palliation only with pericardiocentesis or a pericardial window +/- talc or doxycycline sclerotherapy.

- *Dressler's syndrome.* This syndrome can occur about 2 weeks following an acute MI when a diffuse pericarditis ensues. While it portends a worse prognosis for an acute MI it does not generally cause effusions that require drainage and is treated supportively with NSAIDs +/- colchicine.

- *Metabolic causes.* Uremic pericarditis usually resolves within 2 weeks of aggressive dialysis. It may result in bloody effusions and lead to tamponade. Drainage is reserved for large, symptomatic or refractory effusions.

- *Other causes.* Rheumatoid arthritis and RT exposure may also result in acute pericarditis +/- associated effusions but are generally more important in their contribution to constrictive pericarditis.

Cardiac tamponade

Tamponade is a feared complication of open heart procedures, trauma, or complex pericarditis. It may result from either an acute or chronic accumulation of pericardial fluid. Elevated diastolic filling pressures are transmitted to all cardiac chambers beginning with the RA and RV. This causes a reduction in blood flow into the atrial and ventricular chambers resulting in venous congestion and low cardiac output. Acute compensatory measures include tachycardia and elevated systemic and pulmonary venous tone.

The diagnosis is readily made in a postoperative patient with a drop in cardiac index, elevated filling pressures, hypotension, narrowed pulse pressure, and oliguria. Other findings include jugular venous distention (JVD), *pulsus paradoxus* (exaggerated decrease in systolic blood pressure of more than 10 mmHg with inspiration), and equilibration of diastolic pressures. In addition, there may be a loss of the y-descent on the venous tracing suggesting a loss of passive flow from the atrium to the ventricle during early diastole. Echocardiography may reveal a pericardial effusion with a lack of IVC collapse with inspiration. Treatment requires evacuation via pericardiocentesis (subacute/chronic thin effusions), pericardial window (loculated effusions) or median sternotomy (acute post-op) depending on the clinical situation and urgency.

Constrictive pericarditis

Constrictive pericarditis (CP) can develop as a late sequelae of acute pericarditis. The most common etiology in Western countries is idiopathic, followed by prior cardiac surgery and mediastinal RT. It may also result from hemorrhagic effusions, which leave excessive scar tissue over time as well. The most common cause of CP in the developing world is TB.

Patients with constrictive pericarditis present with signs of low cardiac output (fatigue, hypotension, tachycardia) and/or elevated venous pressures (hepatomegaly, edema, ascites, shortness of breath on exertion). There are important differences between CP and tamponade physiology. While there is an increase in filling pressures with CP they occur much later in diastole. There is usually a steep y wave descent followed by a plateau that forms a "square root sign" on venous pressure tracings (due to rapid early diastolic filling of the ventricle followed by lack of additional filling due to compression in late diastole). Echocardiography will show a septal bounce as an abrupt end to ventricular filling occurs. The patient may also have Kussmaul's sign where inspiration causes a paradoxical increase in venous pressure and JVD.

It is important to distinguish constrictive pericarditis from restrictive cardiomyopathy (RCM) since the latter is not amenable to surgery. This may be difficult since both entities produce similar symptoms and patterns on pressure tracings and echocardiography. Restrictive cardiomyopathy may be caused by amyloidosis, sarcoidosis, RT, carcinoid, hemochromatosis, or anthracycline toxicity. On echocardiography, a myocardial speckling pattern may be seen with amyloidosis. An endomyocardial biopsy may be necessary if the patient's history suggests RCM. Heart transplantation is the only option for RCM leading to heart failure.

The surgical approach to CP includes surgical stripping usually through a median sternotomy or left antero-lateral thoracotomy. The pericardium is resected anteriorly from phrenic nerve to phrenic nerve and down to the diaphragmatic reflection.

III. Congenital Cardiac Surgery

59. Cardiac embryology and segmental approach

T. K. Susheel Kumar, Daniel J. DiBardino

The heart develops from the splanchnopleuric mesoderm lying immediately cranial to the prochordal plate (also called the "cardiogenic" area). The two cardiogenic areas on either side of the primitive streak have intrinsic differential growth characteristics and are the determinants of sidedness, which is the first fundamental choice the primitive heart makes (*situs solitus* or *situs inversus*). The formation of the heart begins as a pair of endothelial tubes that fuse with each other and develop a series of dilatations termed the *bulbus cordis*, primitive ventricle, primitive atrium, and *sinus venosus*. The *bulbus cordis* lying at the arterial end has a distal portion called the *truncus arteriosus* and a proximal portion called the *conus*. The *truncus arteriosus* in turn is continuous with the aortic sac, which communicates with the bilateral pharyngeal arch arteries. The *sinus venosus* lying at the venous end has recognizable right and left horns. Each horn in turn receives a vitelline vein (from yolk sac), an umbilical vein (from placenta), and a common cardinal vein (from body wall). Thus by the 3rd to 4th week, the blueprint for future development of the heart has been laid out. The fate of various early structures is summarized in Table 59-1.

Table 59-1. Fate of early structures in cardiac development.

Structure	Fate of structure
Distal portion of *bulbus cordis* (*truncus arteriosus*)	Forms ascending aorta and pulmonary trunk
Proximal portion of *bulbus cordis* (*conus*)	*Conus* gets absorbed into primitive ventricle
Primitive ventricle	Partitions into right and left ventricles
Primitive atrium	Partitions into right and left atria
Sinus venosus	Gets absorbed into right atrium. Left horn regresses to form part of coronary sinus

Formation of the interatrial septum

Early in development, the primitive atrium is divided partially by the appearance of an invagination of its roof called the *septum primum*. This grows downwards and ultimately fuses with the AV (atrioventricular) cushions obliterating the gap between them (called for*amen primum*). However, well before this fusion can happen, the upper portion of the *septum primum* breaks down to create a gap called *foramen secundum*. This is essential for the oxygenated blood from placenta reaching the right side of the heart to enter the left side and rest of the body. A second partition now grows downward from the roof to the left of the primary septum and overlaps the free upper edge of the *septum primum*. The slit-like gap between the two septa is called the *foramen ovale* and allows unidirectional flow of blood from the right to left.

Development of the right atrium

The *sinus venosus* gets absorbed into the right half of the primitive atrium and gives rise to the smooth portion of the RA (*sinus venarum*). The left horn of the *sinus venosus* regresses and takes part in formation of the coronary sinus. The veins emptying into the right horn of the *sinus venosus* give rise to terminal part of the IVC (right vitelline vein) and the SVC (right common cardinal vein). The opening of the *sinus venosus* into the RA is guarded by the right and left venous valves. The right venous valve expands greatly and forms the *crista terminalis*, the Eustachian valve (guarding the opening of the IVC) and the Thebesian valve (guarding the opening of the coronary sinus). The *crista terminalis* delineates the pectinate portion of the RA (arising from the primitive atrium) from the *sinus venarum* (arising from the sinus venosus).

Development of the left atrium

The LA develops from the left half of the primitive atrium. The lungs develop as outpouchings of the primitive foregut and initially lack any connection to the embryonic heart. They carry the arteries and veins investing the foregut, which are connected to splanchnic (systemic) arterial and systemic venous circulations. Around the 30th day of gestation, a dorsal eventration of the LA (the common pulmonary vein) appears and joins the pulmonary venous plexus surrounding the lung buds. With this, the pulmonary-systemic connections regress. The common pulmonary vein gets absorbed into the LA during growth so that the four pulmonary veins open separately into the LA.

Development of the AV canal

The primitive atrium and primitive ventricle are connected by a narrow AV canal. Mesodermal tissue at this junction called AV cushions appear on the dorsal and ventricular wall. They proliferate and fuse forming what is called the *septum intermedium*. Proliferation of this tissue contributes to the formation of the lower part of the atrial septum, the inlet portion of interventricular septum, the septal leaflet of the tricuspid valve, and the anterior leaflet of the mitral valve. The rest of the AV valve leaflets arise by a process of delamination.

Development of the ventricles

The *conus* gets absorbed into the primitive ventricle and gives rise to both the outflow tracts. Initially, the heart is a straight tube but differential growth results in a rightward loop called D-loop. Bulboventricular loop-ing is a morphogenetic process independent of the one that leads to cardi-ac situs determination. In normal D-loop, the primitive RV and the aorta lie on the right side. In L-loop, the primitive RV and aorta lie to the left.

The right half of the primitive ventricle connects with the outflow tract while the left half is connected to the primitive atrium. The right and left halves communicate through a primitive VSD called bulboventricular defect. The acquisition by the early loop heart of the final ventricular morphology requires a widening of the AV canal to the right and shift of the *conus* to the left with disappearance of the bulboventricular flange.

The formation of the interventricular septum is a complex process and partition of the ventricle proceeds in such a way that each half communi-cates with the corresponding atrium and the RV opens into the pulmonary tract while the LV opens into the aorta. The primitive ventricular septum develops as an infolding of the floor of the primitive ventricle and grows upward. Bulbar ridges arising in the floor of the conical portion of the bulboventricular cavity give rise to the bulbar septum. This grows downward towards the primitive interventricular septum. The gap be-tween the upper edge of the interventricular septum and lower edge of the bulbar septum is filled by proliferation of tissue from the AV cushions. Thus the proper development of the ventricular septum depends on the convergence and fusion of various components. The final section of the ventricular septum to close is composed of fibrous tissue (membranous septum), whereas the rest of the septum is composed of thick muscular tissue.

Development of the outflow tract

The distal part of the *bulbus cordis* (called *truncus arteriosus*) gives rise to the great arteries. A spiral septum arises from fusion of right and left truncal swellings and divides the *truncus arteriosus* into relatively equal-sized great vessels, namely pulmonary trunk and aorta. As the name sug-gests, the septum is a spiral structure such that the pulmonary trunk lies ventral to the aorta at the lower end and comes to lie to the left of the aor-ta as it is traced upwards.

Development of the major arteries

The right and left primitive aortae are the first arteries to appear in the embryo. These are connected with the endothelial heart tubes ventrally and arch backwards to continue as the dorsal aorta. Following fusion of the heart tubes, the ventral portions of the primitive aorta fuse to form the aortic sac that communicates with the primitive *truncus arteriosus*. A series of arteries appear in the pharyngeal arches on either side and connect the dorsal aortae to the aortic sac (Table 59-2). The origin of the major arteries is summarized in Table 59-3.

Table 59-2. Fate of the pharyngeal arch arteries.

Pharyngeal artery	Fate of artery
1st arch artery	Greater part disappears. Remnants form the maxillary artery
2nd arch artery	Greater part disappears. Remnants form the stapedial artery
3rd arch artery	Common carotid and internal carotid arteries on either side
4th arch artery	Subclavian artery on right and aortic arch on left
5th arch artery	Disappears
6th arch artery	Artery to developing lung bud on either side. Form the pulmonary artery on either side and *ductus arteriosus* on left

Table 59-3. Summary of development of main arteries.

Structure	Origin
Ascending aorta and pulmonary trunk	Primitive *truncus arteriosus*
Aortic arch	Ventral portion of aortic sac, left horn of aortic sac (proximal arch) and left 4th arch artery (distal arch)
Descending aorta	Left dorsal aorta
Brachiocephalic	Right horn of aortic sac
Carotid	3rd arch artery
Subclavian	Right from the right 4th arch + right 7th cervical intersegmental artery Left from the left 7th cervical intersegmental artery
Pulmonary artery	6th arch between the pulmonary trunk and branch to lung bud
Ductus arteriosus	6th arch between the branch to lung bud and dorsal aorta

Valves of the heart

The leaflets and tensor apparatus of the AV valves are formed by a process of delamination of the inner layers of the inlet zone of the ventricles. The AV cushions also contribute to formation of the septal leaflet of the tricuspid valve and anterior mitral leaflet. The aortic and pulmonary valves are derived from endocardial cushions formed at the junction of *truncus arteriosus* and *conus*. Initially, two cushions, the right and left, appear in the wall of the *conus* and fuse with each other. Following division of the primitive *truncus*, these get subdivided. Subsequently, an anterior and posterior cushion appear. Thus each opening has 3 cusps.

Development of the coronary arteries

Normal development of the coronary arteries occurs by connection between buds that arise from the aortic sinuses of Valsalva and the epicardial arterial plexus. Buds also grow from the pulmonary sinuses as part of normal development and later regress.

Segmental nomenclature to describe congenital heart disease

The heart and great vessels can be viewed as three separate segments: the atria, the ventricles, and the great arteries. These segments can each individually vary from their normal positions, resulting in many different concordant and discordant connections. Van Praagh's segmental approach is the most commonly used nomenclature for describing the relative relationship of each segment for any given cardiac specimen. The following symbols are used for each of the three segments:

- *Visceroatrial relationship*

    - S – solitus. The normal anatomic arrangement

    - I – inversus. Mirror image of normal

    - A – ambiguous. Ambiguous appearance; description not possible

- *Ventricular loop*

    - D-loop. The normal "right handed" arrangement leading to a morphologic RV on the right side and a morphologic LV on the left side. Note that the AV valves always follow the appropriate ventricles.

    - L-loop. The mirror image of normal; a "left handed" arrangement leading to a morphologic RV on the left side and a morphologic LV on the right side. Note that the AV valves always follow the appropriate ventricles.

    - X. Uncertain or indeterminate

- *Great arteries*

    - S – solitus. The normal anatomic arrangement of an anterior and leftward PA and a posterior and rightward aorta.

- I – inversus. The mirror image of the normal arrangement, leading to a rightward and anterior PA and a leftward and posterior aorta.

- D – dextro transposition. Rightward and anterior aorta with leftward and posterior PA.

- L – levo transposition. Mirror image of D-transposition, leading to leftward and anterior aorta with rightward and posterior PA.

With these symbols, the segmental relationship of the heart can be expressed by three letters. This segmental approach is independent of the location of cardiac apex and thus applies to both dextrocardia and levocardia, which must be expressed separately when describing the anatomy.

The embryologic basis of several congenital heart lesions is summarized in Table 59-4.

Table 59-4. Embryologic basis of basic congenital heart lesions.

Defect	Embryologic basis
ALCAPA	Failure of establishment of connection between left aortic bud and the epicardial arterial plexus.
Aortopulmonary window	Incomplete development of spiral septum
Cleft mitral valve	Defect in AV cushion contribution to formation of anterior mitral valve
Coarctation of the aorta	Flow theory: Blood flow through cardiac chambers and great arteries during fetal life determines their size. Coarctation occurs as a consequence of lack of blood flow across aortic isthmus (either because of VSD or left-sided obstructive lesions). Ductal sling theory (Skoda): Abnormal extension of contractile ductal tissue into the aorta. Contraction and fibrosis of this tissue at time of ductal closure leads to coarctation.
Common AV canal	Failure of contribution of AV cushion towards formation of atrial and ventricular septa
Common pulmonary venous atresia	Common pulmonary vein gets obliterated after pulmonary systemic connections have disappeared.
Common ventricle	Severe lack of ventricular septation most likely caused by total absence of both primitive ventricular septum and component of AV cushion
Congenital aortic stenosis	Failure of normal development of cusps resulting in primitive gelatinous masses guarding aortic opening.
Cor triatriatum	Abnormal connection between the common pulmonary vein and the LA
Cor triatriatum dexter	Persistence of right venous valve resulting in membranous obstruction of the tricuspid valve, RVOT or IVC.

Corrected transposition (I-TGA)	Reverse looping of the heart tube (l loop rather than d loop) with malseptation of truncus resulting in both AV and VA discordance.
d-TGA	Failure of septum to spiral in usual fashion resulting in ventriculoarterial discordance. Alternative theory: underdevelopment of subpulmonary *conus* resulting in pulmonary mitral continuity (Van Praagh)
DILV	Persistence of primitive arrangement where both AV valves empty into LV.
DIRV	Rightward shifting of AV canal exceeds normal shifting resulting in both AV valves emptying into RV.
DOLV	Leftward shifting of *conus* exceeds the normal shifting leading to inclusion of both conal derivatives into LVOT.
DORV	Persistence of primitive arrangement where RV empties into both outlets. Abnormality of spiral septation such that aorta becomes dextroposed. This is greater dextroposition than seen in TOF but lesser than that of TGA.
Ebstein's anomaly	Failure of delamination of the septal and posterior leaflets of the tricuspid valve resulting in downward displacement of these leaflets.
Gerbode defect	Defect in AV cushion contribution to formation of septal component of tricuspid valve resulting in LV to RA communication
Hypoplastic left heart syndrome	Leftward displacement of *septum primum* deflects usual volume of blood away from left heart leading to its underdevelopment Alternative theories: 1) Premature narrowing of *foramen ovale* leading to faulty transfer of blood from IVC to LA. 2) Severe underdevelopment of LVOT leading to altered flow pattern in fetus.
Inlet VSD	Failure of normal contribution of AV cushion towards formation of ventricular septum
Interrupted aortic arch	Failure of normal fusion between the various segments. Type of interruption depends upon level of failure of fusion.
Ostium primum defect	Failure of septum primum to reach the AV cushions. Alternate theory: Defective formation of AV cushions.
Ostium primum defect	Failure of normal contribution of AV cushion towards lower part of atrial septum
Ostium secundum defect	Resorption of the *septum primum*, which normally provides floor of *fossa ovalis*.
Patent *ductus arteriosus*	Persistent patency of *ductus arteriosus*
PFO	Persistence of oblique valvular passage between *septum primum* and *secundum*.
Pulmonary atresia / intact ventricular septum	Failure of pulmonary valve leaflets to open resulting in decreased flow through the tricuspid valve and RV and consequent hypoplasia. Variable degree of RV hypoplasia depending on the stage at which fault occurs.

Pulmonary vein stenosis	Abnormal connection between the individual pulmonary veins and the common pulmonary vein.
Shone's complex	Premature narrowing of *foramen ovale* or improper angulation of *limbus* leads to hypoplasia of left heart structures (flow theory)
Subaortic stenosis	Malseptation of conal septum with primitive interventricular septum. May be associated with posterior malaligned VSD when conal septum projects into LVOT. Subaortic membrane develops as a result of turbulence in abnormally shaped LVOT.
TAPVR	Failure of the common pulmonary vein to connect to the pulmonary venous plexus of the lung buds.
TOF	Classic theory: Faulty septation of *bulbus cordis* resulting in unequal sized great vessels (i.e. large aorta and small pulmonary trunk). Alternative theory: Underdevelopment of subpulmonary *conus* with consequent rightward and superior shift of the aortic valve (Van Praagh).
TOF / pulmonary atresia	Failure of 6th arch arteries to connect with the systemic arteries carried by the lung bud from the primitive foregut and persistence of connections from aorta (aortopulmonary collaterals). Variable degree of development of true PA depends on stage at which defect sets in.
Tricuspid atresia	Failure of normal development of the tricuspid valve resulting in hypoplasia of the RV.
Truncus arteriosus	Complete failure of septation of distal portion of *bulbus cordis*.
Vascular rings	Disturbance of normal development of pharyngeal arch arteries. Double aortic arch: Persistence of right dorsal aorta with incomplete resorption of left. Right aortic arch: Persistence of right dorsal aorta with resorption of left aortic arch.
VSD – Conoventricular	Defect between the conal and primitive interventricular septum usually associated with some degree of malalignment.
VSD – inlet (type 3)	Defect of the endocardial AV cushion, most likely the medial cushions
VSD – muscular (type 4)	Defect in the primitive interventricular septum
VSD – outlet (type 1)	Defect in development of the bulbar septum
VSD – perimembranous (type 2)	Failure of membranous septum to form completely and may occur because of inadequacy of any of the three contributors.

ALCAPA: Anomalous left coronary artery from the pulmonary artery, AV: Atrioventricular, DILV: Double inlet left ventricle, DIRV: Double inlet right ventricle, DOLV: Double outlet left ventricle, DORV: Double outlet right ventricle, IVC: Inferior vena cava, LA: Left atrium, LV: Left ventricle, LVOT: Left ventricular outflow tract, PA: Pulmonary artery, PFO: Patent foramen ovale, RA: Right atrium, RV: Right ventricle, RVOT: Right ventricular outflow tract, TAPVR: Total anomalous pulmonary venous return, TGA: Transposition of the great arteries, TOF: Tetralogy of Fallot, VA: Ventriculoarterial, VSD: Ventricular septal defect.

60. Congenital cardiac evaluation and physiology

John C. Lin

Physiology

At birth, the lung becomes the primary organ for gas exchange. With the expansion of the lung, the pulmonary arterial bed dilates, decreasing the PVR. The RV blood volume then enters the lung rather than the ductus arteriosus. The increase in pulmonary venous return to the LA typically shuts the *foramen ovale* and ends the prenatal physiologic right-to-left shunt. Both the increase in oxygen and the reduction in prostaglandin E lead to vasoconstriction of the ductus and its eventual closure.

The congenital cardiac lesions are compatible with life while in utero due to the compensatory circulation in the heart and in the great vessels. In addition, the low level of oxygen in utero (50% O_2 saturation) allows for additional adaptation initially after delivery.

Evaluation

Each individual cardiac lesion will be discussed separately and in detail in the subsequent chapters. In general, infants with congenital cardiac findings can be asymptomatic or can exhibit respiratory discomfort to distress, failure to thrive, arrhythmia, and frequent infections. CXR with cardiac enlargement is possible. More importantly, the use of echocardiography has become the gold standard for congenital cardiac diagnostic workup.

Pulmonary resistance

At birth, the pulmonary resistance is 8 Wood units (i.e., 8 mmHg • min/L), but drops to the normal level of 2 Wood units at about 8 weeks. A pulmonary/systemic vascular resistance ratio of less than 0.2:1 is considered normal. With the expansion of the lungs at birth, the dilation of the existing pulmonary arteries along with the development of new arteries/arterioles follows, contributing to the drop in PVR. In the setting a left-to-right shunt, the normal maturation of the pulmonary arterial bed is disturbed.

The most reliable way to evaluate the pulmonary vascular bed is a cardiac catheterization. The response of the PVR to pulmonary vasodilators (i.e., oxygen, prostacyclin, and nitric oxide) is often tested. A pulmonary-to-systemic resistance ratio of 0.7:1 or a pulmonary resistance of 8-10 Wood units is used as the cutoff point when surgical intervention for a congenital lesion will no longer reverse the pathologic disease process. Therefore, any intervention for cardiac lesions with pulmonary vascular disease should take place prior to the first year of life and/or before the PA pressure exceeds more than half of the systemic arterial pressure.

61. Palliative operations

Bret A. Mettler, Ibrahim Abdullah

A palliative operation is one that provides symptomatic relief but leaves the main pathophysiology uncorrected. In congenital heart surgery, the two classic palliative procedures are the aortopulmonary shunt and the PA band. The goals of palliative procedures are to alter the hemodynamic physiology in a manner making the cardiac malformation more tolerable, providing an improvement in the patient's condition, and permitting growth until the child has complete correction. In addition to the more commonly performed palliative procedures above, historically an atrial septectomy was performed to improve mixing for d-transposition of the great vessels until an atrial level repair could be performed. More complex palliative procedures include the Norwood operation for hypoplastic left heart syndrome and the Glenn operation. As these operations are specific procedures associated with defined pathology, they will be discussed elsewhere.

Pulmonary artery band

Historically, PA banding was performed in small children with large left-to-right shunts and increased pulmonary blood flow. As advancements have been made in performing neonatal cardiac surgery, PA banding is sometimes indicated for a few defined lesions.

- "Swiss-cheese" muscular ventricular septal defects

- Single ventricle physiology with increased pulmonary blood flow in preparation for future Fontan procedure (i.e., tricuspid atresia type IIc)

- To prepare and retrain the ventricle in patients with transposition of the great arteries for future arterial switch procedure

In patients with normally related great vessels, PA banding may be performed either through a left thoracotomy or a median sternotomy. While banding material is chosen by surgeon preference, the most common materials include ePTFE (Gore-Tex®) and Silastic® tubing. Anatomically, PA bands are placed circumferentially around the mid-PA. Proximal placement may lead to pulmonary valve dysfunction. More commonly, band placement too distal or band migration can impinge upon the right PA leading to ostial stenosis. Safe generalizations regarding the degree of band tightening include:

- Elevation in the systemic systolic blood pressure by 10-20 mmHg.

- The main PAP should be reduced to 50% systemic in patients scheduled for a future biventricular repair.

- For patients in whom a completion Fontan procedure is anticipated, the lowest possible distal main PAP is most acceptable.

- Oxygen saturations for anticipated biventricular repair should be left at 90%; if final pathway is a Fontan procedure then oxygen saturations 80-85% is most acceptable.

- Trusler's rule can be used to guide the initial circumference of the band. For simple defects (VSD, tetralogy of Fallot): 20mm + 1 mm for each kg body weight. For mixing defects (single ventricle, transposition): 24mm + 1 mm for each kg body weight.

As the patient undergoes somatic growth, band tightness increases, further decreasing distal PA pressure and oxygen saturations.

Aortopulmonary shunts

Classic Blalock-Taussig shunt

The classic Blalock-Taussig shunt is a direct end-to-side anastomosis of the transected subclavian artery to the PA. The classic shunt does not require prosthetic material and provides a precise amount of pulmonary blood flow limited by the orifice of the subclavian artery. In addition, the shunt enlarges with somatic growth providing more pulmonary blood flow. Adversely, the shunt sacrifices a subclavian artery, which in a small number of patients has lead to devastating extremity ischemia. In addition, the affected arm is often shorter than the contralateral limb and will not have a palpable pulse. Due to the limited length of the subclavian artery and the distance required for translocation, the PA is easily distorted complicating further palliative procedures reliant on passive pulmonary blood flow.

Modified Blalock-Taussig shunt

The modified Blalock-Taussig shunt uses a synthetic conduit to create an aortopulmonary connection and is considered by most centers the shunt of choice. Benefits of the modified shunt include preservation of the affected arm circulation, regulation of shunt flow by the size of the systemic inflow, high patency rate, guarantee of adequate shunt length and ease of shunt takedown. In some patients, serous fluid will leach through the synthetic conduit leading to prolonged chest tube drainage. The size of the graft is selected by the size of the patient. Historically, a 5 mm graft has been used directly from the subclavian artery, relying on the size of the artery to limit inflow. Currently, most use a 3-4 mm shunt originating on the innominate artery. As a general rule for children less than 3 kg, a 3 mm shunt should be adequate while children larger than 3 kg require a 3.5 mm shunt. Some choose to place a larger shunt in all children and if pulmonary blood flow is excessive, shunt flow is externally restricted. Using this method, percutaneous procedures can be used to remove restriction and increase pulmonary blood flow as required with somatic growth.

Waterston/Cooley shunt

The Waterston/Cooley shunt is created by performing a direct anastomosis between the posterior aspect of the ascending aorta and the anterior right PA. Benefits of this shunt are the ease of construction not requiring prosthetic material and the preservation of the subclavian artery. The impediment of creating this shunt is distortion of the right PA and the inability to reliably regulate pulmonary blood flow. The shunt is infrequently used today due to the success of the modified Blalock/Taussig shunt.

Potts shunt

The Potts shunt is a direct anastomosis between the descending thoracic aorta and the left PA. This shunt is no longer used today due to complications of left PA aneurysm formation, frequent excessive pulmonary blood flow leading to pulmonary hypertension and the difficulty in taking down the shunt.

62. Patent ductus arteriosus

Robroy H. MacIver

A PDA is the result of patency of the fetal ductus arteriosus. It makes up 5-10% of congenital heart disease. The communication that forms between the upper descending aorta and proximal left PA creates a left-to-right shunt. Two times more common in females, it is associated with Rubella in the first trimester.

Derived from the 6th aortic arch, in normal development the PDA closes in two stages at birth. Release of histamine, catecholamines, bradykinin, and acetylcholine are factors that facilitate closure. The most important stimulus for closure is an increase in oxygen tension that begins with breathing. The first stage of closure is completed in the first 24 hours of life and is instigated by smooth muscle contraction. The second stage is completed at 2-3 weeks and involves fibrous proliferation of the intima and necrosis of inner layer of media. Unlike the first stage, the second stage is irreversible. Closure of the PDA begins at the PA towards the aorta; incomplete closure can cause a diverticulum on the aortic side.

Closure of the PDA depends on both intrinsic and extrinsic factors. pH, release of PGE_1/ PGE_2 / prostacyclin and PaO2 all affect the rate of closure. A decrease in oxygen tension can occur in children with congenital malformations that cause hypoxia. In addition, congenital malformations that cause the ductus to supply systemic circulation such as interrupted aortic arch, coarctation, and hypoplastic left heart syndrome all can be associated with a PDA. In these settings, a PDA can be kept open or closure reversed in the first week with the use of PGE_1.

Presentation

Most pre-term infants with a birth weight below 1,500 grams will have a PDA. A third of these patients will have a hemodynamically significant PDA. Most commonly, patients present with increased incidence of respiratory infections. On exam, a "machinery" murmur can be auscultated. Findings of heart failure, pulmonary infection, LV volume overload, and increased pulmonary blood flow by CXR markings can also occur in later stages. The increased blood flow through a PDA can eventually lead to pulmonary endothelial injury and subsequent pulmonary hypertension. Irreversible pulmonary changes (Eisenmenger's Syndrome) can be seen by 2 years of age. CHF accounts for 30% of deaths in children with an untreated PDA. PDAs can be classified as small, moderate, or large depending on a Qp:Qs of <1.5, 1.5 to 2.2, and >2.2, respectively.

Diagnosis

The workup of a PDA after physical exam involves an EKG, a CXR, and echocardiography. The EKG can be normal or show left, right or biventricular hypertrophy. The degree of hypertrophy is dependent on other malformations, amount of shunting, and associated pulmonary hypertension.

CXR can reveal cardiomegaly and increased pulmonary vascular markings. The changes in pulmonary vasculature can be difficult to interpret in the setting of intrinsic lung disease, which can be common in the premature infant. A prominent aortic knob is sometimes seen. In adults, calcification of the ductus can be seen.

Echocardiography is the main test to diagnose and guide treatment of a PDA. Doppler is used to assess the size of the shunt and to measure mean PA pressure. PA pressure is measured by calculating the mean left-to-right reading and subtracting it from the mean blood pressure. Diagnosis of other congenital cardiac malformations is key so as not to close off a physiologically necessary left-to-right shunt.

Treatment

Indications for closure of a PDA include respiratory distress, a large hemodynamically significant PDA (depending on the difference between pulmonary and systemic vascular resistance), failure of 2 courses of indomethacin or ibuprofen, necrotizing enterocolitis, and intracranial hemorrhage. A PDA does not necessarily need intervention. Approximately 90% are closed by 8 weeks. Roughly 1 of every 2000 infants will have a persistent PDA. High altitude, hypoxia, inheritance, low gestational age, and other associated cardiac malformations are associated with PDA.

Treatment of a PDA can be surgical, endovascular, or medical. Initial treatment of a PDA is focused on treatment of symptoms with the use of digoxin, diuretics, ventilator support, inotropes, and antibiotics, as appropriate. Medical closure of a PDA is achieved with indomethacin $0.1 - 0.2$ mg/kg Q8H for 3 doses. Indomethacin treatment is discouraged in the setting of renal failure. Medical treatment fails approximately 10% of the time, requiring surgical closure.

The surgical management of a PDA involves either a left thoracotomy or thoracoscopic approach. The ductus is closed by either or placement of a clip. Excessive dissection of the ductus can lead to significant morbidity. The recurrent laryngeal nerve takes off from the vagus nerve lateral to the ductus, curves under the arch of the aorta and then courses in the tracheoesophageal groove. In some series, a thoracotomy may be associated with the rate of future scoliosis in patients. Care must be taken prior to ligation in order to identify the subclavian artery, transverse aorta, and descending aorta. Common complications are related to surrounding anatomy. Phrenic and recurrent laryngeal nerve injury, and chylothorax can all occur, with recurrent laryngeal nerve injury being most common.

Endovascular treatment of a PDA mainly involves placement of an occlusion device such as the Rashkind umbrella. Transcatheter treatment can have closure rates of around 85% in ducts 8 mm or smaller.

Endocarditis prophylaxis recommendations are unclear. Prophylaxis is recommended for patients with device closure of the PDA or those with some residual defect.

63. Atrial septal defect, partial anomalous pulmonary venous return, and cor triatriatum

Carlos M. Mery

ASD is a communication of any size between both atria.

Embryology

The common atrium begins to divide on the 4th week of gestation by a semilunar mesenchymal *septum primum* that grows from the dome of the common atrium. The space between the *septum primum* and the inferior-ly-located endocardial cushions that create the ventricular septum is called the *ostium primum*. As the *septum primum* advances to close the *ostium primum*, its superior part gets reabsorbed with multiple fenestra-tions that coalesce to form the *ostium secundum*. The *septum secundum* then emerges from the dorsal part of the common atrium parallel and to the right of the *septum primum*. The *septum secundum* circumscribes the *foramen ovale* that forms a flap valve with the edge of the *ostium secun-dum*, thus allowing flow from right to left during fetal circulation. After birth, the higher pressure of the LA compared to the RA closes the *fora-men ovale*. Fibrous adhesions then seal the communication in most peo-ple by the first year of life.

Types of ASD

* *PFO.* Not technically an ASD. Present in 30% of normal hearts. The *septum primum* and *septum secundum* fail to fuse leading to a patent natural valve in the *fossa ovalis* that may allow intermittent shunting.

* *Ostium secundum.* 80% of ASDs. Located in the *fossa ovalis* and due to incomplete coverage of the *ostium secundum* by underdevel-opment of the *septum primum*.

* *Ostium primum.* 10% of ASDs. Due to persistence of the *ostium primum*. Associated with atrioventricular canal defects.

* *Sinus venosus.* 2-10% of ASDs. Located in the posterior atrial sep-tum and associated with partial anomalous pulmonary venous return (PAPVR). Most commonly, one or both right pulmonary veins drain (right upper most commonly) to either the RA or the SVC, just lat-eral to the ASD. Less commonly, the pulmonary veins may enter the RA close to the IVC-RA junction.

- *Coronary sinus defect.* 1-2% of ASDs. Due to complete or partial unroofing of the coronary sinus onto the posterior wall of the LA.

Pathophysiology

The magnitude of the shunt in ASDs is dependent on the size of the defect and the compliance of the ventricles. In the neonatal period, the compliance of the ventricles is similar and the magnitude of the shunt is small. As life progresses, the LV becomes less compliant with resulting higher left-sided pressures and increasing left-to-right shunt. Volume overload of the RV eventually leads to impaired systolic and diastolic RV function. The increase in pulmonary blood flow leads in turn to pulmonary hypertension in early adulthood. As many as 50% of patients with untreated ASDs will develop pulmonary hypertension by the age of 40. If the defect remains untreated, it can lead to irreversible pulmonary vascular changes (Eisenmenger's syndrome). ASDs less than 6 mm in diameter usually regress during the first years of life. On the contrary, defects greater than 8 mm in diameter usually enlarge.

Clinical presentation

Most ASDs are asymptomatic, especially during childhood. The clinical presentation depends mainly on the magnitude of the shunt and the age of the patient. Clinical symptoms usually appear when the Qp:Qs (pulmonary flow : systemic flow) exceeds 2:1.

Symptoms of ASDs include reduced exercise capacity and history of recurrent respiratory infections in children and adolescents. Adults may present with palpitations, atrial fibrillation, and CHF. Patients with advanced pulmonary hypertension may present with cyanosis due to reversal of the shunt across the ASD (Eisenmenger's syndrome).

On exam, patients may present a prominent RV impulse and leftward displacement of the apex with left chest wall prominence. Auscultation reveals a systolic flow murmur on the left upper sternal border (from increased flow through the pulmonary valve), fixed split S2, and apical mid-diastolic murmur (from increased flow through the tricuspid valve).

Diagnostic studies

- *EKG.* RV hypertrophy with a prominent R' wave on right precordial leads, right axis deviation, incomplete or complete right bundle branch block, atrial fibrillation or atrial flutter on adults.

- *CXR.* Cardiomegaly with prominent lung markings.

- *Echocardiography.* Modality of choice for most ASDs. Bubble contrast (from agitated saline injection) can be used to improve detection.

- *MRI and CT.* Used for complex ASDs, mainly those involving anomalous venous return.

- *Cardiac catheterization.* Rarely necessary. A step-up in oxygen saturation can be observed from the SVC to the RA.

Indications for treatment

Elective closure is recommended for all ASDs with a Qp:Qs of 1.5:1 or greater. Ideally, closure is performed between 2 and 5 years of age. In adults, ASDs associated with RV volume overload, arrhythmias, and heart failure should be treated.

Fixed pulmonary hypertension, defined as a PVR of 8-12 Wood units/m^2 despite aggressive vasodilator challenge (with inhaled nitric oxide, oxygen, and prostacyclin analogues) is a contraindication for surgery. PVR should fall below 7 Wood units/m^2 for the patient to be considered candidate for closure.

Treatment

Catheter-based devices can be used to close simple ASDs up to 3.8 cm in size. ASDs with larger size, small septal rim, or associated PAPVR are not candidates for catheter-based closure. Complications occur in 1.5% of patients with the most common being device malposition or embolization.

Surgical therapy is usually performed through a median sternotomy with bicaval cannulation, caval snares, and right atriotomy. The ASD is closed either primarily or with a patch (bovine pericardium, autologous pericardium +/- glutaraldehyde treatment, Dacron, or ePTFE), depending on the size and location.

Sinus venosus defects associated with PAPVR are treated with an intra-atrial patch that baffles the right-sided pulmonary vein flow through the ASD into the LA. Care must be taken to enlarge the ASD, if needed, to avoid obstruction of the baffle. When the anomalous veins drain high into the SVC and the baffle would narrow the SVC lumen, the SVC can be patched open or transected above the anomalous pulmonary veins and anastomosed to the RA appendage. Alternately, a Warden procedure can be performed. Here, the SVC is transected and oversewn just above the entry of the anomalous vein into the SVC. The orifice of the SVC-RA junction is then baffled through the ASD into the LA. Finally, the distal end of the SVC is anastomosed to the RA appendage to re-establish superior systemic venous continuity with the right heart. Isolated coronary sinus defects are treated by closing off the coronary sinus.

Complications of surgical repair of ASDs include patch dehiscence, heart block or sinus node dysfunction (up to 55% of patients with sinus venosus ASD/PAPVR undergoing baffle treatment), atrial fibrillation or flutter, thromboembolic events, late cardiac failure, or residual shunt (up to 2%). A potential important complication is baffling the IVC to the LA by mistakenly including the Eustachian valve in the repair, in which case cyanosis and desaturation will be found after weaning off CPB.

Cor triatriatum

Cor triatriatum sinistrum is a separation of the LA into two chambers by a fibromuscular membrane: a common pulmonary venous chamber and a chamber containing the LA appendage and the mitral valve. The communication between both chambers is limited to one or multiple perforations on the membrane. Clinical manifestations depend on the degree of pulmonary venous obstruction and whether there is an ASD between the RA and the common pulmonary venous chamber. Signs and symptoms are those of pulmonary venous congestion such as poor growth, pulmonary edema, pulmonary infections, pulmonary hypertension, and right-sided heart failure. Diagnosis is made by echocardiography, although MRI can also be useful. The treatment is surgical with complete excision of the membrane. The repair is usually performed through a trans-septal approach via a right atriotomy, although a left atriotomy can be used for older children and adults.

Cor triatriatum dexter (subdivision of the RA) is a much rarer occurrence with a clinical presentation that varies from asymptomatic, to cyanosis from shunting through an ASD, to right-sided heart failure. Treatment is surgical excision of the membrane.

64. Ventricular septal defects

Ravi K. Ghanta, Bryan M. Burt

A ventricular septal defect (VSD) is an abnormal opening between the RV and LV. A VSD develops from congenital malformation, trauma, or MI. Surgical management of VSD is dependent on anatomic location, size, shunt flow, hemodynamic sequelae, and patient age (infant vs. adult).

Anatomy

The 4 anatomic types of VSDs are based on RV septal anatomy and outlined in Table 64-1. For each of the 4 types there are alternative terminologies also listed in the Table. The membranous septum is a fibrous structure located below the septal leaflet of the tricuspid valve (TV). It should be noted that the Bundle of His descends within the membranous septum and must be accounted for during repair. The inlet is the posterior region of the RV septum below the septal leaflet of the TV. Inlet VSDs are often associated with mitral valve defects, which may require concomitant repair. The outlet is located below the pulmonic valve and superior to the crista supraventricularis. Outlet VSDs are in close association with the aortic valve cusps, which may be incompetent and require repair. The muscular septum is located along the trabecular septum.

Table 64-1. Types of VSDs and surgical indications.

Type [Frequency]	Description	Surgical Indications*
Membranous (conoventricular, Type 2) [80%]	Membranous septum defect located below septal leaflet of TV	*Infants:* symptoms, ↑ PA pressure $\geq$ ½ systemic at 1 year *Adults:* symptoms, $Q_p:Q_s > 1.5$
Outlet (Conal, Subarterial, Supracristal, Type 1) [8%]	Outlet septum, beneath pulmonary valve annulus	*Infants:* repair when discovered *Adults:* symptoms, AI, $Q_p:Q_s > 1.5$
Inlet (AV canal, endocardial cushion, Type 3) [6%]	AV canal below septal leaflet of TV	*Infants:* Repair when discovered *Adults:* symptoms, $Q_p:Q_s > 1.5$ & $PVR < 6$ units/m^2
Muscular (Type 4) [10%]	Muscular interventricular septum	Same as membranous

*Absolute contraindications for repair are fixed pulmonary hypertension: PVR > 8 Woods units not responsive to pulmonary vasodilators (infants) & PVR > 6 Woods units (adults). AV: atrioventricular, TV: tricuspid valve.

Hemodynamics and pathophysiology

VSD resistance to blood flow is characterized as restrictive ($Q_p:Q_s < 1.5$), moderate ($Q_p:Q_s$ 1.5 – 2.5), or nonrestrictive ($Q_p:Q_s>2.5$). Shunt flow is dependent on relative ventricular compliance and contractile properties, PVR, and SVR. VSDs lead to a left-to-right shunt, which increases pulmonary blood flow and elevation of PVR. This increase in PVR decreases shunt flow, but over time the classic Eisenmenger's complex results in which RV hypertrophy and fixed pulmonary hypertension results, followed by right-to-left shunting and cyanosis.

Infants

Isolated congenital VSDs are the most common recognized congenital lesion. They are found in 2 out of every 1,000 births. VSDs are present with other congenital defects in 50% of cases and commonly include tetralogy of Fallot, PDA, and aortic coarctation. The presence of VSD is often detected as a harsh pansystolic murmur on physical exam. Symptomatic patients present with growth failure, tachypnea, and hepatomegaly.

Most VSDs will close spontaneously, however 30% of infants will require surgery due to development of heart failure during the first year of life. Outlet and inlet type VSDs are unlikely to close spontaneously and should be repaired when discovered. All symptomatic membranous or muscular VSDs should be repaired if medical management fails regardless of age. Asymptomatic membranous or muscular VSDs should be followed with serial echocardiography as most will close spontaneously. The development of increased PVR, increased PA pressures, or symptoms is an indication for VSD repair. At 1 year, PA pressure greater than half systemic pressure is an indication for repair.

An important contraindication to surgery is development of fixed pulmonary hypertension. A PVR > 8 woods units that does not decrease with inhaled nitric oxide or 100% oxygen is a contraindication to surgery. However, patients less than 1 year of age with a PVR to SVR ratio of < 0.75 and responsive to pulmonary vasodilators are candidates provided a PVR < 12 woods units.

Specific steps to repair are dependent on location of VSD and concomitant pathology. In general, repairs are transatrial with a patch (Dacron, Gore-Tex, or pericardium) closure of the defect. In patients with VSD and associated AI (usually from prolapse of one of the aortic cusps into the VSD), VSD closure alone is sufficient if the AI is mild-moderate and there is only limited fibrosis of the cusps. Patients with more than moderate AI and cusp retraction usually require aortic valvuloplasty through an aortotomy, in addition to VSD closure.

Results of surgical repair are excellent with minimal mortality. Right bundle branch block is common after VSD repair but is usually well tolerated. Atrioventricular block may occur in < 3% of cases. Small residual VSDs around the repair tend to close spontaneously during the following few months after surgery.

Adults

Adults present with VSDs secondary to congenital, traumatic, or post-ischemic etiologies. Congenital VSDs in adults tend to be restrictive VSDs or patch leaks from childhood repair. Appropriate evaluation of the VSD includes transthoracic and transesophageal echocardiography, right heart catheterization, and left heart catheterization in patients over 40 years age or significant risk factors for CAD. Indications for surgical repair include $Q_p:Q_s$ >1.5 with or without symptoms. Contraindications to repair are a calculated PVR > 6 woods units.

65. Atrioventricular septal defects

Stephanie Mick

Atrioventricular (AV) canal defects ("canal defect" or AV septal defect) are a spectrum of anomalies with physiologies ranging from that of a simple ASD to single ventricle physiology. The below will focus on defects amenable to two-ventricle repair.

Embryology

After primitive tube formation and looping, septation of the heart and development of the AV valves (AVVs) occurs. Endocardial cushion tissue at the heart's core grows toward the posterior wall of the common atrium, forming the atrial part of the AV septum. Note that this is *not* the *septum primum* (the tissue that forms the bottom of the *fossa ovalis*.) If this development fails, a *primum* ASD results. As endocardial cushion tissue grows in the direction of the apex, the ventricular part of the AV septum (the muscular tissue just under the septal leaflet of the tricuspid valve (TV)) is formed. If this proceeds in a faulty manner, an inlet VSD results (typically a pressure restrictive, diminutive VSD). If there is also a defect in inlet septum formation, a large unrestrictive VSD is produced. The septal leaflet of the TV and the anterior leaflet (AL) of the mitral valve (MV) are created as the endocardial tissue grows rightward and leftward. Failure here can cause abnormalities ranging from a cleft in the AL of the MV to a single AVV. In this case, the septal portions of the MV and TV fuse, and superior and inferior bridging (or "common") leaflets are formed.

Anatomy and associated anomalies

A *partial canal defect* is just an *ostium primum* ASD, typically with a complete cleft of the AL of the MV, although this may be incomplete or not present. A solitary AL cleft without an ASD is not considered a canal defect. There may be a "gooseneck deformity" of the LVOT, which is an elongation of the LVOT owing to the apical displacement of the AVV plane. This displacement occurs because usually there is at least some deficit of the ventricular part of the AV septum. The elongation does not automatically result in LVOT obstruction (LVOTO) but chordal attachments or accessory tissue in this region may be present and cause LVOTO in time.

A *transitional AV canal* is a partial AV canal with a pressure restrictive VSD and may also be associated with LVOTO due to chordal attachments from the AL of the MV to the septum.

A *complete AV canal defect* (CAVC) consists of a *primum* ASD, an unrestrictive inlet VSD, and a common AVV. There are three types of CAVC:

- *Rastelli A* (75%). Defined by a complete division of the superior common leaflet over the septal crest with chords attaching the right and left portions of this leaflet to the appropriate side of the septum. In this type, the VSD is often small.

- *Rastelli B.* Rare and almost never seen with balanced ventricles. Straddling chords extend from the TV component into the LV (usually in cases of LV dominance) or from the MV component into the RV (usually in cases of RV dominance).

- *Rastelli C* (25%). There is an undivided superior common leaflet, usually without any chordal attachment of the central part of the leaflet to the septum. This is the type most often associated with tetralogy of Fallot.

Associated cardiac anomalies include tetralogy of Fallot (10%), PDA (10%), LVOTO, multiple VSDs, double orifice MV, single papillary muscle, and double outlet right ventricle. Transposition of the great vessels is also rarely associated. The most important associated non-cardiac anomaly is Down's syndrome; ~50% of Down's children have a canal defect (typically CAVC) and 75% of children with CAVC have Down's. Interestingly, it is rare for partial AV canal to be associated with Down's. Also, Down's patients with canal defects do not frequently have associated LVOTO.

Pathophysiology and clinical presentation

The pathophysiology flows from the left-to-right shunting with resultant increased pulmonary blood flow and the AVV regurgitation (moderate 20%, severe 15%). Therefore, medical therapy consists of anti-congestive measures and afterload reduction if AVV insufficiency is significant.

CAVCs have large left-to-right shunts and elevated RV and PA pressures owing to the unrestrictive VSD. They present early (4-6 weeks) with symptoms of pulmonary hypertension and CHF (difficulty feeding, tachypnea, and failure to thrive). CHF symptoms are more pronounced and presentation is earlier when MV insufficiency, LV underdevelopment or LVOTO are present. These lesions will result in the development of pulmonary vascular occlusive disease if not repaired in infancy. When there is little or no AVV insufficiency, partial and transitional canal defects present later and have a similar presentation and natural history to simple ASDs. It is important to note that patients with Down's have reduced peripheral bronchi and vasculature, increased secretions and bronchiolar plugging, and a tendency to hypoventilation due to small "floppy" airways. Thus in these children, there is a pronounced tendency to accelerated pulmonary vascular disease when pulmonary hypertension is present.

Diagnosis

CXR shows increased pulmonary blood flow (increased pulmonary markings) and may reveal dilation of cardiac chambers (e.g. LA dilatation +/- elevation of the left main bronchus when MR is pronounced). EKG reveals a counterclockwise axis shift axis owing to the inferior displacement of the His bundle (there is a clockwise shift with secundum ASD). Echocardiography is diagnostic and also important in the intraoperative and postoperative assessment of mitral valve competence after repair. Altered loading conditions in the postoperative period can manifest in acute MR days to weeks after repair. Cardiac catheterization may show a "gooseneck deformity."

Surgical treatment

The timing of repair is based around preventing obstructive pulmonary vascular disease and chamber dilatation (which can cause additional pathological changes to AVV tissue). If the AVVs are competent, partial canals are repaired at 1-2 years of age (earlier if there is AVV regurgitation). CAVCs should be repaired at 2-4 months (if left unrepaired, 30% will have pulmonary hypertension at 1 year and 90% at 3-5 years) and earlier if there is heart failure. Postoperative pulmonary hypertension without a residual defect should ideally be managed with nitric oxide. Partial AV canal repairs consist of pericardial patch closure of the *primum* ASD. The patch is sewn to the region of continuity between the MV and TV (care should be taken not to injure the underlying bundle of His lying in crest of the ventricular septum), cleft closure, and possible annuloplasty in the case of annular dilation (often accomplished by suture commissuroplasty). Repair of a transitional canal is similar. As for the VSD in this type of canal defect, it is most commonly located at the level of the MV cleft and a single horizontal pledgeted mattress suture placed at this location obliterates it during cleft closure.

In addition to cleft closure and possible annuloplasty as in the above, patch ASD and VSD closure is necessary in CAVCs. One patch or two patches can be used to accomplish this with no major difference in outcomes. A one-patch repair can be performed in the "Australian" manner or traditional manner.   In the Australian repair, multiple interrupted pledgeted sutures are placed on the right side of the crest of the interventricular septum (to avoid the His Bundle and branches).   The sutures are passed through the superior and inferior bridging leaflets and then through an autologous pericardial patch.   Tying these sutures closes the VSD by bringing the common AVV leaflets down to the crest of the septum.   The traditional one patch repair is similar except that it involves incising the superior and inferior bridging leaflets instead of leaving them intact during patch placement.

66. Interrupted aortic arch and aortic coarctation

John C. Lin

Interrupted aortic arch

Pathophysiology

Interrupted aortic arch is a rare defect, comprising 1% of all congenital heart defects. It is the absence of continuity between the ascending and the descending aorta. Typically, a VSD (80%) or a PDA is present.

- *Type A:* distal to the left subclavian artery (30%)

- *Type B:* between the left subclavian artery and the left common carotid artery (65%)

- *Type C:* between the left carotid and the brachiocephalic artery (5 %)

Untreated, the median survival is 4 days.

Clinical presentation

Most patients present with metabolic acidosis and hemodynamic collapse with the closure of PDA. CHF presentation is also possible. Diagnosis is achieved with echocardiogram.

Treatment

IV PGE$_1$ infusion can keep the *ductus* open and correct the acidosis. Mechanical ventilation and inotropic support are used to optimize the patient.

The treatment is surgical. Aortic arch reconstruction is achieved by direct anastomosis or patch aortoplasty, associated with closure of the VSD. Mortality is around 30%.

Coarctation of the aorta

Pathophysiology

Coarctation of the aorta is a hemodynamically significant narrowing of the aorta, usually present just proximal to the site of insertion of the *ductus arteriosus*, distal the left subclavian artery. A deformity of the aortic media causes the narrowing of the lumen. Associated lesions include a bicuspid aortic valve (50-80%), VSD (30-60%), aortic stenosis (30%), a PDA (20%), and hypoplasia of the aortic arch. Compensatory collaterals are characteristic in children and adolescents; the internal mammary arteries, the posterior intercostal arteries, and the anterior spinal arteries can be significantly dilated.

Both systolic and diastolic pressures are elevated above the coarctation. Below the coarctation, the systolic pressure is lower than that of the upper extremities, but the diastolic pressure tends to be normal.

Aortic coarctation represents 4% of congenital heart lesions (4/10,000 live births). Male to female ratio is about 3:1. 45% of patients with Turner's syndrome have coarctation.

Clinical presentation

Clinical presentation and timing depend on the degree of coarctation. 50% of patients present in the first month of life with signs of CHF, dyspnea, distal organ malperfusion, absent femoral pulses, and metabolic acidosis, as the *ductus* starts to close. Older children with milder forms of the disease may present with failure to thrive, irritability, diaphoresis, and poor feeding. Adults may present with unexplained hypertension, lower extremity claudication, or for workup of an incidentally found murmur.

Without intervention, severe hypertension (25%), heart failure (25%), aortic rupture (20%), stroke (10%) can develop. The mean age of survival for untreated disease is less than 20 years.

Diagnosis

- *Physical exam.* Gallop rhythm with a systolic and a diastolic murmur, prominent carotid pulsation, diminished or absent femoral pulses, differential in arterial pressure and oxygen saturation between upper and the lower extremities

- *CXR.* Cardiomegaly, rib notching in chronic cases (due to erosion of the ribs by hypertensive intercostal arteries)

- *EKG.* Biventricular hypertrophy, T-wave inversion

- *Echocardiogram.* Diagnostic. Clearly delineates the coarctation (especially with Doppler gradients) and other associated cardiac lesions

- *Cardiac catheterization.* Useful for evaluation of the exact site of coarctation. MRI is a non-invasive alternative technique.

Treatment

IV PGE$_1$ infusion can keep the *ductus* open and can provide perfusion to the descending aorta in neonates. Some inotropic support might be necessary.

Balloon angioplasty can be performed but carries a significant restenosis rate (75%). Therefore, it is preferentially used for treatment of critically ill neonates that are poor surgical candidates or for relief of recurrent co-arctation following repair. Stent placement can be used, especially for older children and adults.

Surgical intervention is indicated for symptomatic neonates or infants and for older children and adults that are not candidates for catheter intervention. The procedure is performed via a left posterolateral thoracotomy with direct end-to-end anastomosis or a subclavian flap aortoplasty. A tubular vascular interposition graft may be used in adults.

Complications include chylothorax, paraplegia (<1%), and phrenic/recurrent laryngeal nerve injuries. Post-coarctation syndrome (ileus, abdominal pain, mesenteric vasculitis, and visceral infarction) is possible. Good postoperative blood pressure control is essential.

67. Tetralogy of Fallot

Carlos M. Mery

Tetralogy of Fallot (TOF) represents 5% of all congenital heart defects and is characterized by:

- Large anterior VSD

- *RVOT obstruction.* Obstruction is mainly due to infundibular sub-valvar pulmonary stenosis but patients may present with pulmonary valve stenosis (75%) or supravalvar stenosis.

- *Dextroposition of the aorta* (overriding and clockwise rotation of the aorta)

- RV hypertrophy

However, all four manifestations of TOF can be ascribed to a single embryological defect: the anterior and leftward displacement of the infundibular septum.

Other associated anomalies include coronary artery anomalies (5%), right-sided aortic arch (25%), multiple additional VSDs (15%), and ASD (10%). The most common coronary artery anomaly is an LAD originating from the RCA and crossing over the RVOT, which puts it at risk for injury during surgery. An RCA originating from the left coronary or large conal branches contributing to the LV may also cross the RVOT.

TOF can be associated with other syndromes (30%) such as DiGeorge's / velocardiofacial syndrome (microdeletion of 22q), and trisomies 13 (Patau), 18 (Edwards), and 21 (Down).

Pathophysiology

Shunting across the VSD is usually bidirectional and its main direction depends on the degree of RVOT obstruction. When the obstruction is mild, the shunt is predominantly left-to-right resulting in pulmonary overcirculation and CHF symptoms ("pink" tetralogy). As the obstruction increases, the shunt becomes right-to-left and the child presents with variable degrees of cyanosis.

Clinical presentation

Most children are not cyanotic at birth. The degree of cyanosis and age at presentation depends on the degree of RVOT obstruction. If the obstruction is severe, the neonate may present within a few days with cyanosis and metabolic acidosis. When the obstruction is moderate, cyanosis may become evident at the end of the first year of life.

On exam, in addition to cyanosis, children present with a mid-systolic ejection murmur at the $2^{nd}/3^{rd}$ intercostal spaces, radiating to the axilla, and associated with a single S2. Older children that are untreated may present with stigmata of long-standing hypoxemia (e.g., digital clubbing), constant squatting (to increase SVR and therefore increase pulmonary blood flow), polycythemia that can lead to cerebrovascular thrombosis, and hemoptysis from enlarged bronchial arteries.

Children with TOF may present hypercyanotic episodes ("tet spells"). These are episodes of intense cyanosis that can last from minutes to hours and can be precipitated by dehydration, upper respiratory infections, crying, straining, feeding, or any physical stress. These episodes may lead to loss of consciousness and their occurrence is an indication for semi-urgent repair.

Diagnosis

Some modalities useful for the diagnosis of TOF include:

- *EKG.* Usually normal at birth and afterwards shows RV hypertrophy.

- *CXR.* Boot-shaped heart from RV hypertrophy. Lung fields are oligemic (if the lung markings are normal, suspect other sources of pulmonary blood flow such as aortopulmonary collaterals).

- *Labs.* Polycythemia.

- *Echocardiogram.* Mainstay of diagnosis. Important to assess associated defects, number and location of VSDs, nature of RVOT obstruction, anatomy of proximal PAs, and coronary artery anatomy.

- *Cardiac catheterization.* Rarely necessary. Useful if there is a suspicion of multiple sources of pulmonary blood flow.

Treatment

The treatment of TOF is surgical. In asymptomatic patients, repair is delayed until 4-6 months of age. Children should be kept adequately hydrated and every effort made to protect them from viral infections. Balloon pulmonary valvuloplasty can be attempted for palliation in high-risk, low-weight symptomatic children in order to defer surgery.

Surgical repair is performed under CPB with bicaval cannulation, moderate hypothermia, and cardioplegic arrest. The repair includes:

- Patch closure of the VSD with Dacron / Gore-Tex® / pericardium

- Resection of the obstructing parietal muscle bands from the infundibular septum

- Inspection and measurement of the pulmonary valve diameter with Hegar dilators. If the valve is small (according to the "Z-value" or normal diameter based on BSA), a transannular incision of the PA is performed and a transannular patch placed. This will lead to free pulmonary insufficiency likely requiring a pulmonary valve replacement in adulthood, once the patient develops decreased exercise tolerance or a decline in RV function.

The VSD closure and the resection of the parietal muscle bands can be performed through a right atriotomy, a RV infundibulotomy, or a combination of both.

68. Transposition of the great arteries
John C. Lin

In transposition of the great arteries (TGA), the aorta arises from the RV and the PA arises from the LV. It occurs in 1/4000 live births and is the most common of the cyanotic lesions (3%). Male to female ratio is about 2:1.

Pathophysiology

When the aorta is to the right of the PA, the transposition is called dextro (d) transposition. When the aorta is to the left of the PA, the transposition is called levo (l) transposition.

A patent foramen (PFO), a PDA, and pulmonary stenosis are very common, and about 50% of patients have a VSD. These are obligatory for survival in order to allow for mixing of the systemic and the pulmonary circulations. The coronary arteries arise from the pulmonary trunk.

Clinical presentation

The infants with no other cardiac lesions to allow mixing exhibit severe cyanosis early on after birth. Those with PDA, VSD, or PFO exhibit some cyanosis but will gradually develop heart failure in the first month.

Diagnosis

- *Physical exam.* Tachypnea, dyspnea, gallop rhythm, and a diastolic flow rumble at the apex.

- *CXR,* Initially normal to eventual cardiomegaly.

- *EKG.* Peaked p waves (intact ventricular septum), upright T waves in lateral leads (pulmonary hypertension), right axis deviation, RV hypertrophy.

- *Echocardiography:* Diagnostic. Clearly delineates the transposition and the associated cardiac lesions.

- *Cardiac catheterization:* Useful for evaluating coronary arteries, associated lesions, pressure gradients between ventricles, and allows for possible balloon atrial septostomy (to increase mixing).

Treatment

About 50% of patients die within the first month without intervention. If needed, balloon atrial septostomy creates an interatrial opening increasing the systemic arterial oxygen saturation above 60%. IV PGE₁ infusion increases systemic-pulmonary shunting; intubation is often necessary due to prostaglandin-induced apnea.

Senning (1958) and Mustard (1963) initially described an *atrial* switch. Post-operative pulmonary stenosis and arrhythmias have been documented.

The *arterial* switch repair (1975) is now the standard and is typically performed within the first 3 weeks of life. Beyond 3 weeks, the left/right ventricular pressure ratio can go below 0.6, and a pulmonary arterial band is applied first (to condition the LV to the future systemic circulation.) The switch operation is then performed a week later.

The arterial switch is performed the following way:

- The aortic cannula is placed and the PDA is ligated. The PA is freed out to the hilum for mobilization.

- The great arteries are transected.

- The coronary buttons are excised and reanastomosed to the neoaorta.

- The Lecompte maneuver: The PA is moved to be anterior to the aorta.

- A pericardial patch is used for the neo-PA.

10-year survival after the arterial switch operation is 80%. Most patients achieve good exercise tolerance. Neo-pulmonary stenosis with RVOT obstruction is the most common indication for reintervention. Balloon dilation and/or stenting have been employed to correct the stenosis. In addition, neo-aortic root dilatation can be seen and is sometimes associated with AI.

Those with TGA, pulmonary stenosis, and VSD undergo the Rastelli procedure. A patch is used to close the VSD and to direct the blood in the LV to the aorta. The pulmonary valve is surgically closed and an artificial conduit and valve are constructed from the pulmonary bifurcation to the RV. 10-year survival is 60%.

69. Total anomalous pulmonary venous return

Bret A. Mettler, Ibrahim Abdullah

Total anomalous pulmonary venous return (TAPVR) is a pathologic entity in which all of the pulmonary venous effluent from the lungs drains to the systemic venous system, creating a large left-to-right shunt. An obligatory right-to-left shunt must be present to allow blood to reach the LV and contribute to systemic cardiac output. Most commonly this occurs at the level of the atrial septum, but may present as a VSD or a PDA. The absence of a right-to-left shunt is incompatible with survival.

Anatomy

TAPVR is classified by the site of connection to the systemic venous system into:

- *Supracardiac* (50%). Most common. The ascending vertical vein most often drains into the innominate vein.

- *Cardiac* (20%). The venous confluence drains directly into the right heart, most commonly the coronary sinus.

- *Infracardiac* (25%). The pulmonary vein confluence drains via a descending vertical vein to the portal vein, *ductus venosus* or IVC. Infracardiac TAPVR is the most common subset to present with obstruction and occurs at the junction of the vertical vein with the systemic venous drainage.

- *Mixed* (5%). Multiple sites of systemic venous return.

All patients with TAPVR exhibit a varying degree of lymphangiectasia and media hypertrophy in both the pulmonary arterial and venous circulation. In patients with complete obstruction, pulmonary hypertension will be present.

Presentation

Patients without significant obstruction present in infancy or childhood with symptoms of heart failure due to their large left-to-right shunt. These patients have dyspnea, poor feeding, and poor growth.

Patients presenting with complete pulmonary venous obstruction constitute a surgical emergency. Expeditious medical measures should be taken to resuscitate the patient including intubation and mechanical ventilation with 100% oxygen, hyperventilation, correction of acidosis and inotropic support. Medical measures are minimally effective and surgically correction is required. In patients who present with severe end organ dysfunction, some centers choose a period of ECMO support prior to operative repair. At this time, most centers choose to perform a complete repair with use of ECMO post-operatively if required.

Pathophysiology

The most important anatomic factors in determining the clinical status of the patient include the presence and location of the right-to-left shunt and the presence or absence of obstruction in the pulmonary venous pathway. As pulmonary venous blood is diverted from the LA, blood is unable to reach the LV in the absence of a right-to-left shunt. In the presence of a shunt, the cardiac output is limited to the amount of blood passing through the right-to-left shunt. A second important anatomic factor determining the clinical status is the presence or absence of obstruction in the pulmonary venous pathway. With obstruction, egress of blood from the lungs is limited resulting in pulmonary venous congestion and impairment of oxygenation, leading to life threatening neonatal cyanosis. If associated with a restrictive right-to-left shunt and reduced cardiac output, the patient's precarious clinical status is worsened.

An important subset of obstructed TAPVR is patients in whom the vertical vein ascends between the left PA and the left mainstem bronchus. As the degree of pulmonary vein obstruction worsens, PAP increases, causing further distension of the PA and vertical vein compression, ultimately leading to circulatory collapse due to the physiologic vice.

Diagnostic techniques

CXR shows varying degrees of pulmonary venous congestion dependent upon the degree of obstruction. A prominent RA border and PA vasculature may also be seen.

Echocardiography is the study of choice for identifying TAPVR. The pulmonary venous confluence, pulmonary veins, and connection to the systemic venous system can typically be defined. Intraoperative echocardiography is the best modality to evaluate the anastomosis between the venous confluence and the LA. Echocardiography is also the best modality for long-term follow-up.

Cardiac catheterization is infrequently used in a preoperative setting. Indications for angiography include ambiguous anatomy requiring further delineation or should intervention be required for preoperative stabilization (i.e., balloon atrial septostomy). A classic finding at catheterization is identical oxygen saturations in all chambers of the heart. MRI is emerging as an important diagnostic modality when anatomical clarification is needed and allows a non-invasive method to determine Qp:Qs.

Surgical repair

The treatment of TAPVR is surgical. In asymptomatic patients whose venous outflow is unobstructed by echocardiography, repair is delayed several weeks or until symptoms of dyspnea and feeding intolerance develop. Most children will develop symptoms within 6 months of age. Patients presenting with complete obstruction are considered a surgical emergency and after attempted medical stabilization, operative repair is performed. The conduct of the operation is indistinguishable when performed emergently or electively. Cannulation is performed with a single arterial and venous. If other intracardiac work is expected, bicaval cannulation is likely required. The patient is cooled to 18°C and if present, the patent *ductus* is immediately ligated after initiating CPB. Both supracardiac and infracardiac TAPVR require a direct anastomosis between the pulmonary vein confluence and the LA. With the low-pressure of newborn pulmonary venous blood flow, it cannot be overstated that the anastomosis must be meticulously performed, free of both torsion and tension to permit unimpeded blood flow. For cardiac variant TAPVR, repair requires unroofing of the coronary sinus into the LA with patch closure of the ASD. In this setting, the drainage from the coronary sinus will be into the LA directly. For patients who have small pulmonary veins or a small venous confluence, a sutureless repair may be required. In a sutureless repair, the anterior wall of the venous confluence is widely opened to the pericardial well. The posterior aspect of the LA is incised and sewn directly to the pericardial well. The pulmonary venous drainage is collected in the newly created pericardial-LA reservoir. The sutureless repair is often the procedure of choice for re-operative pulmonary vein stenosis.

70. Tricuspid atresia

Ahmet Kilic

Tricuspid atresia is the congenital absence of any identifiable tricuspid valve tissue resulting in a disconnect between the RA and RV. It is estimated to occur in between 1 to 3% of all congenital heart lesions and is the most common type of single ventricle pathology.

It is associated with other anomalies including altered relationship with the great vessels, VSD, and a persistence of a left-sided SVC. Although different classification systems for tricuspid atresia have been published, most surgeons use the classification system proposed by Tandon and Edwards:

- *Type I.* Normal anatomy (~70%)

  - A: pulmonary atresia with almost nonexistent RV

  - B: pulmonary stenosis with small VSD

  - C: large VSD, pulmonary stenosis

- *Type II.* d-transposition of great arteries (TGA) (~30%)

  - A: pulmonary atresia

  - B: pulmonary/subpulmonary stenosis

  - C: normal / enlarged pulmonary valve and artery with no stenosis

- *Type III.* l-TGA (rare)

Pathophysiology

The underlying problem in tricuspid atresia is that there is no communication between the RA and RV. As such, a right-to-left shunt exists for the circulation of blood. The degree of obstruction to pulmonary blood flow, the relationship of the great arteries, and the restrictiveness of the VSD determine the exact pathophysiology and clinical sequelae of tricuspid atresia. Like other congenital anomalies, the concept of pulmonary overcirculation vs. pulmonary undercirculation dictates symptoms. The less blood flow into the pulmonary circulation, the more cyanotic and hypoxic the child becomes. Conversely, the more blood flow into the pulmonary circulation the more CHF symptoms the child presents.

Clinical presentation

Most patients with tricuspid atresia present with cyanosis in the first month of life, the severity of which depends upon the underlying patho-physiology. In the severe form of obstruction, neonatal pulmonary blood flow is dependent on a PDA and requires continued infusion of prosta-glandin and/or a systemic to pulmonary shunt. Children with less obstruc-tive types can be asymptomatic for a period of time, however, most will need an operation before the age of one. Patients with pulmonary over-circulation will present with signs and symptoms consistent with CHF. Both groups can show growth retardation.

In addition to cyanosis (clubbing) and/or CHF (jugular venous distension, edema, ascites), physical examination may reveal abnormal heart sounds (~80% of all patients):

- Crescendo – decrescendo holosystolic ejection murmur at left sternal border (VSD / pulmonary stenosis)

- Apical diastolic rumble (flow across mitral valve)

- Fixed splitting of S2 (TGA)

Diagnosis

The diagnosis of tricuspid atresia is strongly suggested by the history, physical examination, and timing of symptoms in conjunction with imag-ing modalities (most useful being an echocardiogram). Other useful di-agnostic modalities are:

- *Laboratory data.* Polycythemia from long standing cyanosis.

- *CXR.* Small RV with decreased pulmonary vascular markings (~80%). In cases of increased pulmonary blood flow, cardiomegaly and pulmonary congestion may be present.

- *EKG.* Tall p waves indicative of RA hypertrophy and left axis devia-tion.

- *Echocardiogram.* Best method for diagnosis. Hallmark is absence of the right atrioventricular valve. Additional information that is use-ful includes: relationship of the great vessels, size and presence of atrial / ventricular septal defects, anatomy of great vessels, size of the RV, presence of atrioventricular valve regurgitation, ventricular function, and degree of pulmonary blood flow.

- *Cardiac catheterization.* Can be used for both diagnostic as well as therapeutic reasons in infants. Confirms anatomy, looks at function of RV as well as size of PAs and source of pulmonary blood flow. Balloon septostomy can be carried out if ASD is small / restrictive. Good for pre-operative planning and to measure PA resistance and mitral valve competency.

Treatment

The treatment of tricuspid atresia is dictated in large part by the symptoms for which the infant presents (increased vs. decreased pulmonary blood flow).

The child with decreased pulmonary blood flow can present in extremis with cyanosis and acidemia requiring prompt surgical intervention or can present in a more chronic, compensated manner. Palliation for high-risk, low birth neonates can include infusion of prostaglandin as well as balloon septostomy with the hope of getting them to surgery. The surgical treatment is aimed at getting more pulmonary blood flow through a series of staged procedures culminating in a final single ventricle physiology:

1. Systemic to pulmonary shunt: classic Blalock-Taussig shunt (subclavian to PA) or modified Blalock-Taussig shunt (graft from innominate artery to PA).

2. Cavopulmonary anastomosis (Glenn shunt vs. hemi-Fontan shunt).

3. Fontan procedure for complete separation of systemic and pulmonary blood circulation (lateral tunnel vs. extracardiac conduit).

Numerous complications can arise from the above procedures including arrhythmias, emboli, stroke, polycythemia, valvular insufficiency, ventricular dysfunction, and end-stage heart failure. Patient selection is the key to ensure success for the Fontan procedure and some parameters to follow are:

- Age > 4 years

- Sinus rhythm

- Normal caval drainage, no impairing effects of previous shunts

- Normal RA volume, competent mitral / left atrioventricular valve

- Normal ventricular function (EF $\geq$ 60%)

- Mean PA pressure $\leq$ 15 mm Hg, pulmonary arterial resistance < 4 units / m2

- PA to aorta diameter ratio $\geq$ 0.75

Indeed, even without strict adherence to these guidelines success rates nearing 99% have been reported in the modern era once a child is able to be bridged to the final Fontan palliation procedure.

Infants with increased pulmonary blood flow present with CHF. The symptoms are often treated with diuretic therapy and digitalis while surgical therapy is aimed at restricting pulmonary blood flow (i.e. PA banding).

71. Ebstein's anomaly

Carlos M. Mery

Anatomy and pathophysiology

Ebstein's anomaly is a rare malformation of the tricuspid valve characterized by:

- Downward displacement of the posterior and septal leaflets into the RV. The leaflets are dysplastic and tethered to the ventricular wall by shortened chordae.

- The anterior leaflet is attached to the tricuspid annulus in the normal position but is redundant, "sail-like", with abnormal tethering to the ventricular wall, and with variable number of fenestrations.

- The area of the RV between the tricuspid annulus and the lower attachment of the displaced septal and posterior leaflets is "atrialized", i.e., extremely thin and dysplastic.

- Small functional RV (infundibulum) below the atrialized portion.

Variable degrees of RVOT obstruction from the redundant anterior leaflet and its tethering attachments.

Ebstein's anomaly is associated with an ASD in most cases. Wolff-Parkinson-White (WPW) accessory pathways are common.

Ebstein's anomaly can be divided in several types according to Carpentier's classification:

- *Type A:* Adequate-sized RV

- *Type B:* Large atrialized RV but with free movement of the anterior leaflet

- *Type C:* Large atrialized RV and severely restricted movement of the anterior leaflet which may cause significant RVOT obstruction

- *Type D:* Almost complete atrialization of the RV with the only communication between the atrialized ventricle and the infundibulum (functional RV) being through the anteroseptal commissure of the valve

Ebstein's anomaly causes significant tricuspid regurgitation. In addition, the atrialized portion of the RV bulges out during atrial systole decreasing forward flow, and contracts during ventricular systole impeding venous filling of the RA. As a consequence, the RA becomes massively enlarged. Most patients exhibit a right-to-left shunt through an ASD.

There is an association between Ebstein's anomaly and maternal lithium exposure. Other potential associations include maternal viral exposure. There have been some familial cases described.

Clinical presentation

The clinical course and timing of presentation depends on the degree of tricuspid regurgitation, RVOT obstruction, and associated anomalies. Severe cases present early in life with milder cases presenting in adulthood.

In the neonatal period, since PVR is high, tricuspid regurgitation tends to be significant producing a right-to-left shunt that results in deep cyanosis. If the malformation is not severe, the shunt and cyanosis decrease as the PVR naturally falls over the next few days. Patients with severe malformation of the valve will continue with cyanosis and may go on to develop CHF and hemodynamic instability. It is not uncommon for older children and adults to present with milder forms of the disease. In these cases presentation may be with an incidentally-found heart murmur, new arrhythmia (atrial or ventricular), or signs of heart failure (fatigability, decreased exercise tolerance, dyspnea).

Physical exam findings include:

- Cyanosis and clubbing

- Chest wall deformity due to cardiomegaly

- Systolic murmur from tricuspid regurgitation

- Gallop rhythm with split S1 (from delayed tricuspid closure) and split S2 (from delayed ventricular conduction and pulmonary valve closure)

- Atrial and ventricular filling sounds

- Large v wave in the jugular vein

Diagnostic studies

- *CXR.* Massive cardiomegaly (from enlargement of the RA and atrialized RV) with a globular-shaped silhouette and a narrow waist, similar to that seen on pericardial effusion. CXR may be normal in mild cases.

- *EKG.* Right-axis deviation, PR prolongation, complete or incomplete right bundle branch block, atrial arrhythmias, WPW.

- *Echocardiogram.* Test of choice. The main characteristic that differentiates Ebstein's anomaly from other causes of tricuspid regurgitation is the degree of apical displacement of the septal leaflet. It allows measurement of degree of right-to-left shunt, tricuspid regurgitation, anatomy of the leaflets, size of RA, size and function of the atrialized portion of the RV, and right and left ventricular function.

- *MRI.* Being increasingly used to study anatomy and ventricular size and function.

- *Electrophysiologic (EP) studies.* Holter monitoring is needed for patients with palpitations. Invasive EP studies should be performed on any patient with evidence of WPW on EKG, arrhythmias, or syncope.

Treatment

Symptomatic neonates with CHF and significant cyanosis require surgical intervention. Asymptomatic patients with mild forms of Ebstein's anomaly can be managed medically until they develop symptoms (cyanosis, heart failure, arrhythmias).

There are multiple different surgical techniques. They usually include a combination of:

- Closure of ASD

- Tricuspid valve repair (preferable) or replacement

- Plication of the atrialized portion of RV

- Reduction atrioplasty of the RA

- Anti-arrhythmia procedures as indicated

The valve repair may be achieved by using the anterior leaflet to construct a monocusp valve that coapts with the ventricular septum. A relatively recent technique with good results is the *cone* repair where part of the anterior and posterior leaflets are detached and mobilized from their abnormal ventricular attachments. The septal edge of the posterior leaflet (still attached to the anterior leaflet) is then rotated clockwise and sutured to the septal edge of the anterior leaflet at the level of the tricuspid annulus. The annulus is then plicated and the leaflets sutured to the annulus.

Other techniques include fully reimplanting the leaflets onto the tricuspid annulus and/or reconstructing them with pericardium. A tricuspid annuloplasty may be added to any of these techniques in older children and adults to improve coaptation. Patients at high risk due to poor ventricular function may benefit from the addition of a bidirectional superior cavopulmonary shunt (Glenn) in order to decrease the volume overload on the RV, so called "1.5-ventricular repair".

An alternative management strategy (Starnes procedure) is to perform a single-ventricle repair by closing the tricuspid valve orifice with a fenestrated patch (to allow decompression of blood from Thebesian veins draining into the RV), excising the atrial septum, plicating the atrialized portion of the RV, and creating a systemic-pulmonary shunt. The child is then placed on a single-ventricle pathway that will lead to a Glenn and eventually a Fontan circulation.

Heart transplantation is an alternative treatment for patients with biventricular dysfunction.

72. Double outlet right ventricle
Keki R. Balsara

Introduction

Double outlet right ventricle (DORV) is an anomaly in which both great vessels arise from the RV. The spectrum of presentation, in both anatomy and physiology, spans from tetralogy of Fallot to transposition of the great vessels. In the United States, the incidence of DORV is 0.09 cases per 1000 live births. DORV comprises about 1-1.5% of all congenital heart disease.

Classification

DORV is virtually always associated with a ventricular septal defect (VSD). The accepted means of classification usually hinges on the location of the VSD relative to the great vessels. It is generally divided into four categories: subaortic, subpulmonary, doubly-committed or non-comitted.

- *Subaortic*

    - The VSD is positioned below the aortic valve

    - No subaortic conus

    - Superior margin of VSD is the aortic annulus

    - Blood from the LV flows through the VSD to the aorta and blood from the RV flows mainly to the PA

- *Subpulmonary*

    - VSD is positioned below the pulmonary valve

    - Presence of subaortic conus

    - Blood from the LV flows through the VSD to the PA and blood from the RV flows mainly to the aorta

- *Doubly-committed*

    - VSD is positioned nearly equally below the aortic and pulmonary valves

    - Blood from both ventricles is substantially mixed in the RV, yielding physiology that resembles a large VSD

- *Non-committed*

    - VSD is positioned remote from the conal septum or aortic valve

    - Also includes midmuscular and apical muscular VSDs

Preoperative evaluation

Symptoms are determined primarily by the degree of pulmonary stenosis. Preoperative evaluation, including echocardiography and catheterization, should provide clear information on the anatomically-relevant aspects of the repair. Important points to consider include the location of the VSD, development of conal septum, degree of pulmonary stenosis, coronary anatomy, orientation of the great vessels, and associated anomalies. Several associated cardiac anomalies are associated with DORV. Many of these affect the clinical presentation and the limits of the repair. Occurrence rates of associated cardiovascular anomalies are as follows:

- *Pulmonary stenosis*: 21-47% (most commonly observed with subaortic VSD)

- *ASD:* 21-26%

- *PDA:* 16%

- *Atrioventricular canal:* 8%

- *Subaortic stenosis:* 3-30%

- *Coarctation, hypoplastic arch, and interrupted aortic arch:* 2-45%

- *Mitral valve anomalies:* 30%

Management

Because DORV does not resolve spontaneously, all cases must be surgically repaired. The selection of surgical repair options in DORV is a complex decision, which depends less on the anatomy than upon the underlying physiology. There are a multitude of surgical options depending on the specific anomaly that exists. Patients can be temporized with an infusion of PGE_1. When the contrary clinical picture of CHF is present, careful diuresis, digoxin, inotropic support, and control of pulmonary blood flow by means of intubation and manipulation of blood gases may be indicated.

- *Repair of DORV with subaortic VSD.* A baffle is created, which facilitates a path of flow from the LV to the aorta and the RV outflow path passes around the baffle. The subpulmonary stenosis is relieved by division of the septal and parietal extensions of the conal septum. The VSD is ultimately closed with a pericardial patch.

- *Repair of DORV with subpulmonary VSD* (i.e., Taussig-Bing heart). The preferred surgical repair is anatomic repair (i.e., the arterial switch operation).

- *Repair of DORV with doubly-committed VSD*. Surgical correction is performed in a fashion similar to that described above for DORV with subaortic VSD.

- *Repair of DORV with non-committed VSD*. This is the most difficult to correct. Its correction is a high-risk procedure that often involves univentricular repair. However, an intraventricular tunnel that connects the VSD to the aorta is the operation of choice.

73. Aortic stenosis and left ventricular outflow tract obstruction
Jennifer S. Nelson

LVOT obstruction is the obstruction of blood flow from the systemic ventricle to the ascending aorta due to a congenital anatomic defect. Consisting of subvalvular, valvular, and supravalvular components, the LVOT is a complex anatomic structure (Table 73-1). Obstruction may occur at one or more levels, promoting the development of concentric left ventricular hypertrophy (LVH).

Aortic valve stenosis

The most common congenital cardiac anomaly is a bicuspid aortic valve (AV), occurring in 1-2% of the population and in 70% of those patients who present with aortic valve stenosis (AS) beyond the neonatal period. The fusion in bicuspid AV usually occurs at the intercoronary commissure. Most patients are male and are typically asymptomatic in childhood. A minority of patients will have "critical" neonatal AS, and are ductal-dependent. These children rely on retrograde blood flow from the PDA for perfusion of the heart and brain, and will suffer ischemic injury in the case of ductal closure. In this category, most neonates will have immature, myxomatous valve tissue that is difficult to classify as bicuspid or unicuspid. Associated hypoplasia of other left heart structures such as the mitral valve (MV), LV, LVOT, ascending aorta, and aortic arch is common. Increased impedance to LV ejection leads to concentric LVH. Also, LV compliance may be significantly decreased due to endocardial fibroelastosis. This replacement of myocardium by fibrous tissue is due in part to chronic subendocardial ischemia *in utero*.

Clinical presentation is largely dependent on the severity of AS and the degree of associated LVH. In critical neonatal AS, a PGE_1 infusion must be instituted at birth to prevent closure of the PDA and avoid hypoperfusion and circulatory collapse. In children beyond the neonatal period, some will be asymptomatic while others may present with respiratory distress secondary to pulmonary edema.

Management of critical neonatal AS is primarily by balloon dilation. Balloon dilation promotes growth of the aortic annulus and is indicated when echocardiography shows a peak gradient > 30-40 mmHg, or catheterization shows a peak-to-peak gradient of > 20-30 mmHg. Surgical approaches include: open valvotomy with inflow occlusion, open valvotomy on CPB, and transventricular (closed) dilatation with or without CPB.

Table 73-1. Overview of LVOT obstruction

Lesion Anatomy	Clinical presentation	Diagnostic studies	Intervention
Critical neonatal aortic stenosis Smaller-than-normal and/or hypoplastic valve	Poor perfusion, cyanosis, lethargy, murmur, circulatory collapse	• Prenatal US • TTE	• Mechanical ventilation • Inotropic support • PGE$_1$ infusion • **Balloon valvuloplasty**
Post-neonatal aortic stenosis Adequate aortic annulus; bicuspid valve in >75%	Dependent on severity of LVH. Respiratory distress, angina and/or syncope with exercise, harsh SEM	• EKG (may show ischemia) • TTE	One ventricle (Norwood) vs. two ventricle pathway
Subaortic stenosis See Table 73-3			
Supravalvar aortic stenosis Thickening of sinotubular ridge; narrow coronary ostia	• 50% of asymptomatic patients have Williams syndrome • SEM • Late cardiac symptoms: syncope, angina, CHF, VF, cardiac arrest, sudden death • Death by 2nd decade	• TTE (gradient of >40mmHg + narrowing of STJ = indication for surgery) • Cardiac cath • Possibly MRI	Surgery

EKG: Electrocardiogram, LV: Left ventricle, LVH: Left ventricular hypertrophy, MRI: Magnetic resonance imaging, MV: Mitral valve, PA: Pulmonary artery, PGE$_1$: Prostaglandin E$_2$, SEM: Systolic ejection murmur, STJ: Sinotubular junction, TTE: Transthoracic echocardiogram, US: Ultrasound, VSD: Ventricular septal defect.

Among neonates with non-critical AS, an attempt to discontinue PGE$_1$ is made. Children who are able to feed and grow without respiratory distress may not require any intervention in the short-term. For children who do not tolerate discontinuation of PGE$_1$, a one- versus two- ventricle surgical approach is chosen. Generally within days, infants with severe hypoplasia of left-sided heart structures will require a Norwood procedure. Aortic valve replacement (AVR) for isolated AS is almost never indicated in children with a normal aortic annulus size. In the case of pediatric AS with annular hypoplasia, several surgical options exist and are displayed in Table 73-2. In general, AVR with annular enlargement

(Nicks, Manougian, or extended aortic root replacement with aortic homograft) is used when a modest degree of annular enlargement is needed. An anterior annular enlargement (Ross/Konno, classic Konno, or combined anterior/posterior enlargement) is employed for severe aortic annular hypoplasia.

Table 73-2. Operations for the treatment of congenital aortic stenosis.

Procedure	Description	Special considerations
Nicks	Incision between left and non-commissures into area of fibrous continuity between AV and MV. Dacron patch used to enlarge annulus.	Can be used with mechanical AVR or as part of a homograft root replacement
Manougian	Similar to Nicks, but incision carried into the anterior leaflet of the MV.	Postop MR seen in 0-14%
Extended aortic root replacement with aortic homograft	Uses Nicks incision, coronary buttons reimplanted.	Risk of early calcification of homograft and valve failure
Ross/Konno	Replacement of AV with pulmonary autograft + anterior enlargement of aortic annulus.	Risks: neoaortic root dilation, AI, aneurysm formation at subaortic patch Need for life-long homograft conduit changes in RVOT
Classic Konno	Subaortic region and annulus enlarged using patch. 2nd patch used to close infundibulum.	Oversizing mechanical prosthesis can cause projection into RVOT as well as distortion of the coronary arteries resulting in ischemia. Glutaraldehyde-treated pericardium used in younger patients; Dacron used for older children.
Combined anterior and posterior annular enlargement	Uses elements of both the Manougian and Konno procedures. Mechanical AVR.	

AI: Aortic insufficiency, AV: Aortic valve, AVR: Aortic valve replacement, MR: Mitral regurgitation, MV: Mitral valve, RVOT: Right ventricular outflow tract.

Subaortic stenosis

There are several main forms of subaortic stenosis. Their pathophysiology and treatment is presented in Table 73-3.

- *Discrete subvalvular stenosis.* Most cases are seen in older children and young adults and are likely acquired. It is associated with other congenital defects like VSD in 60-70% of cases. It is characterized by a circular or crescent-shaped fibrous membrane positioned proximal to the aortic valve. Membrane development is likely the result of shear stress and turbulent blood flow in the LVOT secondary to abnormal angles between the septum and the aorta. Surgical resection is approached via aortotomy. The aortic valve leaflets are retracted and the membrane is enucleated. Many times, septal myectomy will also be undertaken to reduce the chance of recurrence. Operative mortality is extremely low. Left bundle branch block (LBBB) is a post-operative complication, but complete heart block is infrequent.

- *Diffuse subaortic stenosis (tunnel-like stenosis).* Much more complex lesion, characterized by muscular or fibromuscular subvalvar stenosis extending for more than one third of the aortic diameter. It is frequently best approached with septoplasty via a right ventriculotomy or right atriotomy using bicaval cannulation. Major risks are complete heart block requiring permanent pacemaker and inadequate relief of obstruction.

- *Muscular obstruction / hypertrophic obstructive cardiomyopathy.* Dynamic form of obstruction resulting from muscle hypertrophy, commonly involving the septum. The pathophysiology is the development of concentric LVH, which, in severe cases, may lead to subendocardial ischemia as coronary arterial neovascularization is unable to meet increasing demands. Because muscular hypertrophy outpaces the availability of coronary blood flow, the child is predisposed to ventricular fibrillation and sudden death. Rarely, subaortic stenosis may become symptomatic causing angina, exercise intolerance, or syncope. Sudden cardiac arrest may unfortunately be the first clinical symptom.

- *Other structural lesions.* Obstruction of the LVOT can also occur from posterior malalignment of the conal septum or accessory endocardial and MV tissues. There should be a low threshold to repair these cases. Indications include peak aortic gradients of 30-40 mmHg and presence of AI.

The diagnosis of subaortic obstruction is made with echocardiography. The gradient across the outflow tract, degree of LVH, and presence of AI are of particular interest. New onset AI is generally an indication for surgery. CXR and cardiac catheterization are not usually helpful. EKG may show evidence of LVH, when present.

Medical therapy for subaortic obstruction with resultant LA hypertension is not usually required. Catheter-based interventions may give short-term improvement, but carry the risk of complete heart block and damage to the aortic valve. Indications for surgical intervention are listed in Table 73-3. Recurrence risk is highest in children under 10 years, so many surgeons will follow these lesions with echocardiography every 6 months until the child is > 5-10 years of age or other generally accepted indications are met.

Table 73-3. Lesions associated with subaortic stenosis.

Type Anatomy/physiology	Indications for surgery	Surgical options
Discrete subaortic (fibro-muscular membrane) • Acquired • Result of turbulence in an abnormally-shaped LVOT causing endocardial injury and subsequent fibrosis. • Membrane causes further turbulence, perpetuating fibrosis. • May lead to AI as leaflets become thick and distorted	• AI or ↑ AI • 40-50mmHg gradient • ↑ LVOT gradient • ↑ LVH	Aortotomy +/- valvotomy with enucleation of subaortic membrane and septal myectomy
Diffuse subaortic (LVOT tunnel) • Fibromuscular proliferation involving more than 1/3 aortic diameter • Contraction of bands connecting the septum to the anterior leaflet may pull the MV anteriorly.	• Peak gradient > 50-60 mmHg • Moderate to severe LVH • New onset AI	• Aggressive resection of obstructing tissues • Aortoventriculo-plasty (i.e., Konno, Rastan) vs. aortoapical conduit vs. septal myectomy and septoplasty
Hypertrophic cardiomyopathy (HCM) • Autosomal dominant disease of sarcomere proteins. • 70-80% of mutations in familial HCM involve β-myosin heavy chain, myosin-binding protein C and troponin T. • LVH with loss of LV cavity volume • May be associated with SAM	• Symptoms (syncope, angina, exercise intolerance) • No response to medical therapy (beta-blockade, calcium channel blockers, and dual chamber pacemaker implantation)	• Resection of subaortic muscle (septal myectomy / Morrow procedure) • MVR with bileaflet prosthetic valve (low profile)

AI: Aortic insufficiency, AV: Aortic valve, LV: Left ventricle, LVH: Left ventricular hypertrophy, LVOT: Left ventricular outflow tract, MV: Mitral valve, MVR: Mitral valve replacement, SAM: Systolic anterior motion of the mitral valve.

Supravalvular aortic stenosis

Supravalvular aortic stenosis is the least common type of LVOT obstruction and represents narrowing at the sinotubular junction (STJ). There are three forms:

- *Williams syndrome.* Supravalvular aortic stenosis, mental retardation, elfin facies, hypercalcemia, pulmonary stenosis.

- *Sporadic form.* From a spontaneous inherited mutation of the elastin gene 5,7.

- *Autosomal dominant familial form.* Most common form in symptomatic infants.

Due to a lack of elastin, the great vessels are less-compliant. Subject to greater wall stress, they become progressively narrowed by medial smooth muscle fibrosis. In a progressive cycle, the narrowed vessels are exposed to even greater sheer stress as blood flow becomes more turbulent. Over time, this process causes endothelial damage, and further thickening of the media. In the diffuse form, the entire ascending aorta becomes thickened and stenotic. As a result, arch vessel origins may also have focal stenoses. As expected, operative mortality, risk of re-operation, and late survival is much better in the localized form compared to the diffuse form. Associated supravalvular narrowing of the main PA, and/or stenosis of branch PAs and peripheral PAs is possible, but uncommon.

In supravalvular aortic stenosis, the narrowed STJ draws the AV commissures closer to each other. Aortic valve leaflets are typically normal, though they may adhere to the sinotubular ridge as distance between the leaflet free edges and the STJ is decreased. If restricted movement of the right and left coronary cusps limits blood flow into the sinuses of Valsalva, or if there is coronary ostial narrowing, blood flow to the hypertrophied LV myocardium may be insufficient, and predispose the patient to ventricular fibrillation and sudden cardiac arrest.

Children with supravalvular stenosis are at an additional risk for sudden death due to degenerative changes in the coronary arteries. Because the coronary ostia are below the level of the obstruction, they are subject to higher pressures and fill during systole rather than diastole. Coronaries may therefore become aneurysmal and tortuous.

Supravalvular stenosis is progressive and treatment is recommended before the development of severe LVH. Prognosis is good with an aggressive surgical approach. Catheter-based interventions are generally limited to peripheral pulmonary stenosis and mediastinal branch pulmonary stenosis. Medical therapy is not usually needed because heart failure is a late finding. Afterload reducing agents should be avoided.

Two-dimensional echocardiography showing a narrowed STJ and gradient of >40mmHg is an indication for surgery, especially with progressive AI. With a less significant gradient and no LVH, the child may be followed with semi-annual echocardiography. In the case of Williams syndrome, children with evidence of a small lumen in the distal ascending aorta extending into the arch vessels should be further imaged with MRI or cardiac catheterization. These studies can help determine the extent of the reconstruction needed. It is also necessary to preoperatively evaluate for the presence of associated supravalvular pulmonary stenosis or branch or peripheral PA stenoses.

Discrete (localized) supravalvular stenosis is generally repaired in the method of Doty whereby an incision is made through the area of stenosis and extended into the sinuses of Valsalva on either side of the RCA. This allows for expansion of the ascending aorta without distortion of the AV. An inverted Y-shaped Gore-Tex patch is placed to complete the reconstruction.

74. Hypoplastic left heart syndrome

Nicholas D. Andersen, Joseph W. Turek

Anatomy and pathophysiology

Hypoplastic left heart syndrome (HLHS) denotes a continuum of congenital heart defects characterized by underdevelopment of the systemic ventricle occurring alone or in combination with abnormalities of the aorta, aortic valve, and/or mitral valve. HLHS accounts for approximately 4% of congenital heart defects yet is responsible for 25% of cardiac deaths in the first week of life. Left-sided structures are inadequate to support the systemic circulation, placing the work of both pulmonary and systemic circulations solely on the RV. Left-to-right shunting at the atrial level allows pulmonary venous return to enter the RA, and right-to-left shunting through an enlarged PDA allows for systemic perfusion. Retrograde flow to the arch and ascending aorta provides cerebral and coronary blood flow. Oxygenation and perfusion are therefore critically dependent on an interatrial communication, ductal patency, and the balance between pulmonary and systemic blood flow. Cyanosis, CHF, and systemic hypoperfusion result as PVR decreases and pulmonary blood flow increases at the expense of systemic blood flow.

Four morphologic subtypes of HLHS can be defined based on the status of the left heart valves:

- Aortic and mitral atresia (AA/MA)

- Aortic atresia and mitral stenosis (AA/MS)

- Aortic stenosis and mitral atresia (AS/MA)

- Aortic and mitral stenosis (AS/MS)

AA/MA is the most common, AS/MA is the least common, and AA/MS is the highest risk subtype. Varying degrees of endocardial fibroelastosis are seen within the LV, and the RV is enlarged with uniform hypertrophy and an increase in size to approximately three times normal. The main PA trunk is large and continues directly into the large PDA.

Presentation

Infants with HLHS are born at gestation and may appear normal at birth or present with mild cyanosis, tachypnea, and tachycardia. A singe S2, left parasternal systolic murmur, and RV lift can be appreciated on physical exam. EKG reveals RA enlargement and RV hypertrophy. CXR reveals cardiomegaly and increased pulmonary vascular markings. Echocardiography is diagnostic. Ductal closure is followed by overt heart failure and rapid circulatory collapse. An intact or restrictive atrial septum requires urgent intervention to create an interatrial communication. Extracardiac malformations or genetic disorders occur in 10-28% of children with HLHS.

Diagnosis

Echocardiography allows for definitive diagnosis and detailed characterization of the involved heart structures. Although HLHS is clinically silent in utero, prenatal diagnosis is increasing in frequency due to the advent of fetal US and the absence of the normal four-chamber heart on ultrasonography leading to further evaluation.

Management

HLHS was historically considered a non-survivable lesion, and treatment involved supportive care until death. Modern surgical therapy now includes staged palliation to a univentricular circulation or cardiac transplantation. If considered for transplantation, procedures to stent the ductus arteriosus or enlarge the interatrial communication may be required. Patients with borderline left-heart function may be considered for a biventricular repair through primary correction of the involved cardiac lesions. Fetal aortic valvuloplasty has been performed in fetuses with aortic stenosis and evolving HLHS and may increase the likelihood of biventricular repair.

Upon birth, infants require infusion of an E-type prostaglandin to maintain ductal patency. Urgent balloon septostomy or surgery is required in patients with an intact atrial septum to allow for left-to-right shunting and systemic flow via the PDA. An adequate balance between pulmonary and systemic blood flow must be maintained by altering PVR and SVR. Low inspired oxygen concentrations and the addition of carbon dioxide to inspired gas are effective in raising PVR in response to pulmonary overcirculation and systemic hypoperfusion. Alternatively, α-adrenergic agonists and antagonists can be used to augment SVR to optimize Qp:Qs and systemic oxygen delivery.

Stage I

For infants selected for univentricular palliation, high neonatal PVR prohibits an immediate Fontan procedure. Instead, the three-staged Norwood sequence is utilized to accommodate the changes in PVR during infancy until a Fontan-type circulation can be constructed. Stage I reconstruction is performed shortly after birth via median sternotomy and deep hypothermic circulatory arrest (DHCA). The aims of the procedure are to provide unobstructed systemic and coronary arterial blood flow, a stable and balanced source of pulmonary blood flow, and unobstructed pulmonary venous return to the systemic RV. These goals are achieved by:

- Performance of an atrial septectomy

- Construction of a neoaorta from the pulmonary valve by division of the PA at the bifurcation and anastomosis of the aorta to the proximal PA

- Placement of a systemic-to-pulmonary modified Blalock-Taussig shunt (mBTS)

The classic mBTS was interposed between the right subclavian artery and the right PA. However, a central shunt from the bifurcation of the innominate artery to the central PA is now preferred to promote symmetrical growth of the pulmonary arteries. More recently, RV-to-PA conduits (Sano modification) have been used as the source of pulmonary blood flow and are thought to improve coronary perfusion by reducing the systemic runoff into the pulmonary circulation and coronary steal that occurs when the arteriopulmonary shunt is placed distal to the pulmonic valve.

At specialized centers, hospital survival after stage I reconstruction and survival to stage II operation can now approach 90% and 80%, respectively. Postoperative management of patients after stage I reconstruction is difficult since these patients tend to be very hemodynamically labile. The cardiovascular system after stage I consists of parallel circulations that are competing with each other in terms of blood flow. The balance between both circulations depends on the pulmonary and systemic vascular resistances with the amount of flow into that circulation being inversely proportional to its vascular resistance. PVR can be modified by changing the FiO_2, allowing hypercapnia, or administering inspired CO_2. Hypoxia and hypercapnia increase the PVR and therefore increase systemic blood flow. Similarly, SVR can be controlled pharmacologically using α-adrenergic agonist and antagonists. The goal is to provide adequate blood supply to both circulations.

Ductal stenting and bilateral PA banding (deemed the "hybrid" procedure) has been employed at some centers for high-risk neonates to achieve stage I palliation without the early morbidity of CPB and DHCA. A comprehensive stage II procedure is then performed at 4-6 months of age at which time the neoaorta and bidirectional cavopulmonary shunt are constructed. Disadvantages of the hybrid procedure include the unrepaired hypoplastic aortic arch, which carries the risk of cerebral and coronary malperfusion due to retrograde arch obstruction, restrictive interatrial communication requiring intervention, mechanical distortion of the branch PAs, and greater surgical requirements during stage II palliation.

Stage II

The second stage procedure (hemi-Fontan or bidirectional Glenn) is performed between 2-6 months of age and aims to reduce the volume load on the RV once PVR has fallen sufficiently to accommodate passive venous return into the pulmonary circulation. The systemic and pulmonary circulations are partially divided by performing a bidirectional cavopulmonary anastomoses whereby the SVC is divided and anastomosed end-to-side to the right PA, in conjunction with takedown of the prior mBTS. Hospital survival after stage II reconstruction approaches 95%. Complications are rare; stenosis of the cavopulmonary anastomosis may occur, causing face and bilateral upper extremity edema.

Stage III

The Fontan operation is performed at 2-4 years of age and entails redirecting IVC flow to the PA/SVC confluence to complete the division of the pulmonary and systemic circulations. The RV is relieved of systemic venous return allowing for pressure and volume offloading of the ventricle and improved oxygenation from abolishment of right-to-left shunting. The two common techniques for Fontan construction are the lateral atrial tunnel or the extracardiac interposition graft. The lateral atrial tunnel uses an intraatrial patch to partition the RA and reroute IVC flow to the PA/SVC confluence. This operation leads to a higher rate of postoperative arrhythmias due to the presence of atrial suture lines. The extracardiac Fontan uses a tube graft sewn directly from the IVC to the PA/SVC confluence. This provides a simpler operation with reduced postoperative arrhythmias. However, shortcomings include thrombogenicity and lack of growth potential. A "fenestration" or communication between the intraatrial tunnel or interposition graft and the RA can be created in high-risk patients to serve as a residual right-to-LA shunt. This modification is intended to decompress high pulmonary venous pressures in the setting of transient increased postoperative PVR. The fenestration may be closed electively at a later date by transvenous catheterization. Hospital survival after stage III reconstruction can reach 98%. Long-term complications of the Fontan circulation include protein-losing enteropathy, thromboemboli, arrhythmia, heart failure requiring re-intervention or transplantation, and sudden cardiac death.

75. Truncus arteriosus and aortopulmonary window

Ibrahim Abdullah, Bret A. Mettler

Truncus arteriosus

Anatomy and classification

In truncus arteriosus, a single great vessel arises from the base of the heart, which supplies the systemic, pulmonary, and coronary circulations. According to the Edwards-Collet classification, truncus arteriosus is classified in four types:

- *Type I.* The branch PAs arise from a segment of the main PA arising from the common trunk. The segment of main PA arises almost always from a site distal to the truncal valve.

- *Type II.* The branch PAs arise in close proximity from the posterior aspect of the common trunk.

- *Type III.* The branch PAs arise from separate, widely spaced origins.

- *Type IV.* There are absent true PAs and pulmonary blood flow is supplied by aortopulmonary collaterals.

A VSD is almost always present. The truncal valve may be tricuspid (70%), quadricuspid, bicuspid or, rarely, unicuspid or pentacuspid.

Pathophysiology

There is mixing of blood at the level of the VSD and a left-to-right shunt at the level of the truncus. This is primarily due to the declining PVR compared to the SVR as the neonate ages. As a result, babies will develop pulmonary over-circulation and signs of CHF. If this persists then the patient may develop irreversible pulmonary vascular disease. In addition, there is both systolic and diastolic shunting, which can lead to poor systemic and coronary perfusion. If there is any truncal valve regurgitation, this can further compromise systemic and coronary perfusion.

Diagnosis

Generally, babies will present with mild cyanosis at birth. As PVR falls, pulmonary over-circulation ensues with a decrease in cyanosis but increasing signs of CHF. Truncal valve regurgitation exacerbates the signs and symptoms of CHF. These typically include tachypnea, tachycardia, poor feeding and diaphoresis.

A CXR will generally show cardiomegaly and increased pulmonary vascular markings. Diagnosis is confirmed by an echocardiogram. If a patient presents late, a catheterization may be needed to assess PVR. A cardiac MRI can also be obtained to further delineate complex anatomy.

Treatment

Neonatal repair has become the treatment of choice. The patient is typically placed on CPB with arterial cannulation high in the aorta and bicaval venous cannulation. The branch PAs are snared to prevent cardioplegia runoff into the pulmonary circulation once the cross-clamp is applied. The branch PAs are then separated from the aorta, taking care to identify the takeoff of the coronaries so as to avoid them. The defect in the aorta is repaired using a patch of pericardium. Any truncal valve insufficiency is addressed. The VSD is closed. This is then followed by construction of a RV-to-PA conduit.

Aortopulmonary window

Anatomy and classification

Aortopulmonary (AP) window is a malformation characterized by a communication between the ascending aorta and main PA. A VSD is usually present. Both semilunar valves are also present.

According to the Congenital Heart Surgery Nomenclature and Database Project, there are four types of AP windows:

- *Type I (proximal).* Defect between adjacent portions of the ascending aorta and main PA.

- *Type II (distal).* Defect near the origin of the right PA.

- *Type III (total).* Large defects with poorly defined margins. Combination of types I and II.

- *Intermediate defects.* Similar to type III but are smaller and have well-defined superior and inferior rims.

Pathophysiology

An AP window is characterized by a non-restrictive left-to-right shunt. As PVR falls following birth, there is even more flow to the lungs with equalization of aortic and pulmonary pressures. The LV gets volume overloaded while the RV gets pressure overloaded. The pulmonary overcirculation leads to interstitial pulmonary edema and eventually will lead to pulmonary vascular obstructive disease.

Diagnosis

As in truncus arteriosus, patients will typically present with signs and symptoms of CHF - tachypnea, diaphoresis, failure to thrive or recurrent respiratory tract infections. There is usually a loud continuous systolic murmur heard best at the left upper heart border. A CXR may demonstrate cardiomegaly with increased pulmonary vascular markings. The gold standard diagnostic study is an echocardiogram. If a child presents later in life, a catheterization may be necessary to quantify PVR.

Treatment

All symptomatic patients should undergo repair. Asymptomatic patients should undergo repair before 3 to 4 months of age. When beyond 6 months of age, consideration should be given to a catheterization before repair. A ratio of PVR/SVR greater than 0.4 has been shown to be a risk factor for perioperative death. Repair is usually contraindicated when the PVR is greater than 8 to 10 Wood units or when the PVR/SVR ratio is greater than 0.7.

Repair is accomplished via a median sternotomy and usage of CPB with bicaval cannulation. After cross-clamping the aorta and arresting the heart with cardioplegia (while snaring the branch PAs), the aorta is opened by the window, taking care to avoid the coronary arteries. The aorta is separated from the PA and the defects in each are usually reconstructed with autologous pericardium. The crossclamp is released, the heart is de-aired, and the patient is subsequently weaned from CPB.

76. Coronary artery anomalies
Immanuel I. Turner, Joseph W. Turek

There are multiple possible anomalies of the anatomy of the coronary arteries. Patients may have the ostia of a coronary artery arise eccentrically from a Sinus of Valsalva, close to a valve commissure, or high in the tubular aorta above the sinotubular junction. Also, both coronaries may arise from the same sinus either as a joined artery or from two separate ostia. The most common of all coronary anomalies consists of the circumflex coronary artery arising from the RCA. While many such anomalies are inconsequential, others have profound implications. For example, an anomalous coronary crossing the RVOT in a patient with tetralogy of Fallot significantly alters the surgical approach. In anomalous origin of the left coronary artery from the PA (ALCAPA), the condition is uniformly fatal without an operation. The risk of exercise-induced sudden death in anomalous aortic origin of a coronary artery (AAOCA) is managed with either exercise-restriction or surgical intervention. This chapter will focus on the latter two coronary abnormalities, ALCAPA and AAOCA, both of which employ surgical therapy as the mainstay for management.

Anomalous origin of a coronary artery from the pulmonary artery

ALCAPA is a rare congenital anomaly with an incidence of 1 in 300,000 live births (0.25-0.50%). It usually presents as an isolated lesion. It carries up to 90% mortality in infancy if left untreated and is the most common cause of MI in children. A RCA arising from the PA is much less frequent and may also present with ischemia or sudden death.

Pathophysiology

Elevated PVR ensures antegrade flow from the PA to the anomalous left coronary artery. Along with ductal closure, the PVR decreases and the LV becomes perfused with low-pressure desaturated blood. The perfusion of the LV becomes dependent on intercoronary collaterals from the RCA. Even though patients may have collaterals to sustain LV perfusion, as the PVR drops further, flow through the left coronary artery reverses causing left-to-right shunting into the PA.

The combination of inadequate collateralization and coronary steal lead to subsequent ischemia and infarction of the LV. If the papillary muscles are involved in the ischemic distribution, MR can result. In addition, an LV aneurysm may form as a result of infarction

Clinical presentation

ALCAPA can be labeled as *infantile-type* if there are poorly-developed coronary collaterals, or *adult-type* when a more developed collateral system allows patients to live until adolescence or adulthood before diagnosis.

Symptoms are usually a result of ischemia or progressive LV dysfunction and can include: distress during feeding or crying, CHF, tachypnea, poor weight gain, poor exercise tolerance, and chest pain. The syndrome also can mimic infantile conditions such as colic, reflux and respiratory infections.

Diagnosis

- *EKG.* Non-diagnostic.

- *CXR.* Cardiomegaly.

- *Echocardiogram.* Most useful study. It will show a dilated ventricle, ventricular dysfunction, and visualization of the abnormal origin of the artery.

- *Cardiac catheterization.* Reserved for cases where the origin of the artery is not clearly visualized on echocardiography.

Treatment

Due to the high mortality associated with medical therapy, surgical intervention is indicated at the time of initial diagnosis. The surgical strategy is restoration of a two-coronary system for patients with ALCAPA while minimizing the extent of ischemic damage to ventricular myocardium.

Severe LV dysfunction and mitral insufficiency are not contraindications to revascularization in infants because of the significant recovery that can occur after the repair. In fact, ECMO will frequently be used as a bridge to recovery in the postoperative period. Mitral valve repair and aneurysmectomy are usually not indicated at the time of the initial procedure.

The most common orientation of the ALCAPA is from the rightward posterior sinus (facing). The dual coronary system is achieved by direct re-implantation of the anomalous coronary into the aorta. Surgical repair is performed under CPB with moderate hypothermia or deep hypothermic circulatory arrest in very small infants. The steps for the procedure are:

- PA is opened transversely above the level of the sinotubular junction.

- Identification of the orifice of the anomalous coronary artery and excision of the ostium   with a general button of PA wall.

- Aorta is opened transversely (above sinotubular junction) and the incision is carried to above the left posterior sinus, which is incised vertically.

- Anastomosis of the coronary button beginning at inferior most aspect, followed by closure of the aorta.

- PA closure (primarily) unless there is tension in which case the *ligamentum arteriosum* is divided to achieve more mobility and/or the PA is closed with a patch of autologous pericardium.

Anomalous aortic origin of coronary artery (AAOCA)

AAOCA from an ectopic sinus occurs with an overall incidence of 0.1-1%. The most common anomaly is the circumflex artery originating from the right coronary sinus or the RCA, which is of no real clinical significance. The next most common anomaly is the RCA arising from the left coronary sinus (ARCA), occurring 6 times more frequently than an anomalous left coronary arising from the right coronary sinus (ALCA). In its most common form, the artery assumes an interarterial course between the aorta and main PA and may or may not have an intramural segment, acute angle of origin, and an associated slit-like ostium. This anatomical configuration has been implicated in exercise-induced sudden death in children and young adults. A single coronary artery is very rare.

Pathophysiology
Postulated mechanisms of ischemia include ostial obstruction due to a slit-like coronary orifice, compression of the anomalous coronary between the great vessels, anomalous coronary vasospasm, dynamic flattening or kinking of the anomalous coronary with aortic distention, or obstruction of the intramural segment, particularly at the level of the commissure, with aortic expansion. An anomalous left coronary carries a higher risk of sudden death.

Clinical presentation
Symptoms of chest pain and syncope appear in 37% of sudden death victims prior to the sentinel event. 63% of AAOCA-attributed deaths occur in previously asymptomatic individuals. There are no characteristic physical exam findings. Diagnosis must be considered in any patient with exercise-induced myocardial ischemia or sudden death.

Diagnosis

Noninvasive imaging techniques used to assess the anomalous course include echocardiography, CTA, and cardiac MRI. Echocardiography remains the best initial test for determining arterial course, including whether there exists an intramural segment and the relationship of this segment to the commissure. In cases of diagnostic dilemma, cardiac MRI appears to be the best confirmatory imaging modality. In some cases, coronary arteriography may be necessary to delineate the anatomy and rule out other associated coronary disease.

Treatment

Surgical intervention is indicated for patients with angina, syncope, or sudden death event found to have AAOCA. The indications for surgery in asymptomatic patients are not clearly defined. Given the higher risk of sudden death with an anomalous left coronary, surgery is often performed in these patients. Any patient with an asymptomatic AAOCA should be excluded from all competitive sports and strenuous activities. This recommendation has led to surgical repair in many cases of asymptomatic ARCA in order to lift the exercise restriction and allow the child to participate in competitive athletics.

The coronary unroofing procedure and modifications of this procedure have been shown to be safe and effective for treatment of AAOCA with an interarterial and intramural course. Surgical repair is performed under CPB with mild hypothermia and antegrade cardioplegia. The interarterial morphology dictates surgical approach. A transverse aortotomy is performed. If the vessel is extramural, the coronary is translocated and re-implanted into the appropriate sinus. If the vessel is intramural, the particular management depends on its relationship with the commissure. Intramural vessels located above the commissure are treated by unroofing the coronary vessel through the aorta. Intramural vessels located below the commissure require creation of a higher neo-ostium or coronary unroofing with detachment and resuspension of the commissure.

Coronary unroofing can be performed concomitantly with other necessary cardiac procedures (CABG, aortic valve replacement, etc.) with minimal additional risk.

77. Vascular rings, pulmonary artery sling, and associated tracheal anomalies
Stephanie Mick

Introduction and review of normal embryology

Vascular rings are congenital malformations of the aortic arch causing tracheal and esophageal encirclement with symptoms related to their compression. A PA sling is the name for a vascular ring formed around the trachea when the left PA passes over it from an anomalous origin off the right PA, associated with respiratory symptoms. Tracheal anomalies such as complete tracheal rings are often associated with PA slings, and are often the cause of the symptoms, rather than physical compression itself.

The embryo begins to form a system of blood vessels consisting of paired dorsal aortae (DAs) at ~21 days. One of these will eventually form the descending thoracic aorta (TA). After the DAs form, 6 paired branchial ("pertaining to gills" as they recall the blood supply of gill-breathing animals) arteries form. On each side, each of these branchial arteries communicates with the DA on that side forming an arch on each side. Normally, the 1st and 2nd arches undergo near-complete resorption and form only facial arteries. The 3rd arches form the carotid arteries. The left 4th arch normally forms the distal aortic arch and aortic isthmus from the origin of the left common carotid (LCC) to the descending TA (which itself is formed from the left dorsal aorta) and joins the conotruncus, which forms the ascending aorta. The right DA resorbs almost completely and contributes to the formation of the right subclavian artery (RSC).

Anatomic variants: vascular rings

The great majority (~95%) of rings have a dominant (larger) right aortic arch (RAA) with ring formation on the left. Therefore surgical division of rings is nearly always performed through a left thoracotomy.

Dominant RAA anomalies (~95%)

- *Double aortic arch.* Two aortic arches, one leftward and anterior (giving off the LCC and left subclavian artery (LSC)) and one rightward and posterior (giving off the right common carotid artery (RCC) and LSC), both attached to the (usually left sided) descending aorta. The esophagus and trachea run between/are encircled by these two AAs. *Origin:* persistent RAA without full resorption of the left aortic arch (LAA).

- *RAA, aberrant LSC and left ligamentum.* The RAA gives off the LCC, RCC, RSC, and LSC in this order. To get to the left side, the LSC goes behind the esophagus and gives off the *ligamentum arteriosum,* which passes anteriorly to get to the LPA, forming a ring. *Origin:* Persistence of the right 4th arch and resorption of the left 4th arch.

- *RAA, mirror-image branching and retroesophageal ligamentum.* The RAA gives off a left innominate, RCC, RSC, and the *ligamentum arteriosum* (which often arises from a prominent diverticulum of the ductus, the diverticulum of Kommerell). The ligament goes behind the esophagus and attaches to the PA anteriorly, forming a ring. *Origin:* persistence of the right 4th arch with resorption of the left 4th arch. Note that if the *ligamentum* arises from the left innominate artery, it can reach the PA without forming a ring (i.e. no *ligamentum* from Kommerell, no ring).

Dominant LAA anomalies (very rare)

If present, the surgical approach will need to be from the right.

- *LAA, mirror-image branching, right DA, and atretic RAA.* Essentially a normal LAA with normal arch vessels and an atretic RAA. The LAA must curve around the esophagus and trachea to get to the right descending TA. The atretic RAA forms a connection between the LAA and descending arch and completes the ring.

- *LAA, right DA and right-sided ligamentum to right PA.* The LAA gives off the RCC followed by the LCC and LSC. The LAA loops around the esophagus and trachea to get to the right descending aorta, gives off the RSC and then the *ligamentum arteriosum.* The *ligamentum* attaches to the right PA, forming the ring.

PA sling and tracheal anomalies

In a PA sling, the (often hypoplastic) left PA arises from the right PA, passes over the esophagus and under the trachea. The *ligamentum arteriosum* arises from the main PA, passes over the trachea to the aorta. The trachea, then, is surrounded by a ring. Approximately 50% of patients with this anomaly have (often hypoplastic) rigid O-shaped ("complete") tracheal rings and the pliable membranous trachea is absent. There is often a localized segment of tracheal stenosis adding to any anatomic or functional stenosis from left PA+*ligamentum* compression.

Pathophysiology, clinical presentation and diagnostic studies

Symptoms from vascular rings are caused by compression of the esophagus and/or the trachea. Respiratory (stridor, wheezing, infections) or esophageal (reflux, dysphagia) symptoms and/or failure to thrive may occur. With severe compression, presentation is in infancy characterized by slow early feeding, becoming more problematic as solids are introduced. Symptoms from PA slings are generally respiratory in nature.

Barium swallow shows a posterior indentation of the esophagus in vascular rings and an anterior indentation in PA sling. Echocardiography is useful in defining the type of vascular ring, if present. CT (or MRI) and bronchoscopy are necessary for tracheal assessment in PA slings but are not absolutely necessary to manage rings. CXR may be useful in defining tracheal and bronchial stenosis in PA slings.

Management

For vascular rings, surgical division is indicated when symptomatic and may be deferred in asymptomatic patients. Good nutritional status and respiratory care should be ensured preoperatively. Unless there is a patent segment of a double arch that is more than 2-3 cm in diameter, the procedure of choice is thoracoscopic ring division. Open, it is performed via a 4th interspace thoracotomy. The ring is divided and the ends are oversewn or ligated. Some degree of tracheomalacia and respiratory symptoms is to be expected but should resolve within a few months.

Most often, PA slings are symptomatic, and therefore surgical intervention is indicated. Surgery consists of anterior translocation of the left PA +/- a tracheal procedure determined by the extent of tracheal anomalies in preoperative workup: segmental (2-3 tracheal ring) resection in cases of localized anatomic stenosis or tracheoplasty in cases of more diffuse tracheal narrowing. Simple compression stenosis will usually resolve following PA relocation alone.

Innominate artery compression of the trachea

This is tracheal compression at the thoracic inlet due to a distally arising innominate artery causing a short segment of tracheomalacia. It presents with stridor (even apneic or syncopal episodes) in infancy. Diagnosis is made with bronchoscopy (pulsatile anterior tracheal compression at the thoracic inlet) and CT/MRI. Surgical approach is through a left anterior thoracotomy and consists of aortopexy to the leftward sternal edge. Confirmatory bronchoscopy should be performed and often shows dramatic improvement but a degree of persistent tracheomalacia should be expected postoperatively.

IV. Cardiothoracic Trauma and Critical Care

78. Cardiac trauma

Ravi K. Ghanta, Bryan M. Burt

Blunt and penetrating traumatic injuries to the heart and great vessels are among the most lethal injuries encountered. Improvements in urban trauma management systems and pre-hospital resuscitation have increased the number of patients with these severe injuries who reach the emergency room alive. In penetrating cardiac injury, the major challenges are rapid *resuscitation* followed by emergent definitive *surgery*. In blunt cardiac injury, the major challenge is *diagnosis*.

Penetrating cardiac trauma

All patients with penetrating wounds between the right midclavicular and left midaxillary lines from the epigastrium to the clavicles should be assumed to have injuries involving the heart until proven otherwise. Based on anatomic position, the RV (35%), LV (25%), RA (24%), and LA (3%) form the order of most common to the least common injured chambers, respectively. The typical patient presents with signs of tamponade or hemorrhage and is often in *extremis*.

Once cardiac injury is suspected, the primary goal is to minimize time in the emergency department and transfer the patient to the operating room. Hemodynamically unstable patients undergo emergent surgical exploration. Hemodynamically stable patients may undergo limited studies to assess the extent of cardiac and non-cardiac injuries. Appropriate studies include CXR, transthoracic echocardiogram, emergent focused assessment for the sonographic examination of the trauma victim (FAST), and chest CT. FAST has a sensitivity of approximately 100% and specificity of 97.3% for pericardial fluid when performed by trained examiners. Pericardiocentesis has *no role* in the diagnosis of cardiac tamponade for *penetrating* cardiac injury, because false positives and false negative rates are high. In patients with occult cardiac injury and other indications for urgent surgical exploration (e.g. ruptured spleen), TEE and subxyphoid pericardial window may be considered.

Initial treatment in the emergency department, as in all trauma, follows the American College of Surgeons Advanced Trauma Life Support (ATLS) protocol. If an impaled object is present, it should be left *in situ* as long as possible, until the pericardium is opened.

An emergent left anterior thoracotomy should be performed in the emergency department in patients who have lost signs of life during transfer to the emergency department or are unresponsive to resuscitative efforts on presentation. The thoracotomy is performed through the fourth inter-costal space, the pericardium is opened anterior to the phrenic nerve, the descending aorta is clamped, and bleeding is controlled. Lacerations should be closed with horizontal mattress pledgeted sutures of 4-0 poly-propylene or vascular clamps if available. If pledgets are unavailable, strips of pericardium are a suitable substitute. For larger lacerations, a Foley catheter may temporarily be inserted into the opening to control bleeding. After primary stabilization and control of bleeding, further exploration and repair should be continued in the controlled setting of the operating room.

The choice of incision (median sternotomy, left anterior thoracotomy, clamshell) in the operating room is made based on the suspected injuries. Median sternotomy incision provides excellent exposure for cardiorrha-phy and repair of the ascending aorta. A cervical extension may be nec-essary for approaching the subclavian or carotid arteries. If additional thoracic injuries are expected, the left anterior thoracotomy provides bet-ter exposure to the heart, lungs, chest wall, and descending aorta. A thor-acotomy may be extended across the sternum to the other side for injuries that traverse the mediastinum. Both thoracotomies together in a "clam-shell" incision provide virtually unlimited access to the entire thorax.

Myocardial free wall injuries are closed primarily with horizontal mat-tress pledgeted sutures. Larger defects may require the use of autologous or prosthetic material with CPB. If an injury is close to a large coronary artery, imbricating pledgets may be used, passing the suture under the coronary vessel. Atrial injuries are controlled with clamps and then closed primarily. Coronary artery injuries are uncommon. Small coro-nary branches may be ligated, but larger vessels should be repaired if possible or bypassed. Bypass grafting should be done with vein grafts; no time should be wasted in dissecting the internal mammary artery from the chest wall.

Missiles should be removed at the time of the primary operation due to the risks of embolization, endocarditis, and erosion.

Blunt cardiac trauma

Blunt cardiac injury occurs when an intense, sudden force is applied to the heart by other structures of the body, most commonly due to motor vehicle accidents. Blunt cardiac trauma can result in the following pa-thology:

• Myocardial contusion

- Pericardial tamponade

- Malignant arrhythmia with cardiac arrest

- Disruption of valves and septum

- Coronary artery injury (thrombosis or laceration)

- Cardiac rupture

The first important step in the diagnostic pathway for patients with blunt cardiac injury is an awareness that such an injury might have occurred. Patients with angina-like chest pain, dyspnea, right-bundle branch block (RBBB) or other type of heart block following blunt chest trauma should be assessed for possible cardiac injury. All patients with blunt chest trauma should undergo a physical examination, CXR, 12-lead EKG and baseline cardiac enzymes. Precordial thrills or murmurs on physical exam should prompt transthoracic echocardiography. Findings on a CXR that raise suspicion of cardiac injury are mediastinal widening, hemothorax, pneumopericardium, or bony fractures. Such findings should prompt additional studies, such as a chest CT and a transthoracic echocardiogram.

Treatment depends on the nature of the injury. Myocardial contusion does not require surgery and is managed similar to an MI. Cardiac rupture or tamponade requires surgical exploration similar to penetrating trauma. For other injures, the timing of the surgery depends on the hemodynamic stability of the patient. If the injuries are well tolerated, a delayed approach is preferred. A delayed approach minimizes bleeding risk from heparinization required for CPB.

79. Thoracic trauma

Lucas M. Duvall

Trauma kills over 150,000 people per year, with one-fourth related to thoracic trauma. Thoracic trauma management is guided by ATLS protocols that allow for prioritization of injuries and provide treatment guidelines. The role of the thoracic surgeon is generally at the request of the trauma surgeon for a specific chest injury. The following is an overview of many of the common thoracic trauma issues, focusing on the chest wall, pleura, lungs and diaphragm.

Initial evaluation of the trauma patient can reveal the need for intubation, needle decompressions, and pericardiocentesis. Specific exam findings include neck veins (distended in tamponade and collapsed in hypovolemia), chest wall motion abnormalities (decreased motion due to fractures and paradoxical due to flail chest), palpation with crepitus, chest percussion (dull with hemothorax and hyperresonance with tension pneumothorax), and breath sounds (decreased in pneumothorax and hemothorax). CXR is often the most common study. FAST scanning is now routine and can help in the diagnosis of pericardial effusion and pneumothorax. CT scanning allows the most detailed imaging and is now standard of care for stable patients.

Chest wall injuries

Rib fractures are the most common thoracic injury. Nearly 40% of all trauma patients have a rib fracture. The most common finding is exquisite pain at the site of injury. One or a few unilateral rib fractures are treated with pain control to avoid splinting and hypoventilation, and good pulmonary hygiene. Pain control methods include oral and IV analgesics, intercostal nerve blocks, intrapleural catheter analgesics, and epidural analgesics. First and second rib fractures are of particular concern due to associated injuries. There is a >50% incidence of head injury and >60% incidence of other thoracic injuries associated with these fractures. Flail chest represents instability of the chest wall. It requires multiple fractures of the ribs and is related to the compliance of the chest wall. Paradoxical motion results in decreased vital capacity and ineffective ventilation. There is also a high incidence of pulmonary contusion. Standard management consists of aggressive pulmonary hygiene with effective epidural anesthesia.

Sternal fractures are not uncommon. They occur generally in a transverse manner at the upper and midportions of the sternum. Treatment is similar to rib fractures and fixation is reserved for severely displaced fragments.

Resection is mandatory for associated infections of the sternoclavicular segment. Scapular fractures are rare, associated with > 70% accompanying injuries, have a higher incidence of brachial plexus deficits and are treated mostly with immobilization followed by range-of-motion therapy. Clavicle fractures are quite common, do not generally affect ventilation, and are primarily treated with immobilization.

Pneumothorax and hemothorax

Penetrating wounds to the thorax can result in a pneumothorax and/or a hemothorax. If there is loss of a portion of the chest wall, it can result in a "sucking chest wound". This can serve as a source of a tension pneumothorax and it is temporarily treated with a three-way dressing that allows air egress but not ingress. During initial assessments, a pneumothorax may not be noted and the CXR is of vital importance. Tension pneumothorax presents with distended neck veins, absent breath sounds, deviated trachea, and respiratory distress. Tension pneumothoraces require needle decompression and then treated as most pneumothoraces in the trauma setting, with tube thoracostomy. Of note, if the lung fails to re-expand, there is a persistent air leak, or the patient sounds excessively stridorous, a tracheobronchial injury should be suspected. The site of bronchial injury will determine operative approach. The right posterolateral approach provides optimal exposure for distal tracheal and bilateral proximal bronchial injuries. An ipsilateral posterolateral thoracotomy is sufficient for more distal bronchial injury. Traumatic tracheal transections should receive a prophylactic tracheostomy during repair to protect the anastomosis.

A hemothorax is associated with penetrating trauma and blunt trauma with bony fractures. CXR is vital. Management mandates evacuation of the blood, usually via tube thoracostomy. Thoracic exploration should be undertaken if there is >1,500 mL at the time of tube insertion or >250 mL/hr for the next 4 hours. Residual hematoma should be evacuated, usually with VATS, to prevent empyema or lung entrapment.

Pulmonary and tracheobronchial injuries

Blunt trauma to the chest wall can cause pulmonary contusions and/or pulmonary hematomas. In pulmonary contusions, the entity consists of hemorrhage into the alveolar and interstitial spaces. They can occur in isolated injuries to children, owing to their chest wall compliance. Clinically significant contusions are usually present on initial CXR. Treatment centers on supporting the patient. Some advocate fluid restriction, as the capillary permeability is increased, but this should be tempered with the overall fluid status of the patient. Massive contusions can produce significant shunt fractions and hypoxemia. A double-lumen endo-tracheal tube with separate ventilation can help. Exogenous surfactants have shown promise, but are not widely used. Pulmonary hematoma is difficult to differentiate from a contusion early on, but after 24-48 hrs, it will coalesce into a discrete mass and identification can be aided by CT scan. Usually, gas exchange is not compromised and the blood is reab-sorbed over time, but secondary infection with abscess formation is a risk.

Major lacerations are infrequent. Local control methods are preferred focusing on correcting coagulopathy, stopping the bleeding, repairing and preventing air leaks, and debriding non-viable tissue. Parenchymal pre-serving, non-anatomic stapled resections are the treatment of choice.

While isolated injuries to the bronchus or pulmonary arteries can be re-paired in the trauma setting, a pulmonary vein tear frequently requires lobectomy due to the high potential for thrombosis of this anastomosis. Only 6-15% of patients with proximal parenchymal or hilar injury sur-vive. Proximal control is essential and if this cannot be done expeditious-ly, stapled pneumonectomy should be performed. This carries a >50% mortality. Air embolism can be seen on penetrating injuries to the hilum and can result in hemodynamic instability, ventricular fibrillation and seizure activity.

Most tracheobronchial injuries occur within 2.5 cm of the carina. While infrequent in blunt trauma (<10%), bronchoscopic exam is essential when there is a high index of suspicion and CT scan is equivocal. Pathophysi-ology is related to rupture of the membranous portion due to rapid in-crease in intraluminal pressure against a closed glottis, rapid deceleration, or avulsion secondary to lateral traction on the lung from crushing chest injuries.

Diaphragmatic injuries

Diaphragmatic injuries occur in about 5% of patients with thoracoab-dominal trauma. They are categorized as acute or late. Blunt diaphrag-matic injury more commonly affects the left diaphragm as it is less pro-tected by the liver mass. Herniation of organs is a concern since the dia-phragm does not spontaneously heal. The stomach, spleen, and small intestine most frequently herniate on the left. Liver and colon can herni-ate on the right. Right-sided hemidiaphragm rupture is often associated with vascular injuries to the vena cava and hepatic veins. Clinical presen-tation includes respiratory distress, bowel sounds in the chest, and trache-al deviation. Operative repair can be done by thoracoscopy, laparoscopy, thoracotomy, or laparotomy. Repair method is geared towards addressing other injuries.

Penetrating diaphragmatic injuries are usually due to gunshot or knife stab wounds. Here, the extent of the diaphragm injury is usually less, and delayed herniation more common than in the acute setting. Symptoms are rare until there is associated visceral hernia. Exploration is warranted if there is a high index of suspicion of a penetrating diaphragm injury. Herniations may even occur remotely from the traumatic injury. Often, these patients present with progressive shortness of breath and partial or complete bowel obstruction. Radiologic studies are the crux of accurate diagnosis and operative strategy planning. Most surgeons advocate a transthoracic approach for repair of chronic injuries due to the marked adhesions between the herniated viscus and the thoracic contents. If visceral strangulation is suspected, an abdominal approach would be more prudent. The most common repair strategy is direct suture closure. Occasionally, a prosthetic is necessary.

Great vessel injuries

Great vessel injuries are not uncommon. By far, the most lethal of these is an aortic injury. The descending thoracic aorta accounts for up to 40% of deaths at the scene involving blunt thoracic trauma. Site of injury is most commonly the medial aorta just distal, or right at the *ligamentum arteriosum*, followed by the aorta at the base of the innominate artery, then the base of the left subclavian, and then finally at the base of the left carotid. These represent relatively fixed attachments of the aorta. Plain CXR is a sufficient screening study. Findings include: widened mediastinum, loss of aortic knob, shift of the endotracheal tube and trachea, elevation of the left mainstem bronchus, apical capping, fracture of the 1st rib, large left-sided hemothorax, and a retrocardiac density. CT scanning of the chest has >96% sensitivity and >98% specificity for blunt injuries. If an emergent laparotomy is needed, a TEE can be performed in the operating room.

The management of these injuries has evolved tremendously in recent years. Once diagnosis is made, invasive blood pressure monitoring and strict management is required. A thorough neurologic exam is needed because these patients almost invariably have a traumatic brain injury. The more recent changes in management include: 1) nonoperative management, 2) delay to definitive treatment, 3) use of endovascular stent grafting, and 4) the use of left heart bypass. The subset of patients most likely treated nonoperatively or with delayed repair includes those with severe head injuries, extensive burns, and hemodynamic instability from other traumatic injuries.

Endovascular stenting has greatly changed the treatment of these injuries. Technical success rates exceed 96% with an endoleak rate of 5.1%. The overall mortality is 7.7%, graft-related mortality of 2%, and a paraplegia rate of 2%, vs. 14.7% mortality and 3.3% paraplegia with open repair. Open repair is via a left posterolateral thoracotomy. With obtaining proximal and distal control, injury to the vagus nerve, recurrent laryngeal nerve, and the thoracic duct needs to be avoided. Traditionally, the "clamp and sew" technique was used but increasing evidence of a decreased paraplegia rate and mortality rate is favoring a left-heart bypass technique. Several systems require very little heparinization, if any. This technique involves cannulation of the LA and the left femoral artery or descending thoracic aorta.

The subclavian vessels are the most frequently injured intrathoracic vessels in penetrating trauma. Surgical approaches include clavicular incision, clavicular incision combined with sternotomy, upper sternotomy with anterolateral thoracotomy through the 4th intercostal space ("trapdoor"), or high anterior thoracotomy. These injuries are usually repaired primarily or with an interposition graft.

Emergent and urgent thoracotomy

There are several indications for emergent or urgent thoracotomy. Often, the cause of hemodynamic instability is not known.

According to the most recent ACS Committee on Trauma report, the overall survival rate for emergency room thoracotomies was only 7.83%. Overall, emergency room thoracotomies should be reserved for patients with penetrating trauma who lose vital signs in the emergency room or in transport. Indications for emergency room thoracotomy are:

• Acute pericardial tamponade

• Exsanguinating intrathoracic hemorrhage

• Need for internal cardiac massage

Indications for urgent thoracotomy include:

• Chest tube drainage >1500 mL initial or >250 mL/hr for 4 hours

• Large unevacuated hemothorax

• Chest wall defect

• Massive air leak or incomplete lung expansion

- Great vessel injury
- Esophageal injury
- Diaphragmatic injury

80. Low cardiac output

Zain Khalpey

Low cardiac output (CO) or cardiogenic shock is defined as an inadequate distribution of blood to end-organs due to a diseased heart. This condition is common in a number of disease etiologies including sepsis, MI (ST-elevation), and CHF.

Factors affecting cardiac output

CO is defined as the amount of blood that the heart pumps out in one minute. Four specific factors determine CO:

- *Heart rate (HR)*. Positively correlated with the amount of blood circulating throughout the body. If the HR is lower than normal, blood will circulate at a slower rate and delivery of oxygen to the tissues will likely be lower than normal.

- *Contractility*. Force with which the heart contracts.

- *Preload*. Extent to which the myocardial cells distend. A patient with decreased preload may have decreased contractility.

- *Afterload*. Force that the ventricles must contract against to eject blood from the heart. Largely determined by the tone of vasculature and blood pressure in the arteries. If the resistance in blood vessels is greater than the force exerted by the ventricles, the heart will pump out less blood resulting in decreased CO.

Measurement of cardiac output

Cardiac index (CI) is the CO indexed to BSA in m^2. The measurement of CO / CI, and hence oxygenation of tissues, is of primary importance in the prognosis and treatment of a patient's condition. For example, patients who are unable to sustain a CI in excess of 2 liters/min per m^2 are more likely to die. Conversely, patients with septic shock who undergo resuscitation measures designed to restore oxygen delivery are less likely to die.

A number of methods are used to monitor CO. A commonly used invasive monitoring technique is the insertion of a PA catheter. The PA catheter is inserted into a major vein (subclavian or jugular vein) through an introducer sheath and guided into the PA through the RA and RV. During PA catheterization, a process called thermodilution is used to determine CO. A cold saline bolus is injected into the catheter to measure change in blood temperature as a function of time; this indicates the rate of blood flow. The area under the time-temperature difference curve is measured to determine the CO. A low area under the time-temperature difference curve indicates high CO.

Other methods such as continuous CO monitoring use electrical impulses to generate heat in coils. These heat signals are used to monitor change in blood temperature in the PA. CO can then be determined by measuring change in temperature over time. The direct Fick method determines CO as a measure of difference in the oxygen content of arterial versus mixed venous blood.

PA catheterization can also provide stroke work index and cardiac power, which are excellent prognostic indicators. In addition, pulmonary capillary wedge pressure (PCWP) can be measured to determine preload of the LV. In recent years PA catheter usage has fallen into disfavor as some studies have shown that it leads to poor outcomes. However, this has not been true for patients with cardiogenic shock and it is still recommended to confirm diagnosis and guide changes in therapy for severely hypotensive patients with MI.

Symptoms of low cardiac output

Clinically, a wide range of symptoms are observed in patients with low cardiac output; symptoms that depend on the degree of hypoperfusion. In cardiogenic shock, often observed in patients after an MI with LV failure, patients present with cool clammy extremities, pulmonary congestion, low to little urine output, and various degrees of altered mental status. Mortality rate is high and varies from 60-90%. Table 80-1 depicts different hypoperfusion / hypotension syndromes.

Treatment

Non-pharmacological
Treatment of low cardiac output due to ventricular infarction is generally supportive with judicious use of fluids for resuscitation, revascularization (CABG, stenting) and mechanical support with IABP and LV support devices.

Pharmacological
Impaired contractility is the fundamental defect in low cardiac output syndrome. Positive inotropes are therefore indicated. Table 80-2 lists the most commonly used vasoactive and inotropic drugs used in low cardiac output syndrome. Catecholamines such as dobutamine, dopamine, and epinephrine stimulate β_1-adrenergic receptors, leading to calcium-

mediated binding of the actin-myosin mechanism with troponin C in cardiac cells, resulting in increased contractility of the cardiac muscle. Norepinephrine (NE), another catecholamine that acts as a β_1 agonist, also increases calcium permeability to enhance aortic contractility. NE is recommended for hypotension by the AHA and ACC because of its potency. Levosimendan, a relatively new inotropic class of drugs known as calcium sensitizers, improves contractility of the heart muscle by increasing sensitivity of calcium to troponin.

Table 80-1. Low cardiac output / hypoperfusion states *(Adapted with permission from Khalpey Z, Ganim GR, Rawn JR. Postoperative care of cardiac surgery patients. In: Cohn LH (ed). Cardiac Surgery in the Adult. 3th edition. New York: McGraw-Hill, 2008: 465-486. Copyright The McGraw-Hill Companies, Inc.).*

MAP	CVP	CO	PCWP	SVR	Strategy
Normotensive	↑	↓	↑	N/↑	Venodilator / diuretic / inotrope
Hypertension	↑	N	↑	↑	Vasodilator
Hypotension	↓	↓	↓	N	Volume
Hypotension	↑	↓	↑	↑	Inotrope / IABP / vasodilator
Hypotension	N/↓	N/↑	N/↓	↓	α-agent

CO: Cardiac output, CVP: Central venous pressure, MAP: Mean arterial pressure, N: Normal, PCWP: Pulmonary capillary wedge pressure, SVR: Systemic vascular resistance

Pressor agents are often used with positive inotropes for greater improvement of symptoms. For example, catecholamines also act on the α_1-adrenergic receptors in arterial muscle cells and cause the cells to contract, resulting in increased vascular resistance. Thus, catecholamines exhibit both inotropic and pressor effects by increasing contractility of cardiac muscle as well as increasing afterload.

Phosphodiesterase inhibitors act on phosphodiesterase, an intercellular enzyme associated with sarcoplasmic reticulum of cardiac cells to mitigate preload and afterload. Vasopressin stimulates V_{1a} receptors in vascular smooth muscle, which results in vasoconstriction. Vasopressin also mediates fluid reabsorption by stimulating V_2 receptors in the renal collecting duct system. Based on the level of stimulation, the renal collecting ducts can become either more permeable or less permeable to fluid.

Positive inotropes have been found useful in treating conditions associated with low cardiac output. However, these agents increase energy demand and oxygen consumption in an already poorly perfused organ. High doses of positive inotropes are associated with poor outcomes due to drug toxicity and to the more serious underlying disease state of the patient. Therefore, they should be used with caution in the lowest possible doses. The use of pressor agents is guided by hemodynamic data obtained from the PA catheter.

Table 80-2. Vasoactive and inotropic drugs *(Adapted with permission from Khalpey Z, Ganim GR, Rawn JR. Postoperative care of cardiac surgery patients. In: Cohn LH (ed). Cardiac Surgery in the Adult. 3rd edition. New York: McGraw-Hill, 2008: 465-486. Copyright The McGraw-Hill Companies, Inc.).*

Pharmacologic agent	HR	PCWP	CO	SVR	MAP	MVO₂
Inotropic agents						
Dobutamine	↑↑	↓	↑	↓	↑↓	↑↔
Milrinone	↑	↓	↑	↓↓	↓	↑↓
Mixed vasoactive agents						
Epinephrine	↑↑	↑↓	↑	↑	↑	↑
Norepinephrine	↑↑	↑↑	↑	↑↑	↑↑	↑
Dopamine	↑↑	↑↓	↑	↑↓	↑↓	↑
Vasopressor agents						
Phenylephrine	↔	↑	↔	↑↑	↑↑	↑↔
Vasopressin	↔	↔	↔	↑↑	↑↑	↑↔
Methylene blue	↔	↔	↔	↑	↑	↑
Vasodilating agents						
Nitroglycerin	↑	↓↔	↔	↓	↓	↓↔
Nitroprusside	↑↑	↓↔	↔	↓↓	↓↓	↓↔
Nicardipine	↔	↔	↔	↓↓	↓↓	↔
Nesiritide	↔	↓↔	↔	↓	↓	↔

CO: Cardiac output, HR: Heart rate, MAP: Mean arterial pressure, MVO₂: Mixed venous oxygen saturation, PCWP: Pulmonary capillary wedge pressure, SVR: Systemic vascular resistance.

81. Pulmonary failure

Samuel J. Youssef

Pulmonary failure may occur secondary to dysfunction in ventilation, intrapulmonary gas exchange, gas transport, or tissue gas exchange. It may occur independent of cardiac performance. Mechanical ventilatory strategies have been shown to improve *intrapulmonary* gas exchange. When pulmonary failure is refractory to these maneuvers, techniques for *extrapulmonary* gas exchange are required as seen in ECMO and PECLA.

Assessment of minute ventilation provides critical insight into the adequacy of the mechanical ventilation. Minute ventilation, or CO_2 removal, is a function of the respiratory rate and the tidal volume. Thus, blood gas parameters measuring CO_2 removal ($PaCO_2$ and pH) are the best determinants of adequate rate and tidal volumes.

The spectrum of pulmonary failure represents a hormonal, parenchymal, and bronchial response to either a primary pulmonary insult or secondary to systemic disease. The phases of injury include *edema* with an increase in lung water and decreased compliance, *proliferation* with an increase cellular response to injury with macrophage and neutrophil migration, and *fibrosis*, which is late and usually irreversible.

Refractory hypoxemia occurs when fluid or cellular infiltrates cause alveolar flooding or collapse. There is peribronchial edema, V/Q mismatching, and microatelectasis. The alveolar-capillary membrane is injured either at the alveolar (smoke inhalation, aspiration) or the blood membrane site (sepsis, fat embolism). An increase in membrane permeability results in protein-rich fluid accumulating in the interstitial and alveolar spaces. Such fluids inhibit surfactant, contributing to widespread microatelectasis. The fluid filled alveoli do not open and do not participate in gas exchange. There is a heterogeneous distribution of alveoli with various degrees of compliance. In later stages, increased PVR and pulmonary hypertension occur.

ARDS is the most severe form of acute lung injury (ALI). Both represent noncardiogenic pulmonary failure characterized by acute onset of symptoms, the presence of bilateral infiltrates, and pulmonary capillary wedge pressure <18 mmHg. The degree of hypoxemia is what distinguishes ALI (PaO_2/FiO_2 <300) from ARDS (PaO_2/FiO_2 <200). The PaO_2/FiO_2 ratio is a reflection of the shunt fraction through the lung and is a barometer of gas exchange. With a ratio <300 as in ALI, there is increased mortality, and in ARDS with ratios <200, there is a predicted mortality of 40-

50%. This high mortality is caused by multiple organ failure, sepsis, stroke, MI, and progressive pulmonary failure.

The focus of treatment strategies is to prevent fibrosis by decreasing the edema and proliferative phases while supporting gas exchange in injured alveoli. Conventional volume-cycled mechanical ventilation can result in alveolar injury due to barotrauma and volutrauma. As such, lung protective ventilation uses a pressure/volume ventilatory management where the goal is to maintain the opening pressures of the alveoli while not exceeding the distension/barotrauma tolerated by the alveolus to achieve gas exchange.

Initial management of ARDS includes:

- *Mechanical ventilation* using the least FiO_2 necessary (goal <60), low tidal volume settings (6-8 ml/kg) with peak inspiratory pressure (PIP) <35 cmH_2O, the use of PEEP between 8-14 cmH_2O to aid oxygenation, fluid restriction, and diuresis

- *Cardiovascular support* with a goal oxygen delivery/consumption >2:1, Hb above 10 mg/dL, and inotrope support

- *Nutrition support* with adequate nitrogen balance and preference for enteral feeding

If the above initial measures fail, further maneuvers include permissive hypercapnea (not excessive), diuresis, prone positioning, late steroids, and extrapulmonary gas exchange with ECMO (standard in children) or PECLA. Some other ventilatory adjuncts that have been used include inverse ratio, high frequency, partial liquid, or intratracheal pulmonary ventilation.

ECMO is the standard treatment of respiratory failure in newborn and pediatric patients who fail conventional therapy. The survival rate is 88% for neonates and 71% in pediatric patients. Based on the experience in children, protocols were established for the management of adults with "severe" ARDS. These patients are characterized by profound hypoxemia (PaO_2/FiO_2 ratio <100 and/or alveolar-arterial oxygen difference (A-a DO_2) >600 mmHg) despite optimal mechanical ventilatory treatment. They have a greater than 80% predicted mortality, and thus require extracorporeal life support measures.

ECMO involves placing a veno-venous (VV) or veno-arterial (VA) life support pump circuit with a membrane oxygenator to temporarily take over the oxygenation and CO_2 removal functions of the lung. VV is the preferred mode of support for isolated respiratory failure. VA access is used when systemic arterial perfusion support is necessary in addition to ventilatory support. The algorithm for ECMO involves maintaining blood flow to meet the goal of SaO_2 >85% (VV) or >90% (VA). Standard heparin is administered to achieve an ACT 160-180 seconds. The ventilator is reduced to "rest" settings with FiO_2 0.3-0.5, rate 6-10, PIP 30 cm, PEEP 10, and inspiratory to expiratory ratio >2:1. High-dose steroids may be given in cases that show no improvement in lung function after 7 days.

Patients are weaned from ECMO when they become hemodynamically stable, clear the sepsis, and have adequate oxygenation at FiO_2 of 0.5 or less. After weaning, patients are maintained on mechanical ventilation until extubation criteria are met.

Results after application of ECMO to severe ARDS patients show decannulation in 67% of patients with 52% survival. ECMO in adult ARDS has not been widely adopted due to specialization in particular centers, misperception of cost, concerns of heparinization, hemolysis and coagulopathy, technical complications, and inexperience.

PECLA is a pumpless extracorporeal lung assist device that uses the blood pressure gradient between arterial and venous circulation as the driving force for blood passing through a low flow resistance oxygenator. It provides gas exchange, but relies on cardiac output for flow. The diffusion membrane has a surface area of 1.3 m^2 to which an oxygen flow of 1-12 L can be administered. The tubing system is coated with high molecular weight heparin and blood maintained with a goal ACT of 130-150 seconds. The arterial cannula is sized from 15-19 Fr based on US measurement of the femoral vessels, and is placed using Seldinger technique; the venous from 17-19 Fr.

Indications for PECLA are similar to ECMO. However, mandatory evaluation of the hemodynamic status of the patient involves placement of a Swan-Ganz catheter or echocardiography. As the PECLA is a pumpless device, a cardiac index >3 L/min/m^2 and a MAP >70 mmHg is necessary because an arteriovenous shunt volume of 1.0-2.5 L/min must be tolerated. Hence, catecholamine support may be required. If this cannot be achieved, a pump-driven device should be used instead.

PECLA therapy is terminated when PaO_2 is greater than 80 mmHg and FiO_2 is less than 0.45 for more than 24 hours. Mean support interval has been reported to be between 7-15 days with significant improvement in oxygenation, reduction in catecholamine demand, improved MAP, decreased serum lactate, and decrease in inflammatory mediators. Elimination of CO_2 improves the ventilation/perfusion matching and has a significant impact on the outcomes of ARDS patients. Survival for all-comers in the largest center was 35%. The design of the unit allows for easier nursing care and facilitates transportation.

82. Postoperative care and perioperative complications

Ramesh Singh, Ashok Babu

Hemodynamic assessment

The principle focus on postoperative care is the assessment and optimization of hemodynamics. This is aided by knowing the patient's comorbidities, preoperative cardiac function, and intraoperative events. The goal is the maintenance of adequate oxygen delivery to vital tissues thus avoiding unnecessary demands on a heart recovering from CPB, ischemia, and surgery. Cardiac output is determined by 3 factors: preload, afterload and contractility.

Preload

For the pump to function adequately, it has to be filled and stretched (no stretch - no contractility). At the most basic level, this is the cellular tension applied. Unfortunately, this cannot be measured in a feasible manner. Hence, markers at the end of filling (end diastole) are used instead. These are (in order of reliability): LV end-diastolic volume (LVEDV), LV end-diastolic pressure (LVEDP), pulmonary capillary wedge pressure (PCWP), PA diastolic pressure (PAD), and CVP.

Right heart filling pressure (CVP) is an unreliable indicator of LVEDV. It can be erroneous in many situations including right heart failure, tricuspid regurgitation, MR, pulmonary hypertension, cardiac tamponade, tension pneumothorax, and pulmonary embolism. Left heart filling pressures (PCWP, PAD) are more accurate in estimating LVEDV provided there is normal PVR. Hence, determining optimal filling pressures is generally empirical. Preload can be manipulated with fluids. It is unclear if colloids are better than crystalloids in cardiac surgery.

Afterload

The afterload is the pressure that has to be overcome for ejection of blood out of the LV (pressure to open the aortic valve). It is dependent on multiple factors including volume status, vascular tone (autonomic nervous system), and atherosclerotic burden. The SVR after CPB can be low due to the systemic inflammatory response that commonly follows CPB. Changes in the peripheral vascular tone stem from the rewarming process and can cause labile hemodynamics. Anesthetic agents and pre-operative ACE inhibitors or ARBs can also contribute to the labile hemodynamics. The afterload can also be high after CPB in the setting of inadequate rewarming, incorrect use of vasopressors, increased sympathetic output caused by pain and anxiety, as well as hypovolemia and pump failure. Afterload is manipulated with vasopressors and vasodilators.

Vasopressors are used in vasodilated patients with normal pump function and unresponsive to volume. Alpha agents (phenylephrine), vasopressin, and methylene blue (for vasopressor-resistant hypotension) can be used in this scenario but caution is advised as peripheral ischemia and vasospasm of native coronary arteries and arterial conduits can develop. Hence, careful EKG and extremity perfusion monitoring is required.

Vasodilators can be used for hypertension or in a normotensive patient with poor pump function. Nitroglycerin and nitroprusside are short acting agents and are easy to titrate. However, hypoxia can develop as they inhibit PA hypoxic vasoconstriction thus increasing blood flow through poorly oxygenated lungs. Nitroglycerin is a stronger venodilator than arterial dilator. It increases intercoronary collateral blood flow but is tachyphylactic. Prolonged use of nitroprusside can lead to cyanide toxicity and methemoglobin levels need to be monitored. If cyanide toxicity is suspected, nitroprusside should be stopped and if severe, medications such as amyl nitrite, sodium nitrite, and sodium thiosulfate (Taylor Cyanide Antidote Package) should be administered. Nicardipine is a calcium-channel blocker with minimal effects on contractility and atrioventricular nodal conduction. It has the efficacy of nitroprusside but without its toxicity. Hypertension can also be treated with beta-blockers but these medications should not be used in patients whose heart function is inotrope dependent.

Contractility
Contractility is difficult to measure since cardiac output, although a useful marker, is dependent also on preload, afterload, and heart rate. Cardiac contractility is manipulated with inotropic agents when the cardiac output is low despite optimized preload and afterload. Dobutamine (β-adrenergic) and milrinone (phosphodiesterase inhibitor) increase myocardial contractility and reduce afterload through peripheral vasodilation. They are arrhythmogenic and can exacerbate coronary ischemia. Epinephrine and norepinephrine have both β- and α- adrenergic agonist effects. They are vasopressors in addition to positive inotropes. Dopamine in low doses also increases cardiac output and causes splanchnic and renal vasodilation.

When required, there are other more invasive methods to help improve perfusion. These include IABP, ECMO, and VADs.

Some important hemodynamic parameters, formulas, and normal ranges can be found in Table 82-1.

Oxygen delivery

The content of arterial oxygen (CaO_2) is determined by the amount of oxygen bound to hemoglobin (hemoglobin saturation, SaO_2) and to a much lesser extent by the amount of oxygen dissolved in the arterial blood (PaO_2). Therefore, increasing the amount of hemoglobin improves CaO_2 much more than increasing PaO_2. Oxygen delivery (DO_2) is the rate at which oxygen is transported to the tissues. It is related to cardiac output and CaO_2 and can therefore decrease in low-cardiac output states or in cases of decreased CaO_2 (e.g., anemia, poor oxygenation).

Oxygen delivery to the tissues is also related to the oxyhemoglobin dissociation curve. This curve plots the relationship between PaO_2 and SaO_2. In general, due to the sigmoidal form of the curve, PaO_2 levels higher than 60 mmHg cause small changes in SaO_2. However, at PaO_2 levels below 60 mmHg, small drops in PaO_2 translate into precipitous decreases in SaO_2. Conditions such as high levels of CO_2, lower pH, higher temperatures, and higher levels of 2,3-diphosphoglycerate (2,3-DPG) produced as a consequence of higher tissue oxygen demands make the curve shift to the right, improving oxygen delivery to the tissues (given a constant PaO_2, SaO_2 will be lower as the oxygen is released more avidly). On the contrary, hypothermia, alkalosis, and decreased levels of 2,3-DPG will shift the curve to the left, indicating more avid binding of oxygen by hemoglobin with less release of oxygen to the tissues.

Oxygen consumption (VO_2) is the rate at which oxygen is removed from the arterial blood by the tissues and can be calculated from the cardiac output and the arterial and venous concentrations of blood.

Stroke after CPB

CABG may be the single largest iatrogenic cause of strokes. The incidence of stroke after cardiac surgery is reported to be about 3-10%. Risk factors include postoperative atrial fibrillation, age > 75, female sex, DM, hypertension, carotid artery stenosis, CHF, recent MI, previous stroke, chronic renal failure, EF < 35%, unstable angina, and emergent CABG. The ROOBY trial did not show a significant difference between off-pump and on-pump CABGs in terms of incidence of stroke. There are significant implications of stroke including increased length of hospital and ICU stay, increased mortality by a factor of 5 (14.4% vs. 2.7%), cardiovascular, pulmonary, and renal complications, as well as higher hospital charges.

Table 82-1. Important hemodynamic parameters, formulas, and normal values.

Parameter	Formula	Normal values
SBP		90 – 140 mmHg
DBP		60 – 90 mmHg
MAP	(SBP + (2 x DBP)) / 3	60 – 90 mmHg
PASP		15 – 25 mmHg
PADP		8 – 15 mmHg
MPAP	(PASP + (2 x PADP)) / 3	10 – 20 mmHg
LAP		6 – 12 mmHg
PCWP		6 – 12 mmHg
CVP		1 – 6 mmHg
RAP		5 – 15 mmHg
CO	SV x HR	4 – 8 L/min
CI	CO / BSA	2.4 – 4.2 L/min/m^2
SVR	80 x (MAP – CVP) / CO	800 – 1200 dynes sec/cm^5
SVRI	SVR / BSA	1600 – 2400 dynes sec/cm^5 m^2
PVR	80 x (MPAP – PCWP) / CO	50 – 250 dynes sec/cm^5
PVRI	PVR / BSA	200 – 400 dynes sec/cm^5 m^2
SV	EDV – ESV	60 – 100 mL/beat
SVI	CI / HR	40 – 70 mL/beat/m^2
LVSWI	SVI x (MAP – PCWP) x 0.0136	40 – 60 g m/m^2
EF	(EDV – ESV) / EDV	60 – 70%
EDV	SV / EF	80 – 150 mL/m^2
ESV	EDV – SV	50 – 100 mL
RVSWI	SVI x (MPAP – RAP) x 0.0136	4 – 8 g m/m^2
SvO$_2$		70 – 75%
CaO$_2$	(1.34 x Hb x SaO$_2$) + (0.0031 x PaO$_2$)	20 mL / dL
DO$_2$	CI x 13.4 x Hb x SaO$_2$	900 – 1100 mL/min
VO$_2$	VO$_2$ = CI x 13.4 x Hb x (SaO$_2$ – SvO$_2$)	200 – 270 mL/min

BSA: Body surface area, CI: Cardiac index, CO: Cardiac output, CVP: Central venous pressure, DBP: Diastolic blood pressure, DO$_2$:Oyxgen delivery, EDV: End-diastolic volume, EF: Ejection fraction, ESV: End-systolic volume, Hb: Hemoglobin concentration, HR: Heart rate, LAP: Left atrial pressure, LVSWI: Left ventricular stroke work index, MAP: Mean arterial pressure, MPAP: Mean pulmonary arterial pressure, PADP: Pulmonary arterial diastolic pressure, PASP: Pulmonary arterial systolic pressure, PCWP: Pulmonary capillary wedge pressure, PVR: Pulmonary vascular resistance, PVRI: Pulmonary vascular resistance index, RAP: Right atrial pressure, RVSWI: Right ventricular stroke work index, SaO$_2$: Oxygen saturation, SBP: Systolic blood pressure, SV: Stroke volume, SVI: Stroke volume index, SvO$_2$: Mixed venous oxygen saturation, SVR: Systemic vascular resistance, SVRI: Systemic vascular resistance index, VO$_2$: Oxygen consumption.

Deep sternal wound infection (mediastinitis)

Mediastinitis complicates 1-2% of all heart surgeries. It is a serious and still prevalent complication that carries a 30% mortality rate. Risk factors include use of bilateral internal mammary grafts in diabetics, emergency surgery, cardiopulmonary resuscitation (CPR), obesity (>20% ideal body weight), postoperative shock (especially with multiple blood transfusions), prolonged CPB and operating room times, reoperation, re-exploration following initial surgery, sternal wound dehiscence, and surgical technical factors (e.g., excessive use of electrocautery, bone wax, paramedian sternotomy). Three main different types of postoperative mediastinitis can be distinguished:

- Associated with obesity, COPD, and sternal dehiscence, typically caused by coagulase-negative Staphylococci

- Following perioperative contamination of the mediastinal space, often caused by *S. aureus*

- Spread from concomitant infections in other sites during the postoperative period, often caused by Gram-negative rods

Adequate debridement and sterilization during the first reoperation is required. Options for closure are immediate rewiring after sternal debridement, delayed closure with the use of vacuum-assisted closure devices, and multiple debridements followed by muscle flap closure.

Arrhythmias

Supraventricular and ventricular arrhythmias occur commonly after cardiac surgery. Risk factors include advanced age, preoperative history of arrhythmias, CHF, duration of CPB, bicaval cannulation, COPD, discontinuation of preoperative β-blockers, and electrolyte disturbances. Atrial fibrillation is the most common arrhythmia after cardiac surgery and occurs in 20-50% of cases. Its peak incidence is during postoperative days 2 and 3. Arrhythmias associated with hemodynamic instability should be treated with cardioversion or defibrillation. Stable patients may be treated with β-blockers or calcium channel blockers. However, amiodarone may be the drug of choice, especially among patients with reduced LV function. The use of prophylactic antiarrhythmics in cardiac surgery is controversial.

Other complications

Other important complications after cardiac surgery include:

- *Renal failure.* Acute renal failure requiring dialysis occurs in 1-4% of cardiac surgery patients. Preoperative renal dysfunction is the most important risk factor. Other risk factors include valve surgery, reduced LV function, COPD, vascular disease, and use of IABP.

Urine electrolytes are useful to determine the cause of renal dysfunction. Acute tubular necrosis is characterized by urinary sodium concentration > 40 mEq/L and a fractional excretion of sodium (FENa) > 2%. On the contrary, hypovolemia (pre-renal state) is associated with urinary sodium < 20 mEq/L and a FENa < 1%.

- *Hyperglycemia.* The stress response after cardiac surgery can cause hyperglycemia, especially among patients with prior history of DM. Tight blood glucose control is associated with a decreased risk of sternal wound infections. The specific glycemia level to achieve postoperatively is controversial but ranges between 110 and 140 mg/dL.

- *Postoperative bleeding.* Coagulopathy is common after CPB due to decreased platelet numbers and function, preoperative use of antiplatelet and anticoagulant medications, hypothermia, persistence of a fibrinolytic state (associated with duration of CPB). In the presence of bleeding, platelets and blood factors should be replaced as needed. Bleeding at a rate of 400 mL/h for one hour, 300 mL/h for 2-3 hours, or 200 mL/h for 4 hours warrants consideration for re-exploration.

- *Heparin-induced thrombocytopenia (HIT).* HIT is a syndrome characterized by a decrease in platelet counts after administration of heparin. HIT type I is a non-immune transitory thrombocytopenia of minimal clinical significance. HIT type II is an immune-mediated disorder due to antibodies against the heparin-platelet factor 4 complex and is characterized by thrombocytopenia and platelet-rich arterial thrombosis (white clot). Platelet antibodies may form in up to 15-20% of cardiac surgery patients although the incidence of the HIT syndrome is much lower. HIT should be differentiated from the common thrombocytopenia seen in 50% of patients during the first 2-3 days after CPB. The serotonin release assay is the gold standard for diagnosis of HIT. The first treatment for HIT is cessation of all heparin-related products including heparin flushes and low-molecular weight heparin (it can cross-react with the antibodies). The use of direct thrombin inhibitors (e.g. lepirudin, bivalirudin, argatroban, fondaparinux) followed by warfarin anticoagulation is recommended.

83. Pediatric cardiac intensive care

Daniel J. DiBardino

There are dramatic differences in the cardiac intensive care of the postoperative pediatric patient in comparison to the adult. One complicating factor in the care of congenital heart patients is extreme variation in the range of normal and expected vital sign values with physiology, age and size. Table 83-1 summarizes age-adjusted blood pressure and heart rate data. One common rule is that smaller animals generally generate (and tolerate) lower blood pressures and have higher baseline heart rates than larger counterparts. Neonates and small infants have less reserve in terms of stroke volume and therefore require higher heart rates to increase cardiac output in times where such is required. This also implies the significance of normal sinus rhythm; loss of atrioventricular (AV) synchrony is not well tolerated in babies and small children.

Table 83-1. Vital signs by age *(Adapted with permission from Mathers LH, Frankel LR. Pediatric emergencies and resuscitation. In: Kliegman RM, Behrman RE, Jenson HB, et al (eds). Nelson Textbook of Pediatrics. 18th edition. Philadelphia: Saunders, 2007: 389. Copyright Elsevier).*

Age	HR (bpm)	BP (mmHg)	RR (breaths/min)
Premature	120-170	55-75/35-45	40-70
0-3 mo	100-150	65-85/45-55	35-55
3-6 mo	90-120	70-90/50-65	30-45
6-12 mo	80-120	80-100/55-65	25-40
1-3 yr	70-110	90-105/55-70	20-30
3-6 yr	65-110	95-110/60-75	20-25
6-12 yr	60-95	100-120/60-75	14-22
> 12 yr	55-85	110-135/65-85	12-18

BP: Blood pressure, bpm: Beats per minute, HR: Heart rate, RR: Respiratory rate.

Tubes, lines and monitoring

The majority of postoperative pediatric cardiac patients, and certainly all neonates and complex infant cases, will return via direct transfer to the ICU and remain intubated on arrival, on sedation and inotropic medication and with an assortment of monitoring tools and drainage catheters. Monitoring, in particular, tends to be more elaborate than in adult cardiac surgery.

Many units utilize real-time in-line end-tidal CO_2 (ETCO$_2$) monitoring, which is a rapid and sensitive initial screening tool for the adequacy of CO_2 exchange. Aside from identifying ventilator circuit issues such as mucus plugging, circuit malfunction or disconnection, sudden decreases in pulmonary blood flow cause immediate and dramatic decreases in

$ETCO_2$. The latter would be the case in a situation such as shunt thrombosis in a shunt dependent pulmonary circulation. In the absence of
complications, the $PaCO_2$ to $ETCO_2$ difference should be < 5-10 mmHg.
Peripheral transcutaneous SaO_2 monitoring (pulse oximetry) is often tak-
en for granted as accurate in adults, who are expected to saturate > 90-
95% in the absence of extreme pathology such as pulmonary embolism or
ARDS. An important limitation in this technology is the increasing inac-
curacy at lower PaO_2 levels and saturations. This is particularly important in pediatric cardiac surgery where many children are expected to
saturate well below adult norms (Table 83-2). As such, corroborative
ABG data is essential. It is also imperative that each patient's residual
anatomy and echocardiogram results be taken into consideration when
interpreting pulse oximetry data. The persistence of a PFO in the face of
RV dysfunction, RV non-compliance, or elements of anatomic RVOT
obstruction would allow obligate right-to-left shunting and desaturation in
the postoperative period. A common example of this would be a neonatal
tetralogy of Fallot (TOF) repair patient with a persistent PFO saturating
80-85% on the first postoperative night.

Table 83-2. Expected oxygen saturation values following various stages
of single ventricle palliation.

Operation	Typical age	Saturation
Norwood Stage I	Neonate	75%
Shunt for ductal-dependent pulmonary blood flow (TOF/PA)	Neonate	75%
Bidirectional Glenn or hemi-Fontan	2-6 months	80-85%
Fontan completion	2-4 years	95% (variable, based on size of fenestration)

TOF/PA: Tetralogy of Fallot/pulmonary atresia

Central access can be difficult to obtain in pediatric cardiac surgery as
size and the redo status of many patients are important constraints. Cut-
down attempts at the groin and wrist are relatively common for arterial
access and must be carefully protected in the ICU. A useful neonatal
option is the placement of an umbilical artery catheter (UAC) and/or venous catheter shortly after birth. These can be used for operative and
postoperative management as long as the team is aware of the limitations.
During coarctation repair, for example, only a post-isthmus value would
be available from a UAC.

The strategic use of intracardiac lines and percutaneous venous access is
a complicated subject with much inter-institutional variation. Many centers avoid internal jugular or subclavian access in patients eventually requiring Glenn or Fontan circulations. On the contrary, patients with TOF

and PA atresia who will require multiple future groin catheter access attempts and PA rehabilitation should preferably have the femoral vessels spared if possible. It is commonplace at some major centers to infuse low-dose heparin through neonatal and infant central lines in the hopes of avoiding clot formation. Swan-Ganz catheters are not used in the care of pediatric cardiac patients in favor of intra-cardiac lines, which are left directly in the relevant cardiac chambers and brought out the subcostal skin at the time of operation.

While convenient and accurate during the immediate postoperative period, the management of such lines is complicated by removal protocols. If the chest is closed at the index operation, the removal should be done in the monitored ICU setting. Platelets and coagulation studies should be normalized as much as possible prior to removal. It is desirable to remove intracardiac lines prior to extubation if possible, as a Valsalva during removal could theoretically result in air entrapment and embolism.

Unlike in adults who are commonly complicated by baseline renal dysfunction and diuretic dependence, hourly urine output (UOP) is considered a sensitive and accurate indicator of the accuracy of cardiac output in the child. This is especially true in neonates and UOP should exceed 1 cc/kg/hr after the first few postoperative hours. The stomach should be routinely decompressed with a NGT. Mediastinal and pleural chest tubes should be frequently stripped and/or cleared with 8 or 10 French suction catheters as needed to maintain patency, particularly if bleeding or a pneumothorax is an issue. Atrial and ventricular pacing wires should be labeled and accessible for use in an emergency. A pacemaker box and a backup battery should be immediately accessible if not already connected to the patient.

Common issues in postoperative care: sedation, ventilation and cardiac output

Sedation and analgesia are related aspects of ICU care, which have an intimately close association with ventilation and cardiopulmonary performance. Regardless of the specific medication infusions chosen, the common goal should be to choose and enforce a "sedation goal," which is appropriate for the child's current physiologic state. This goal is re-addressed on daily rounds and more frequently if needed as the condition changes.

A common ventilation strategy for postoperative pediatric cardiac patients is pressure control mode. Synchronized intermittent mandatory ventilation (SIMV) with pressure control triggering allows the peak inspiratory pressure (PIP) and positive end expiratory pressure (PEEP) to be set at given levels resulting in inspiratory volumes dependent on the pulmonary compliance during the mandatory number of set breaths (set "rate), along with a pressure support (PS) for additional patient initiated breaths. Common initial PIPs are in the 20 mmHg range with a PEEP of 5 and PS of 10 mm Hg and will commonly result in the appropriate tidal volumes of 8-10 cc/kg. Further adjustments are made based on ABG data. Rate setting should vary from 8-10 in larger children to 20-24 in newborns and adjusted as needed for minute ventilation. Although it is common to transport on 100% FiO_2, this should be adjusted in a lesion-dependent fashion and should, in general, be weaned as quickly as possible. Typical weaning in the uncomplicated patient is coordinated with lighter sedation and is commonly done via weaning the SIMV rate in pressure control mode or by the use of 30-minute pressure support "sprints" to assess the adequacy of the breathing mechanism. A final sprint ABG is obtained and the patient is usually extubated after 3 successive sprints, generally 8 hours apart or more frequently. Prior to extubation, lack of a cuff leak or prior failed extubation or other reason for airway inflammation and/or edema should prompt the use of dexamethasone, usually given in 3 doses starting 12-24 hours prior to target discontinuation of mechanical ventilation.

While postoperative pulmonary dysfunction in adults is commonly related to the overwhelming incidence of COPD/emphysema, it is much more commonly the case that otherwise healthy children will acquire pulmonary dysfunction related directly to the cardiac lesion (over-circulation with a left-to-right shunt) or its repair. The latter can include mechanical or technical issues that arise during or immediately after attempted repair or palliation while pulmonary and chest wall edema are common sequelae of all repairs utilizing CPB. Pleural effusions and pneumothoraces are notoriously poorly tolerated in the single ventricle patient and in neonates in general, requiring aggressive pigtail catheter or chest tube placement. Phrenic and recurrent laryngeal nerve dysfunction, obstruction of small endotracheal tubes, atelectasis, pulmonary venous obstruction and recurrent or residual significant left-to-right shunting (elevated Qp:Qs) with or without pulmonary hypertension) are other common causes of failure to wean. Residual VSD after TOF repair is a particularly poorly tolerated form of overcirculation, as preoperative RVOT obstruction results in a pulmonary bed that is not prepared for the resulting elevated Qp:Qs. The incidence of tracheostomy in pediatric patients is somewhat center dependent but in general much lower than in the adult ICU/trauma population.

Evidence of technical or mechanical issues in the postoperative period can be gleaned from saturation, pressure, and waveform tracing data.

Normal RA saturation is between 75-80%, but obviously depends on the presence of mixing, O_2 extraction, and pulmonary function. Increased RA saturation occurs commonly due to residual left-to-right shunting; it is commonly quoted that a 10% "step-up" from RA to PA should draw consideration to significant residual ventricular level shunting. Decreased LA saturation most commonly occurs with right-to-left shunting or pulmonary venous desaturation as would occur with effusion, edema, ARDS or other pulmonary parenchymal process such as pneumonia. The PA is the most accurate site to obtain a true mixed venous value since it reflects all mixing at the atrial and ventricular level. It is commonly taught that PA saturation > 80% on 50% FiO_2 is an independent predictor of significant residual VSD after TOF repair and is associated with a Qp:Qs > 1.5.

The PAP is slightly elevated after CPB but should generally be < 25mmHg in the absence of known preoperative pulmonary hypertension. PAP < 50% systemic pressure is desirable and in general anything higher should cause concern and evaluation. Post-cardiotomy RA and LA pressures are generally 6-8 mm Hg with LA pressure expected to be 1-2 mm Hg higher. The nature of the waveform also carries significant information. New onset or persistent v waves on LA pressure tracing may signify residual regurgitation after canal repair or other type of mitral valve repair. Often the LA pressure tracing may be the first obvious evidence of the loss of AV synchrony, such as junctional rhythm or with ventricular pacing. Echocardiogram and catheterization should be used liberally as needed in order to evaluate the postoperative patient who deviates from the anticipated course.

While searching for post-repair error in the form of mechanical and technical issues in cases of unexpected outcome, concomitant attention should be focused on modifying cardiac output and performance in terms of rate/rhythm, preload conditions, afterload conditions and contractility. Infant stroke volume is generally fixed so that manipulation of heart rate is often necessary to significantly alter cardiac output. Dopamine, dobutamine and isoproterenol are all used in part for chronotropic effects while AV sequential pacing in certain cases of arrhythmia (slow junctional, sinus bradycardia, heart block) has the added benefit of restoring synchrony. If the latter persists as symptomatic arrhythmia and requires persistent pacing, permanent pacemaker implantation should be considered after 7-10 days. Epicardial pacemakers require at least partial redosternotomy but are preferred in neonates and infants as transvenous systems are not generally able to be implanted in patients < 10-15 kg.

Preload conditions vary widely in the perioperative period as a consequence of bleeding, diuresis, insufficient or overaggressive replacement of losses, or conditions like tamponade. Normal circulating blood volume becomes proportionately less volume per kg weight with increasing patient weight; 95 cc/kg in the neonate and 75 cc/kg in the adult, with intermediate size patients being somewhere in between. Volume replacement choices must take into consideration the source of the loss. Most major centers maintain single ventricle patients above hematocrit values of 40% while other complex neonates and infants are maintained above 30-35%. Pack red blood cell transfusions are given in 10-15 cc/kg aliquots and irradiated products are used in suspected DiGeorge syndrome and certain transplant situations. Crystalloid and albumin boluses are given between 10-20 cc/kg in addition to provision of maintenance fluids. Responses are monitored based on the Frank-Starling curve. In general, little gain in output is derived from maintaining filling pressures > 15 mmHg while LA pressure > 20 mmHg is associated with pulmonary edema.

Afterload is taken to include PVR and SVR and aberrancy includes conditions like pulmonary hypertension crises and systemic vasoconstriction and vasodilation. Increases in PVR and SVR reduce stroke volume (and thus cardiac output) and can cause ventricular dysfunction. Any operation involving outflow tract obstruction could harbor residual obstruction as a cause of increased resistance as can any operation involving CPB in addition to the more commonly taught causes such as acidosis, hypoxia, hypercarbia and hypothermia. Milrinone, nitroprusside, and nitroglycerine can decrease SVR and PVR, while vasopressin and agents such as phenylephrine and norepinephrine are used to increase SVR. The latter commonly occurs in sepsis and in the post-CPB patient maintained on a preoperative ACE inhibitor.

Common causes of decreased intrinsic contractility include acidosis, electrolyte disturbances, inadequate myocardial protection, and the effects of cardiotomy and suture lines. As opposed to awaiting the development of low cardiac output, prophylactic separation from CPB with dopamine +/- low dose epinephrine is used for most cardiac operations and the addition of milrinone is at least considered for most complex cases. When all these manipulations have been exhausted and technical error and mechanical issues ruled out, persistent low cardiac output should lend consideration for mechanical circulatory support. In neonates and infants, veno-arterial ECMO support (central cannulation in post-cardiotomy or cervical cannulation) or Biomedicus centrifuge support can provide effective assistance and buy time to find a reversible condition.

References

Chapter 4. Early-stage lung cancer

1. The NCCN Clinical Practice Guidelines in Oncology. Non-Small Cell Lung Cancer (Version 1.2011). National Comprehensive Cancer Network, 2010. Available at: NCCN.org. Accessed November 5, 2010.

2. Ginsberg RJ, Rubinstein LV. Randomized trial of lobectomy versus limited resection for T1 N0 non-small cell lung cancer. Lung Cancer Study Group. *Ann Thorac Surg* 1995; 60: 615-622.

Chapter 27. Esophageal reflux disease

1. Kahrilas PJ. Clinical practice. Gastroesophageal reflux disease. *N Engl J Med* 2008; 359: 1700-1707.

2. Sharma P. Clinical practice. Barrett's esophagus. *N Engl J Med* 2009; 361: 2548-2556.

3. Chiba N. Proton pump inhibitors in acute healing and maintenance of erosive or worse esophagitis: a systematic overview. *Can J Gastroenterol* 1997; 11 Suppl B: 66B-73B.

4. Khan M, Santana J, Donnellan C, et al. Medical treatments in the short term management of reflux oesophagitis. *Cochrane Database Syst Rev* 2007; 2: CD003244.

5. Rice TW, Blackstone EH. Surgical management of gastroesophageal reflux disease. *Gastroenterol Clin North Am* 2008; 37: 901-919.

Chapter 39. Coronary artery disease

1. Smith SC, Allen J, Blair SN, et al. AHA/ACC Guidelines for Secondary Prevention for Patients With Coronary and Other Atherosclerotic Vascular Disease: 2006 Update. *Circulation* 2006; 113: 2363-2372.

2. Serruys PW, Morice MC, Kappetein AP, et al. Percutaneous coronary intervention versus coronary-artery bypass grafting for severe coronary artery disease. *N Engl J Med* 2009; 360: 961-972.

3. Eagle KA, Guyton RA, Davidoff R, et al. ACC/AHA 2004 guideline update for coronary artery bypass graft surgery: A report of the American College of Cardiology/American Heart Association Task Force on Practice Guidelines (Committee to Revise the 1999 Guide-

lines for Coronary Artery Bypass Graft Surgery). *Circulation* 2004; 110: e340-e347.

4. Sellke FW, DiMaio JM, Caplan LR, et al. Comparing On-Pump and Off-Pump Coronary Artery Bypass Grafting. *Circulation* 2005; 111: 2858-2864.

5. Chan V, Sellke FW, Ruel M. Coronary artery bypass grafting. In: Sellke FW, del Nido PJ, Swanson SJ (eds). Sabiston & Spencer Surgery of the Chest. 8th edition. Philadelphia: Saunders Elsevier; 2010: 1367-1395.

Chapter 43. Aortic valve disease

1. Bonow RO, Carabello BA, Chatterjee K, et al. ACC/AHA 2006 guidelines for the management of patients with valvular heart disease: a report of the American College of Cardiology/American Heart Association Task Force on Practice Guidelines (writing committee to revise the 1998 Guidelines for the Management of Patients With Valvular Heart Disease). *Circulation* 2006; 114: e84-231.

Chapter 45. Mitral regurgitation

1. Bonow RO, Carabello BA, Chatterjee K, et al. 2008 Focused Update Incorporated into the ACC/AHA 2006 Guidelines for the Management of Patients with Valvular Heart Disease: A report of the American College of Cardiology / American Heart Association Task Force on Practice Guidelines (Writing Committee to Revise the 1998 Guidelines for the Managamenet of Patients with Valvular Disease). *J Am Coll Cardiol* 2008; 52: e1-e142.

Chapter 46. Mitral stenosis

1. Bonow RO, Carabello BA, Chatterjee K, et al. 2008 Focused Update Incorporated into the ACC/AHA 2006 Guidelines for the Management of Patients with Valvular Heart Disease: A report of the American College of Cardiology / American Heart Association Task Force on Practice Guidelines (Writing Committee to Revise the 1998 Guidelines for the Managamenet of Patients with Valvular Disease). *J Am Coll Cardiol* 2008; 52 (13): e1-e142.

Chapter 48. Endocarditis

1. Vassileva CM, Yuh DD. Surgical management of endocarditis. In: Yuh DD, Vricella LA, Baumgartner VA (eds). The Johns Hopkins

Manual of Cardiothoracic Surgery. 1ˢᵗ edition. New York: McGraw Hill; 2007: 633-662.

Chapter 54. Arrhythmia surgery

1. Fuster V, Rydén LE, Cannom DS, et al. ACC/AHA/ESC 2006 guidelines for the management of patients with atrial fibrillation. *J Am Coll Cardiol* 2006; 48: e149-e246.

2. Calkins H, Brugada J, Packer DL, et al. HRS/EHRA/ECAS expert consensus statement on catheter and surgical ablation of atrial fibrillation. *Heart Rhythm* 2007; 4: 816-861.

Chapter 55. Pacemakers and defibrillators

1. Epstein AE, DiMarco JP, Ellenbogen KA, et al. ACC/AHA/HRS 2008 Guidelines for Device-Based Therapy of Cardiac Rhythm Abnormalities. *J Am Coll Cardiol* 2008; 51: e1-e62.

Sources

Books

Bojar RM. Manual of Perioperative Care in Adult Cardiac Surgery. 4th edition. Malden: Blackwell Publishing; 2005.

Cohn LC (ed). Cardiac Surgery in the Adult. 3rd edition. New York: McGraw Hill; 2007.

Fauci AS, Braunwald E, Kasper DL, et al (eds). Harrison's Principles of Internal Medicine. 17th edition. New York: McGraw Hill; 2008.

Jonas RA. Comprehensive Surgical Management of Congenital Heart Disease. 1st edition. London: Arnold; 2004.

Kaddoura S. Echo Made Easy. 2nd edition. Philadelphia: Churchill Livingstone Elsevier; 2009.

Kaiser LR, Kron IL, Spray TL. Mastery of Cardiothoracic Surgery. 2nd edition. Philadelphia: Lippincott Williams & Wilkins; 2006.

Khonsari S, Sintek CF. Cardiac Surgery: Safeguards and Pitfalls in Operative Technique. 4th edition. Lippincott Williams & Wilkins; 2008.

Kouchoukos NT, Karp RB, Blackstone EH, et al (eds). Kirklin / Barratt-Boyes Cardiac Surgery. 3rd edition. Philadelphia: Churchill Livingstone; 2003.

Marino PL. The ICU Book. 3rd edition. Philadelphia: Lippincott Williams & Wilkins; 2007.

Mavroudis C, Backer C (eds). Pediatric Cardiac Surgery. 3rd edition. Philadelphia: Mosby; 2003.

N/A. UpToDate. Waltham: UpToDate Inc. www.uptodate.com.

Nichols DG, Cameron DE. Critical Heart Disease in Infants and Children. 2nd edition. Philadephia: Mosby; 2006.

Patterson GA, Pearson FG, Cooper JD, et al (eds). Pearson's Thoracic and Esophageal Surgery. 3rd edition. Philadelphia: Churchill Livingstone; 2008.

Reitz BA, Yuh DD. Congenital Cardiac Surgery. 1st edition. New York: McGraw Hill; 2001.

Sellke F, del Nido PJ, Swason SJ. Sabiston and Spencer's Surgery of the Chest. 8th edition. Philadelphia: Saunders Elsevier; 2010.

Shields TW, LoCicero J, Reed CE, Feins RH. General Thoracic Surgery. 7th edition. Philadelphia: Lippincott Williams & Wilkins; 2009.

Singh I. Human Embryology. 5th edition. Madras: McMillan India; 2003.

Sugarbaker DJ, Bueno R, Krasna MJ, et al (eds). Adult Chest Surgery. 1st edition. New York: McGraw Hill; 2009.

Yang SC, Cameron DE. Current Therapy in Thoracic and Cardiovascular Surgery. 1st edition. Philadelphia: Mobsy; 2004.

Yuh DD, Vricella LA, Baumgartner WA. The Johns Hopkins Manual of Cardiothoracic Surgery. 1st edition. New York: McGraw Hill; 2007.

Journal articles

Delahaye F, Wong J, Mills PG. Infective endocarditis: a comparison of international guidelines. *Heart* 2007; 93: 524–527.

Fishman A, Martinez F, Naunheim K, et al. National Emphysema Treatment Trial Research Group A randomized trial comparing lung-volume-reduction surgery with medical therapy for severe emphysema. *N Engl J Med* 2003; 348: 2059-2073.

Flörchinger B, Philipp A, Klose A, et al. Pumpless Extracorporeal Lung Assist (PECLA): A 10-Year Institutional Experience. *Ann Thorac Surg* 2008; 86:410-417.

Gutierrez-Martin MA, Galvez-Aceval J, Araji OA. Indications for surgery and operative techniques in infective endocarditis in the present day. *Infect Disord Drug Targets* 2010; 10: 32-46.

Hemmila MR, Rowe SA, Boules TN, et al. Extracorporeal life support for severe acute respiratory distress syndrome in adults. *Ann Surg* 2004; 240: 595-607.

Honjo O, Caldarone CA. Hybrid palliation for neonates with hypoplastic left heart syndrome: Current strategies and outcomes. *Korean Circ J* 2010; 40: 103-111.

Ishikawa S, Kawasaki A, Neya K, et al. Surgical treatments for infective endocarditis involving valve annulus. *Ann Thorac Cardiovasc Surg* 2009; 15: 378-81.

Kang N, Wan S, Ng CS, et al. Periannular extension of infective endocarditis. *Ann Thorac Cardiovasc Surg* 2009; 15: 74-81.

Mathews L, Singh KRK. Swan-Ganz catheter in hemodynamic monitoring. *J Anaesth Clin Pharmacol.* 2006; 22: 335-345.

McDonald JR. Acute infective endocarditis. *Infect Dis Clin North Am* 2009; 23: 643-664.

McKellar SH, Sundt TM. Valve replacement options in the setting of an ascending aortic aneurysm. *Future Cardiol* 2009; 5: 375-383.

Overgaard CB, Dzavík V. Inotropes and vasopressors: review of physiology and clinical use in cardiovascular disease. *Circulation* 2008; 118: 1047-1056.

Pinsky MR. Why measure cardiac output? *Crit Care* 2003; 7: 114-116.

Rychik J. Hypoplastic left heart syndrome: From in-utero diagnosis to school age. *Semin Fetal Neonatal Med* 2005; 10: 553-566.

Sciurba FC, Ernst A, Herth FJ, et al. VENT Study Research Group. A randomized study of endobronchial valves for advanced emphysema. *N Engl J Med* 2010; 363: 1233-1244.

Silva-Cardoso J, Ferreira J, Oliveira-Soares A, et al. Effectiveness and safety of levosimendan in clinical practice. *Rev Port Cardiol* 2009; 28: 143-154.

Slaughter MS, Pagani FD, Rogers JG, et al. Clinical management of continuous-flow left ventricular assist devices in advanced heart failure. *J Heart Lung Transplant* 2010; 29: S1-S39.

Sohail MR, Uslan DZ, Khan AH, et al. Infective endocarditis complicating permanent pacemaker and implantable cardioverter-defibrillator infection. *Mayo Clin Proc* 2008; 83: 46-53.

Vincent JL. Understanding cardiac output. *Crit Care* 2008; 12: 174.

38211008R00200